INTRAVENOUS MEDICATIONS

a handbook for nurses and other allied health personnel

Intravenous Medications

a handbook
for nurses and
other allied health
personnel

Betty L. Gahart, RN

Director, Inservice Education,
Queen of the Valley Hospital,
Napa, California

Fourth Edition

The C. V. Mosby Company

ST. LOUIS • TORONTO • PRINCETON   1985

MOSBY

A TRADITION OF PUBLISHING EXCELLENCE

Editor: Barbara Ellen Norwitz
Developmental editor: Sally Adkisson
Manuscript editor: Timothy O'Brien
Book design: Jeanne Genz
Cover design: Tom Zigrang
Production: Barbara Merritt, Kathleen L. Teal

FOURTH EDITION

Copyright © 1985 by The C.V. Mosby Company

Previous editions copyrighted 1973, 1977, 1981

Printed in the United States of America

The C.V. Mosby Company
11830 Westline Industrial Drive, St. Louis, Missouri 63146

Library of Congress Cataloging in Publication Data

Gahart, Betty L.
    Intravenous medications.

    Bibliography: p.
    Includes index.
    1. Injections, Intravenous—Handbooks, manuals, etc.
2. Intravenous therapy—Handbooks, manuals, etc.
3. Nursing—Handbooks, manuals, etc. I. Title.
[DNLM: 1. Injections, Intravenous—handbooks.
WB 39 G133i]
RM170.G33 1985   615'.63   84-19015
ISBN 0-8016-1746-4

GW/D/D   9 8 7 6 5 4 3   03/C/322

To

**ALL NURSES, PHYSICIANS, AND
OTHER HEALTH CARE PROFESSIONALS**

who care enough to quickly review
every intravenous medication
before administration

Preface

Our knowledge of pharmacology is compounding almost daily. Additional research finds new, sometimes previously contraindicated, uses for many drugs.

Intravenous drugs are instantly absorbed into the bloodstream, hopefully leading to a prompt therapeutic action, but the risk of an inappropriate reaction is a constant threat that can easily become frightening reality.

In such an intense environment, health professionals expected to administer intravenous medications must have an accurate, accessible, complete, and concise reference tool available to them. This fourth edition of *Intravenous Medications: A Handbook for Nurses and Other Allied Health Personnel* is that tool. All drugs presently approved for intravenous use are included. All information has been revised to incorporate the most current documented knowledge available.

All information presented is pertinent only to the intravenous use of the drug and not necessarily to intramuscular, subcutaneous, oral, or other means of administration. Before preparing any intravenous medication, check all labels carefully to confirm use as an intravenous injection.

At all times the patency of the vein must be determined to avoid extravasation into the surrounding tissue. Accidental arterial injection can cause gangrene and must be avoided.

Knowledgable health professionals need more than dose and dilution; here is what you can expect from *Intravenous Medications:*

The generic name of the drug is in capital letters and boldface type.

Assorted trade names are in parentheses under the generic name. Boldface type and alphabetical order enable you to verify correct drug names easily.

The pH is listed in the upper right-hand corner of the page. Information on drug pH is not consistently available; however, the pH is provided whenever possible. It represents either the pH of the undiluted drug after the addition of diluents supplied by the manufacturer or after initial dilution required for administration.

Usual dose: Doses recommended are the usual range for adults unless specifically stated otherwise. Doses calculated on body weight are usually based on pretreatment weight and not on edematous weight. Impaired renal function increases the blood levels of circulating drugs, and dose reductions are frequently required.

Pediatric dose: Pediatric doses are specifically stated if they vary from mg/kg of body weight or M^2 dose recommended for adults. Not all drugs are recommended for use in children.

Dilution: All diluents and solutions mentioned must be suitable for intravenous use. Sterile technique is imperative in all phases of preparation. Specific directions for dilution are given for all drugs if dilution is necessary or permissible.

Rate of administration: Accepted rates of administration are clearly stated. As a general rule slow is better. A 25-gauge needle aids in giving a small amount of medication over a stretch of time. Life-threatening reactions (time-related overdose or allergy) are frequently precipitated by a too-rapid rate of injection.

Actions: Clear, concise statements outline the origin of each drug, how it affects body systems, length of action, and method of excretion.

Indications and uses: Uses recommended by the manufacturer are listed. An experimental or research use is stated as such.

Precautions: The section on precautions includes the balance of information needed before injecting any drug. All necessary nursing considerations are listed here. Number 15 is as important as number 1.

Contraindications: All contraindications are those specifically listed by the manufacturer. Consultation with the physician is necessary if an ordered drug is contraindicated for your patient. The physician may have additional historical information that alters the situation or may decide that use of the drug is indicated in a critical situation.

Incompatible with: Incompatible drugs are alphabetized by generic name for ease in locating the drugs you are working with. Not all incompatibilities are absolute. They are intended to alert the nurse to a problem requiring consultation with a pharmacist or the physician. It may be that a specific order of mixing is required or that particular drugs are compatible only in a specific solution. The brand of intravenous fluids or additives, concentrations, containers, rate of mixing, pH, and temperature all affect solubility and compatibility. Knowledge is growing daily in this field. After receiving specific directions from the pharmacist on correctly mixing two drugs that have a compatibility problem, write the directions on the patient's medication record or nursing care plan so others will not have to retrace your research steps when the medication is to be given again.

Side effects: Alphabetical order simplifies your confirmation that a patient's symptom could be associated with specific drug use. Where there is a distinct line of tolerance for side effects, they are listed as minor or major and alphabetized after each of these subheadings. Reactions may be caused by a side effect of the drug itself, allergic response, or overdose. Allergic response and overdose are frequently related to the rate of injection.

Antidote: Specific antidotes are listed in this section. In addition, specific nursing actions to reverse undesirable side effects are clearly stated, an instant refresher course for critical situations.

Intravenous Medications is designed for use in critical care areas, at the nursing station, in the office, in the public health field, and by students and the armed services. Pertinent information can be found in a few seconds. Take advantage of its availability and quickly review every intravenous medication before administration.

My sincerest appreciation is extended to my husband,

Bill, for his patience and assistance during the preparation of this manuscript. To my daughter, Debbie, a special thanks for the many hours of accurate typing needed to prepare this revision.

Betty L. Gahart

Change in the page size of this revised reference manual was made by The C.V. Mosby Company to facilitate the use of the manual in the clinical environment. The publisher welcomes comments on this new pocket size by users of previous editions.

INTRAVENOUS MEDICATIONS
*a handbook for nurses and other
allied health personnel*

(Diamox)

Usual dose: 5 mg/kg of body weight/24 hr, or 250 mg to 1 Gm/24 hr. Given in divided doses over 250 mg. Dose in epilepsy may range from 8 to 30 mg/kg/24 hr in divided doses.

Dilution: Each 500 mg should be diluted in 5 ml of sterile water for injection. May then be given directly IV or added to standard IV fluids.

Rate of administration: 500 mg or fraction thereof over at least 1 minute or added to IV fluids to be given over 4 to 8 hours.

Actions: A potent carbonic anhydrase inhibitor and non-bacteriostatic sulfonamide, acetazolamide depresses the tubular reabsorption of sodium, potassium, and bicarbonate. Excreted unchanged in the urine, it produces diuresis, alkalinazation of the urine, and a mild degree of metabolic acidosis.

Indications and uses: (1) Glaucoma, (2) congestive heart failure, (3) increased intracranial pressure, (4) epilepsy (petit mal seizures), (5) migraine headaches, (6) drug-induced edema (steroids, etc.).

Precautions: (1) Chemically related to sulfonamides. (2) May be alternated with other diuretics to achieve maximum effect. (3) Greater diuretic action is achieved by skipping a day of treatment rather than increasing dose. (4) Direct IV administration is the preferred route. (5) Use with caution in severe respiratory acidosis. (6) Potassium excretion is proportional to diuresis. Hypokalemia may result from diuresis, severe cirrhosis, or concurrent use of steroids. Toxicity may occur with digitalis. (7) Use within 24 hours of dilution. (8) Potentiates amphetamines, ephedrine, and quinidine. Inhibits lithium, methotrexate, and salicylates.

Contraindications: Depressed sodium and potassium levels, first trimester of pregnancy, hyperchloremic aci-

---

* NOTE: Information on drug pH is not consistently available; however, the pH will be provided whenever possible.

dosis, marked kidney or liver disease, sensitivity to sulfonamides, adrenocortical insufficiency.

Incompatible with: Specific information not available; note precautions.

Side effects: Minimal with short-term therapy. Respond to symptomatic treatment or withdrawal of drug: acidosis, bone marrow depression, confusion, crystalluria, drowsiness, fever, hemolytic anemia, paresthesias, polyuria, rash, renal calculus, thrombocytopenic purpura.

Antidote: Notify physician of any adverse effects and discontinue drug if necessary. Treat allergic reactions as indicated.

(Zovirax)

Usual dose: 5 mg/kg of body weight every 8 hours for 7 days. Normal renal function is required. Reduce length of treatment to 5 days in severe initial clinical episodes of herpes genitalis. Never exceed these recommendations.

Pediatric dose: 250 mg/M^2 every 8 hours for 7 days.

Dilution: Initially dissolve the 500 mg vial with 10 ml of sterile water for injection (50 mg/ml). Shake well to dissolve completely. Withdraw the desired dose and further dilute in an amount of solution to provide a concentration less than 7 mg/ml (70 kg adult at 5 mg/kg of body weight equals 350 mg dissolved in 100 ml of solution equals 3.5 mg/ml). Compatible with most infusion solutions.

Rate of administration: A single dose must be administered at a constant rate over 1 hour as an infusion. Use of an infusion pump or microdrip (60 gtt/ml) is recommended.

Actions: An antiviral agent with in vitro and in vivo inhibitory action against herpes simplex virus, varicella zoster virus, Epstein-Barr virus, and cytomegalovirus. Onset of action is prompt, and therapeutic levels maintained for 8 hours. Widely distributed in tissues and body fluids. Excreted in the urine.

Indications and uses: (1) Treatment of initial and recurrent mucosal and cutaneous herpes simplex infections in immunosuppressed adults and children, (2) severe initial clinical episodes of herpes genitalis in patients who are not immunocompromised.

Precautions: (1) Confirm diagnosis of herpes simplex virus (HSV-1 or HSV-2) through laboratory culture. Initiate therapy as quickly as possible after symptoms are identified. (2) Renal tubular damage will occur with too-rapid rate of injection. Acyclovir crystals will occlude renal tubules. (3) Maintain adequate hydration and urine flow before and during infusion. (4) Use caution and reduce dose in impaired renal function. (5) Use caution with underlying neurological abnormalities, in patients receiving intrathecal methotrexate or interferon, or with patients who have had previous neurological reactions to cytotoxic drugs. (6) Adjust dose downward based on creatinine clearance. (7) Use extreme caution in pregnancy and lactation. Adequate studies are not available. (8) Side effects are increased by other nephrotoxic drugs. (9) Potentiated by probenecid. (10) Confirm patency of vein: will cause thrombophlebitis. Rotate site of infusion.

Contraindications: Hypersensitivity to acyclovir.

Incompatible with: Blood products, protein solutions.

Side effects: Acute renal failure, agitation, coma, confusion, diaphoresis, hallucinations, headache, hematuria, hives, hypotension, lethargy, nausea, obtundation, phlebitis, rash, seizures, transient increased serum creatinine levels, tremors.

Antidote: Notify physician of all side effects. Discontinue drug with onset of CNS side effects. Treatment will be symptomatic and supportive. Removed by hemodialysis. Treat anaphylaxis and resuscitate as necessary.

(Nisentil)

Usual dose: 10 to 30 mg (0.4 to 0.6 mg/kg of body weight). Repeat one fourth of initial dose after 15 minutes if necessary to achieve desired effect. Maximum dose is 240 mg/24 hr.

Dilution: Each dose should be diluted with 5 to 10 ml of sterile water for injection. May be combined with levallorphan tartrate (Lorfan) to prevent narcotic-induced respiratory depression.

Rate of administration: 20 mg or fraction thereof over 1 minute.

Actions: Alphaprodine is a synthetic narcotic analgesic related to meperidine. It is fast acting (1 to 2 minutes) and has a brief duration of relief (30 to 60 minutes). Pain threshold is elevated, and the reaction of the individual to the painful experience is altered. This drug is rapidly excreted in the urine.

Indications and uses: (1) Obstetrical analgesia, (2) urological procedures, (3) minor surgery analgesia, (4) preoperative sedation, (5) cardiovascular pain, (6) renal or biliary colic.

Precautions: (1) There is no established dosage for children under 12 years. (2) Can produce dependency. (3) Respiratory depressant effects are increased by barbiturates, general anesthetic agents, phenothiazines (prochlorperazine [Compazine], etc.), alcohol, and other CNS depressants. (4) Severe hypotension and death may result in patients receiving MAO inhibitors (pargyline [Eutonyl], etc.). (5) Use during final stages of labor may precipitate respiratory depression in the fetus. (6) Should not be used to relieve chronic pain. Frequent doses increase the possibility of addiction. (7) Patient should be lying down. (8) Use with caution in head injury, increased intracranial pressure, acute asthma, chronic obstructive pulmonary disease, and decreased respiratory reserve. (9) Use caution in supraventricular tachycardias; vagolytic action may increase rate of ventricular response. (10) Cimetidine (Tagamet) may increase CNS toxicity.

Contraindications: First trimester of pregnancy, known sensitivity to alphaprodine, old and debilitated individuals or infants, respiratory depression.

Incompatible with: Specific information not available. Interactions between analgesics and other drugs are common.

Side effects: *Average dose:* Constipation, diaphoresis, dizziness, drowsiness, hypotension, nausea and vomiting, respiratory depression, urinary retention, urticaria. *Overdose:* Respiratory depression, coma, death.

Antidote: With increasing severity of minor side effects or onset of any major side effects, discontinue the drug and notify the physician. Naloxone (Narcan) or levallorphan (Lorfan) will reverse serious respiratory depression. A patent airway, artificial ventilation, oxygen therapy, and other symptomatic treatment must be instituted promptly.

ALPROSTADIL

(PGE$_1$, prostaglandin E$_1$, Prostin VR Pediatric)

Usual dose: Begin with 0.1 µg/kg of body weight/minute. When therapeutic response is achieved, reduce infusion rate by increments to lowest dose that maintains the response (0.1 µg to 0.05 to 0.025 to 0.01 µg/min). If necessary, dose may be increased gradually to a maximum of 0.4 µg/kg/min. Generally these higher rates do not produce greater effects. May be given through infusion into a large vein or if necessary through an umbilical artery catheter placed at the ductal opening.

Dilution: Each 500 µg must be further diluted with normal saline or dextrose for infusion. Various volumes may be used depending on infusion pump capabilities and desired infusion rate. 250 ml provides 2 µg/ml.

Rate of administration: See Usual dose. Infusion pump capable of delivering 0.005, 0.01, 0.02, or 0.05 ml/min/kg of body weight is required. Use for the shortest time possible at the lowest rate therapeutically effective.

Actions: A naturally occurring acidic lipid. Smooth muscle of the ductus arteriosus is susceptible to its relaxing effect, reducing blood pressure and peripheral resistance and increasing cardiac output and rate. Metabolized by oxidation almost instantly (80% in one pass through the lungs). Remainder is excreted as metabolites in the urine.

Indications and uses: Temporarily maintain the patency of the ductus arteriosus until corrective or palliative surgery can be performed on infants with pulmonary atresia, pulmonary stenosis, tricuspid atresia, tetralogy of Fallot, interruption of the aortic arch, coarctation of the aorta, or transposition of the great vessels.

Precautions: (1) Usually administered by trained personnel in pediatric intensive care facilities. (2) Monitor respiratory status continuously. Ventilatory assistance must be immediately available. Will cause apnea, especially in infants under 2 kg. (3) Measure effectiveness with increase of Po$_2$ in infants with restricted pulmonary blood flow and increase of blood pressure and blood pH in infants with restricted sytemic blood flow. (4) Monitor arterial pressure intermittently by umbilical artery catheter, auscultation, or Doppler transducer. Decrease rate of infusion stat if a significant fall in arterial pressure occurs. (5) Prepare fresh solution for administration every 24 hours. (6) Response is poor in infants with Po_2 values of 40 mm Hg or more. More effective with lower Po_2. (7) Use caution in neonates with bleeding tendencies.

Contraindications: None known. Not indicated for respiratory distress syndrome (hyaline membrane disease).

Incompatible with: Specific information not available.

Side effects: Cardiac arrest, cerebral bleeding, cortical proliferation of long bones, diarrhea, DIC, hyperextension of the neck, hyperirritability, hypothermia, seizures, sepsis, tachycardia. Many other side effects have occurred in 1% of less of infants receiving alprostadil. *Overdose:* Apnea, bradycardia, flushing, hypotension, pyrexia.

Antidote: Notify physician of all side effects. Discontinue immediately if apnea or bradycardia occurs. Institute emergency measures. If infusion is restarted use extreme caution. Decrease rate if pyrexia or hypotension occurs. Flushing is usually caused by incorrect intraarterial catheter placement. Reposition.

(Amikin)

Usual dose: Up to 15 mg/kg of body weight/24 hr equally divided into 2 or 3 doses at equally divided intervals. Do not exceed a total adult dose of 15 mg/kg/24 hr in average-weight patient or 1.5 Gm in heavier patients by all routes in 24 hours. Normal renal function is necessary.

Newborn dose: 10 mg/kg of body weight as a loading dose, then 7.5 mg/kg every 12 hours.

Dilution: Each 500 mg or fraction thereof must be diluted with 200 ml of intravenous 5% dextrose in water, 5% dextrose in normal saline, or normal saline. Amount of diluent may be decreased proportionately with dosage for children and infants.

Rate of administration: A single dose over at least 30 to 60 minutes. Infants should receive a 1- to 2-hour infusion.

Actions: An aminoglycoside antibiotic with neuromuscular blocking action. Bactericidal against many gram-negative organisms resistant to other antibiotics including other aminoglycosides such as gentamicin (Garamycin), kanamycin (Kantrex), and tobramycin (Nebcin). Well distributed through all body fluids; crosses the placental barrier. Excreted in the kidneys. Cross-allergenicity does occur between aminoglycosides.

Indications and uses: Short-term treatment of serious infections caused by susceptible organisms resistant to alternate drugs that have less potential toxicity.

Precautions: (1) Use extreme caution if therapy is required over 7 to 10 days. (2) Sensitivity studies are indicated to determine the susceptibility of the causative organism to amikacin. (3) Reduce daily dose commensurate with amount of renal impairment. Increase intervals between injections. (4) Maintain good hydration. (5) Watch for decrease in urine output, rising BUN and serum creatinine, and declining creatinine clearance levels. Dosage may require decreasing. Routine serum levels and evaluations of hearing are recommended. (6) Response should occur in 24 to 48 hours. (7) Use during pregnancy and lactation only when absolutely necessary. (8) Concurrent use topically or systemically with any other ototoxic or nephrotoxic agents should be avoided. May have dangerous additive effects with anesthetics, other neuromuscular blocking antibiotics (kanamycin, streptomycin, etc.), diuretics (furosemide [Lasix]), vancomycin, and many others. All aminoglycosides are also potentiated by anticholinesterases (edrophonium, etc.), antineoplastics (nitrogen mustard, cisplatin, etc.), barbiturates, muscle relaxants (tubocurarine, etc.), phenothiazines (promethazine [Phenergan], etc.), procainamide, quinidine, and sodium citrate. *Apnea can occur.* (10) Superinfection may occur from overgrowth of nonsusceptible organisms.

Contraindications: Known amikacin sensitivity.

Incompatible with: Administer separately as recommended by manufacturer. Note precautions. Amphotericin B, cephalothin (Keflin), chlorothiazide (Diuril), heparin, phenytoin (Dilantin), thiopental (Pentothal), vitamin B complex with C, warfarin (Coumadin). Inactivated by carbenicillin, ticarcillin, and other penicillins.

Side effects: Occur more frequently with impaired renal function, higher doses, or prolonged administration. *Minor:* fever, headache, hypotension, nausea, paresthesias, skin rash, tremor, vomiting. *Major:* albuminuria, anemia, arthralgia, azotemia, oliguria, ototoxicity.

Antidote: Notify physician of all side effects. If minor side effects persist or any major symptom appears, discontinue drug and notify the physician. Treatment is symptomatic, or a reduction in dose may be required. Hemodialysis or peritoneal dialysis may be indicated. Resuscitate as necessary.

AMINOCAPROIC ACID

(Amicar)

Usual dose: 5 Gm initially. Follow with 1 to 1.25 Gm/hr for 6 to 8 hours. Maximum dose is 30 Gm/24 hr.

Dilution: 1 Gm equals 4 ml of prepared solution. Further dilute with compatible infusion solutions (normal saline, dextrose in saline or distilled water, or Ringer's solution). 50 ml of diluent may be used for each 1 Gm.

Rate of administration: 5 Gm or fraction thereof over first hour in 250 ml of solution, then administer each succeeding 1 Gm over 1 hour in 50 to 100 ml of solution.

Actions: A monaminocarboxylic acid with the specific action of inhibiting plasminogen activator substances; to a lesser degree, inhibits plasmin activity. Increases fibrinogen activity in clot formation by inhibiting the enzyme required for destruction of formed fibrin. Onset of action is prompt, but will last less than 3 hours. Readily excreted in the urine. Easily penetrates red blood cells and tissue cells after prolonged administration.

Indications and uses: (1) Hemorrhage caused by overactivity of the fibrinolytic system; (2) systemic hyperfibrinolysis (pathological), which may result from heart surgery, portacaval shunt, aplastic anemia, abruptio placentae, hepatic cirrhosis, or carcinoma of the prostate, lung, stomach, and cervix; (3) urinary fibrinolysis (normal physiological phenomenon), which may result from severe trauma, anoxia, or shock, surgery on the genitourinary system, or carcinoma of the genitourinary system.

Precautions: (1) Use extreme care in cardiac, hepatic, or renal disease. Endocardial hemorrhage, myocardial fat degeneration, teratogenicity, and kidney stones have resulted in animals. (2) Use only in conjunction with general and specific tests to determine the amount of fibrinolysis present. (3) Rapid administration in any form may cause hypotension, bradycardia, and/or arrhythmia. (4) Whole blood transfusions may be given if necessary. (5) Large doses in the presence of anticoagulants may induce incoagulability.

Contraindications: Disseminated intravascular coagulation, evidence of thrombosis, first and second trimester of pregnancy.

Incompatible with: Sodium lactate.

Side effects: Cramps, diarrhea, dizziness, headache, grand mal seizure, malaise, nausea, skin rash, stuffy nose, tearing, thrombophlebitis, tinnitus.

Antidote: Treat side effects symptomatically. Discontinue use of drug if any suspicion of thrombophlebitis.

AMMONIUM CHLORIDE

Usual dose: 10 ml of a 2.14% solution (4 mEq)/kg of body weight for severely alkalotic infants and adults. If edema or hyponatremia not present, the estimated total dose in mEq of chloride ion is equal to 20% of body weight in kg times the serum chloride deficit in mEq/ml. Use minimum effective dose initially. Maximum effect of a single dose not fully apparent for several days.

2.14% solution contains 0.4 mEq NH_4 and 0.4 mEq Cl/ml.

26.75% solution contains 5 mEq NH_4 and 5mEq Cl/ml.

Dilution: 2.14% may be given without further dilution. 26.75% solution should be diluted with normal saline for infusion. Use 10 ml or more of diluent for each ml of ammonium chloride. Add potassium chloride, 20 to 40 mEq/L to the ammonium infusion.

Rate of administration: 1 ml of 2.14% solution/min for adults. Reduce rate for infants.

Actions: Acidifying agent. Ammonium chloride dissociates into an ammonium cation and a chloride anion. Ammonium ions are converted to urea by the liver, freeing hydrogen ions and chloride ions. Hydrogen ion reacts with bicarbonate to form water and carbon dioxide (excreted by the lungs). Chloride ion combines with fixed bases (mostly sodium) to produce diuresis. Combined process reduces the alkaline reserve of the body. A compensatory action occurs within the body to halt this process within 3 days.

Indications and uses: Treatment of metabolic alkalosis due to chloride loss from vomiting, gastric fistula drainage, gastric suction, or excessive alkalinizing medication.

Precautions: (1) Accurate blood chemistry data are required before, during, and after therapy to avoid serious metabolic acidosis and deficiencies. (2) Observe respirations closely (increased ventilation at rest and exertional dyspnea indicate acidosis). Record intake and output. (3) Use caution in impaired renal function, pulmonary insufficiency, or cardiac edema. (4) Inhibits or potentiates many drugs as an acidifying agent. (5) Slow infusion rate for pain along venipuncture site.

Contraindications: Marked hepatic impairment.

Incompatible with: Chlortetracycline (Aureomycin), codeine, dimenhydrinate (Dramamine), levorphanol (Levo-Dromoran), methadone hydrochloride, sulfisoxazole (Gantrisin), warfarin (Coumadin). All alkalies.

Side effects: Most side effects are caused by ammonia toxicity. Bradycardia, calcium-deficient tetany, coma, depression, disorientation, EEG abnormalities, excitability, glycosuria, headache, hyperglycemia, hypokalemia, increased rate and depth of breathing (Kussmaul), irregular respiration, metabolic acidosis, nausea, pallor, skin rash, stupor, twitching, vomiting, weakness.

Antidote: For all side effects reduce rate of administration or discontinue drug and notify the physician. Treat hypokalemia with potassium and tetany with calcium. Sodium lactate or sodium bicarbonate IV may be used to treat acidosis. Resuscitate as necessary.

(Amytal sodium)

Usual dose: 65 to 500 mg (gr 1 to 7½). 1 Gm (gr 15) is the maximum single adult dose.

Pediatric dose: *Children over 6 years:* 65 mg (gr 1) to 250 mg (gr 3¾); 500 mg (gr 7½) is the maximum dose. *Convulsions:* 5 to 8 mg/kg of body weight is usually required.

Dilution: Each 125 mg (gr 2) must be diluted with a minimum of 1.25 ml of sterile water for injection to make a 10% solution. Inject diluent slowly and rotate vial to dissolve powder. Do not shake.

Rate of administration: Each 100 mg or fraction thereof over 1 minute for adults and 60 mg/min for children. Titrate slowly to desired effect.

Actions: A sedative, hypnotic barbiturate of intermediate duration with anticonvulsant effects. Amobarbital is a CNS depressant. Onset of action is prompt by the IV route and lasts about 4 to 6 hours. Pain perception is unimpaired. Rapidly absorbed by all body tissues and excreted fairly quickly in changed form in the urine. Crosses the placental barrier. Excreted in breast milk.

Indications and uses: (1) Control of convulsive seizures due to disease, eclampsia, psychiatric management, and drug poisoning; (2) sedation; (3) narcoanalysis and narcotherapy.

Precautions: (1) IV route is for emergency use only. Use of large veins is preferred to prevent thrombosis. Intraarterial injection causes gangrene. (2) Hydrolyzes in dry or solution form when exposed to air. Use only absolutely clear solutions and discard powder or solution that has been exposed to air for 30 minutes. (3) Use only enough medication to achieve desired effect. Rapid injection may cause symptoms of overdose. (4) Record blood pressure, pulse, and respiration every 3 to 5 minutes. Keep patient under constant observation. (5) Keep equipment for artificial ventilation available. Maintain a patent airway. (6) Treat the cause of a convulsion. (7) Use caution in hypertension, hypotension, pulmonary cardiovascular diseases, depressive states after convulsions, and in the elderly. (8) May be habit forming. (9) Use with extreme caution if any other CNS depressants have been given, such as alcohol, narcotic analgesics, anesthetics, antidepressants, sedatives, neuromuscular blocking antibiotics, tranquilizers. Potentiation with respiratory depression may occur. (10) Inhibits corticosteroids, doxycycline (Vibramycin), griseofulvin, oral anticoagulants, oral contraceptives, quinidine, and beta adrenergic blockers (propranolol [Inderal], etc.). Capable of innumerable interactions with many drugs. (11) Will cause birth defects; use in pregnancy is not recommended. (12) May cause paradoxical excitement in children or the elderly.

Contraindications: History of porphyria, impaired liver function, known hypersensitivity to barbiturates, severe respiratory depression.

Incompatible with: Cefazolin (Kefzol), cephalothin (Keflin), chlorpromazine (Thorazine), cimetidine (Tagamet), clindamycin (Cleocin), codeine, dimenhydrinate (Dramamine), diphenhydramine (Benadryl), droperidol (Inapsine), hydrocortisone sodium succinate (Solu-Cortef), hydroxyzine (Vistaril), insulin (aqueous), levarterenol (Levophed), levorphanol (Levo-Dromoran), meperidine (Demerol), methadone, morphine, oxytetracycline (Terramycin), pentazocine (Talwin), penicillin G potassium, phytonadione (Aquamephyton), procaine, prochlorperazine (Compazine), streptomycin, tetracycline (Achromycin), thiamine (Betalin S), trifluoperazine (Stelazine), vancomycin (Vancocin).

Side effects: *Average dose:* asthma, bronchospasm, depression, dermatitis, facial edema, fever, hypotension, neonatal apnea, respiratory depression (slight), thrombocytopenic purpura. *Overdose:* apnea, coma, cough reflex depression, hypotension, hypothermia, laryngospasm, pulmonary edema, reflexes (sluggish or absent), renal shutdown, respiratory depression.

Antidote: Notify the physician of any side effect. Symptomatic and supportive treatment is most important in overdose. Maintain an adequate airway with artificial ventilation if indicated. Keep the patient warm. IV volume expanders (dextran) will help maintain adequate circulation. Osmotic diuretics (mannitol) or hemodialysis will promote elimination of the drug. Vasopressors (dopamine [Intropin], etc.) will maintain blood pressure.

AMPHOTERICIN B

(Fungizone)

Usual dose: Begin with a test dose of 1 mg in 20 ml of 5% dextrose. Infuse over 10 to 30 minutes. Determine size of therapeutic dose by intensity of reaction over a 4-hour period. Usual is 0.25 mg/kg of body weight/ 24 hr gradually increased to 1 mg/kg/24 hr as tolerance permits. Up to 1.5 mg/kg/24 hr may be given on alternate-day therapy. Several months of therapy are usually required and recommended for cure. Dosage must be adjusted to each specific patient. In some instances higher doses can be used.

Dilution: A 50 mg vial is initially diluted with 10 ml of distilled water for injection (without a bacteriostatic agent); 5 mg equals 1 ml. Shake well until solution is clear. Further dilute each 1 mg in at least 10 ml of 5% dextrose in water for injection. Dextrose must have a pH above 4.2. Do not use any other diluent. Do not wipe vials with alcohol sponges. Use a sterile needle at each step of the dilution. Maintain aseptic technique. Larger-pore 1 μm filters may be used.

Rate of administration: Daily dose over 6 hours by slow IV infusion. Concentration of solution must not be greater than 0.1 mg/ml.

Actions: Antifungal antibiotic agent. It injures the membrane of the fungi. Not effective against other organisms. Remains in the body at a therapeutic level up to 20 hours after each infusion. Excreted very slowly in the urine.

Indications and uses: Treatment of fungal infections that are progressive in nature and potentially fatal, such as cryptococcosis, blastomycoses, and disseminated forms of moniliasis, coccidioidomycosis, and histoplasmosis. Diagnosis must be positively established by culture or histological study.

Precautions:: (1) Use only fresh solutions without evidence of precipitate or foreign matter. (2) Protect from light at all times. (3) Preserve concentrate in refrigerator up to 7 days. (4) Should be used only on hospitalized patients. (5) Monitor vital signs and intake and output. (6) Use caution in concomitant use of corticosteroids, nephrotoxic antibiotics, and antineo-plastic agents (nitrogen mustard, etc.). (7) During therapy, frequent renal and liver function tests, blood counts, and electrolyte panels are necessary. (8) A small amount of heparin added to the infusion may reduce the incidence of thrombophlebitis. (9) Whenever medicine is not given for 7 days or longer, restart treatment at lowest dosage level. (10) Hydrocortisone 0.7 mg/kg of body weight added to the infusion may prevent chills. (11) May potentiate digitalis and skeletal muscle relaxants (succinylcholine [Anectine], diazepam [Valium], etc.).

Contraindications: Known amphotericin B sensitivity and pregnancy, unless a life-threatening situation is present.

Incompatible with: Do not mix with any drug unless absolutely necessary. Amikacin (Amikin), calcium chloride, calcium gluconate, calcium disodium edetate (Calcium Disodium Versenate), carbenicillin (Geopen), chlorpromazine (Thorazine), chlortetracycline (Aureomycin), cimetidine (Tagamet), diphenhydramine (Benadryl), dopamine (Intropin), gentamicin (Garamycin), heparin, kanamycin (Kantrex), electrolyte solutions, metaraminol (Aramine), nitrofurantoin (Ivadantin), oxytetracycline (Teramycin), penicillin G potassium or sodium, polymyxin B (Aerosporin), potassium chloride, preservatives such as benzyl alcohol, prochlorperazine (Compazine), saline solutions, tetracycline (Achromycin), vitamin B with C. Not compatible in any solution with a pH below 4.2.

Side effects: Common even at doses below therapeutic levels: anorexia, chills, convulsions, diarrhea, fever, headache, phlebitis, vomiting. Anaphylactoid reactions, anemia, cardiac disturbances (including fibrillation and arrest), coagulation defects, hypertension, hypokalemia, hypotension, and numerous other side effects occur fairly frequently. Renal function is impaired in 80% of patients. May reverse after treatment ends.

Antidote: Notify the physician of all side effects. Many are reversible if the drug is discontinued. Some will respond to symptomatic treatment. Administration of this drug on alternate days may decrease the incidence of some side effects. Urinary alkalinizers may minimize renal tubular acidosis. Treat allergic reactions and resuscitate as necessary.

(Omnipen-N, Polycillin-N, SK Ampicillin-N, Totacillin-N

Usual dose: 500 to 1,000 mg every 4 to 6 hours. 150 to 200 mg/kg of body weight/24 hr is required in meningitis or septicemia.

Pediatric dose: 50 mg/kg of body weight/24 hr in equally divided doses at 6- to 8-hour intervals, unless this exceeds the adult dose.

Dilution: Each 500 mg or fraction thereof must be diluted with at least 5 ml of sterile water for injection. If necessary, this may be further diluted in 50 ml or more of one of the following solutions and given as an IV infusion over not more than 4 hours: 5% dextrose in water, 5% dextrose in 0.45 sodium chloride solution, 10% invert sugar in water, and ⅙ sodium lactate solution. In isotonic sodium chloride, potency is maintained over 8 hours. After initial dilution, may also be added to the last 100 ml of a compatible IV solution.

Rate of administration: 500 mg or fraction thereof over at least 5 minutes when given direct IV. In 100 ml or more of solution, administer at prescribed infusion rate but never exceed direct IV rate. Too-rapid injection may cause seizures.

Actions: An extended-spectrum penicillin. Bactericidal against many gram-positive and gram-negative organisms. Appears in all body fluids. Appears in cerebrospinal fluid only if inflammation is present. Excreted in the urine.

Indications and uses: Highly effective against severe infections caused by gram-positive and gram-negative organisms, except penicillinase-producing staphylococci.

Precautions: (1) Sensitivity studies are indicated to determine the susceptibility of the causative organism to ampicillin sodium. (2) Individuals with a history of allergic problems are more susceptible to untoward reactions. Watch for early symptoms of allergic reaction. (3) Avoid prolonged use of this drug; superinfection caused by overgrowth of nonsusceptible organisms may result. (4) Use within 1 hour of reconstitution unless diluted in aforementioned solutions. (5) Streptomycin potentiates bactericidal activity against enterococci. (6) SGOT may be increased. Renal, hepatic, and hematopoietic function should be checked during prolonged therapy. (7) Penicillins interact with many drugs; some of these, such as antibiotics (chloramphenicol, erythromycin, kanamycin, and tetracycline), can inhibit the bactericidal activity of the penicillins. (8) False positive glucose reaction with Clinitest and Benedict's or Fehling's solution. (9) Potentiated by probenecid (Benemid); toxicity may result. (10) May potentiate heparin. (11) May inhibit aminoglycosides (gentamycin [Garamycin], etc.).

Contraindications: Known penicillin or cephalothin sensitivity and pregnancy.

Incompatible with: Do not use as an additive with any other drug. Do not mix in any solutions other than those specifically recommended. Some drugs may be administered through the Y tube in small amounts. Consult with the pharmacist.

Side effects: Primarily hypersensitivity reactions such as anaphylaxis, exfoliative dermatitis, rashes, and urticaria. Anemia, leukopenia, and thrombocytopenia have been reported. Thrombophlebitis will occur with long-term use.

Antidote: Notify the physician of any side effect. For allergic symptoms, discontinue drug, treat allergic reaction as indicated or resuscitate as necessary, and notify the physician.

ANTIHEMOPHILIC FACTOR (HUMAN)

(Factorate, Factorate Generation II, Hemofil, Hemofil T, Humafac, Koate, Profilate)

Usual dose: Completely individualized. Suggested doses are as follows.

Prophylaxis of spontaneous hemorrhage: 10 AHF IU/kg of body weight to increase factor VIII by 20%. Minimum of 30% of normal is indicated.

Minor hemorrhage and minor surgery: 15 to 25 AHF IU/kg to increase factor VIII by 30% to 50% of normal. Maintain with 10 to 15 IU/kg every 8 to 12 hours.

Severe hemorrhage: 40 to 50 AHF IU/kg to increase factor VIII to 80% to 100% of normal. Maintain with 20 to 25 AHF IU/kg every 8 to 12 hours.

Major surgery: Sufficient dose to increase factor VIII to 80% to 100% of normal; given 1 hour before surgery. Confirm with AHF level assays just before surgery. Give a second dose one half of the first in 5 hours. Maintain factor VIII at 30% of normal for 10 to 14 days.

Dilution: All preparations provide diluent and administration equipment. Actual number of AHF units is shown on each vial. Use only the diluent provided, and maintain strict aseptic technique.

Rate of administration: Preparations with less than 34 AHF IU/ml—infuse each 10 to 20 ml over 3 minutes. Preparations with more than 34 AHF IU/ml—infuse at a maximum rate of 2 ml/min. Reduce rate of infusion if a significant increase in pulse rate occurs.

Actions: A lyophilized or dried (depending on specific preparation) concentrate of coagulation factor VIII (antihemophilic factor). Obtained from fresh (less than 3 hours old) human plasma and prepared, irradiated, and dried by a specific process.

Indications and uses: (1) Treatment of the congenital deficiency of factor VIII (classical hemophilia A); (2) used to control unexpected hemorrhagic episodes, during emergency or elective surgery, and prophylactically to maintain known hemophiliac patients as necessary to prevent hemorrhage.

Precautions: (1) Identification of factor VIII deficiency with level assays is mandatory previous to administration and during treatment. Adjust dosage as indicated. (2) Must be refrigerated. Give *within* 3 hours of reconstitution. (3) Use a new sterile needle and syringe or administration set for each vial. (Use a plastic syringe to prevent binding to glass surfaces.) (4) Can transmit hepatitis. (5) If AHF does not significantly improve the partial thromboplastin time, increase the dose; factor VIII antibodies are probable. (6) Intravascular hemolysis can occur when large volumes are given to individuals with blood groups A, B, or AB. (7) Type-specific cryoprecipitate has been used to maintain adequate factor VIII levels.

Contraindications: None when used for the specific indications listed.

Incompatible with: Sufficient information not available. Do not mix with other drugs.

Side effects: Occur infrequently: backache, erythema, fever, headache, hepatitis, hives. Consider risk potential of contracting AIDS.

Antidote: All side effects except hepatitis usually subside spontaneously in 15 to 20 minutes. Keep the physician informed.

ANTI-INHIBITOR COAGULANT COMPLEX

(Autoplex, Feiba Immuno)

Usual dose: Range is 25 to 100 Factor VIII correctional units/kg. May be repeated in 6 to 12 hours. Do not exceed 200 units/kg/24 hr. Completely individualized and adjusted according to patient response.

Dilution: All preparations provide diluent for IV infusion. Actual number of Factor VIII inhibitor bypassing activity units shown on each vial. Use only the diluent provided and maintain strict aseptic technique. May be given through Y tube or three-way stopcock of infusion set.

Rate of administration: 10 ml or less per minute. If symptoms of too-rapid infusion (headache, flushing, and changes in blood pressure or pulse rate) occur, discontinue until symptoms subside Restart at 2 ml/min.

Actions: A 1-unit volume of Factor VIII correctional activity (quantity of activated prothrombin complex) will correct clotting time to normal (35 seconds) when added to an equal volume of Factor VIII deficient or inhibitor plasma. A dried or freeze-dried concentrate prepared from human plasma by a specific process.

Indications and uses: To control hemorrhagic episodes in hemophiliacs (hemophilia A) with Factor VIII inhibitors who are bleeding or will undergo elective or emergency surgery. Most frequently indicated if Factor VIII inhibitor levels are above 2 to 10 Bethesda units or rise to that level following treatment with AHF.

Precautions: (1) Identification of Factor VIII inhibitor level is mandatory previous to administration. (2) Monitor prothrombin time before and after treatment; this is the only accurate means of treatment evaluation. Must be two thirds of preinfusion value after treatment if patient is to receive any additional doses. (3) APTT, WBCT, and other clotting factor tests do not correlate with actual results and may lead to overdose and DIC. (4) Could transmit AIDS and hepatitis. (5) Refrigerate before reconstitution. (6) Not recommended for use with antifibrinolytic products (aminocaproic acid, tranexamic acid). (7) Use extreme caution in liver disease. (8) Safety for use in pregnancy is not established.

Contraindications: Disseminated intravascular coagulation, symptoms (signs) of fibrinolysis, known hypersensitivity.

Incompatible with: Specific information not available. Do not mix directly with other drugs.

Side effects: Anaphylaxis, bradycardia, chest pain, chills, cough, decreased fibrinogen concentration, decreased platelet count, fever, flushing, headache, hypertension, hypotension, prolonged partial thromboplastin time, prolonged prothrombin time, prolonged thrombin time, respiratory distress, tachycardia, urticaria.

Antidote: If side effects occur, discontinue the infusion and notify the physician. May be resumed at a slower rate, or an alternate product may be used. Symptoms of DIC (blood pressure and pulse rate changes, respiratory discomfort, chest pain, cough, prolonged clotting tests) require immediate treatment. Treat anaphylaxis (antihistamines, epinephrine, and corticosteroids) and resuscitate as necessary.

ANTIVENIN *(CROTALIDAE)* POLYVALENT

Usual dose: Testing for sensitivity to horse serum is required before use (see precautions).

Dosage is based on severity of envenomation when patient is initially assessed.

No envenomation: None.

Minimal envenomation: 2 to 4 vials (20 to 40 ml).

Moderate envenomation: 5 to 9 vials (50 to 90 ml).

Severe envenomation: 10 to 15 vials (100 to 150 ml).

Additional antivenin need is based on clinical response and progression of symptoms. If condition deteriorates, 1 to 5 additional vials (10 to 50 ml) may be given. Most effective within 4 hours of the bite, less effective after 8 hours, but in the presence of envenomation is to be given even after 24 hours have elapsed.

Pediatric dose: Not based on weight. Small children bitten by large snakes may require larger doses of antivenin.

Dilution: Each single vial must be diluted with 10 ml of sterile water for injection (supplied). Must be further diluted with normal saline or 5% dextrose for infusion for a 1:1 to 1:10 solution (1 ml of antivenin to 10 ml of infusion solution is preferred unless the patient's condition limits fluid intake). Avoid foaming by gently swirling to mix thoroughly.

Rate of administration: Infuse 5 to 10 ml over a minimum of 3 to 5 minutes. If no adverse reaction occurs, give remaining initial dose at maximum rate of administration based on severity of envenomation, and fluid tolerance appropriate for patient's body weight and condition.

Actions: Prepared from the blood serum of horses immunized against the venom of Crotalids (pit vipers) found in North, Central, and South America. Will neutralize the venom of rattlesnakes, copperheads, and cottonmouth moccasins. (See literature for specific species.)

Indications and uses: Treatment of patients with symptoms of envenomation sustained from the bite of a rattlesnake, copperhead, and cottonmouth moccasin or other specific pit viper species of snake.

Precautions: (1) Read drug literature supplied with antivenin completely before use. Essential to evaluate symptoms and individual status of each patient. (2) Determine patient response to any previous injections of serum of any type and history of any allergic type reactions. (3) Hospitalize patient. (4) Test every patient for sensitivity to horse serum without exception (1 ml vial of 1:10 dilution horse serum supplied). Skin test and conjuctival test are recommended for maximum safety.

Skin test: Inject 0.02 ml of 1:10 horse serum into (not under) skin (intracutaneous). A like injection of normal saline can be used as a control. Compare in 20 minutes. An urticarial wheal surrounded by a zone of erythema is a positive reaction.

Conjunctival test: Instill 1 drop of 1:10 horse serum into conjunctival sac for adults (1 drop of 1:100 dilution for children). Itching, redness, burning, and/or lacrimation within 30 minutes constitute a positive reaction. A drop of normal saline in the opposite eye is used as a control and should be asymptomatic. Reverse adverse effects of positive reaction with 1 drop of epinephrine ophthalmic solution.

Other testing methods may be used. Use at least two. (5) A systemic reaction may occur even when both sensitivity tests are negative. (6) In most cases, the sooner a sensitivity reaction occurs, the greater the sensitivity. Observe patient continuously. (7) Monitor all vital signs at frequent intervals. Before antivenin is administered draw adequate blood for baseline studies (type and cross-match, CBC, hematocrit, platelet count, prothrombin time, clot retraction, bleeding and coagulation times, BUN, electrolytes, and bilirubin). (8) Initiate two IV lines as soon as possible, one to be used for supportive therapy, the other for antivenin and electrolytes. (9) Keep emergency equipment available at all times including oxygen, epinephrine, antihistamines (diphenhydramine [Benadryl], etc.), vasopressors (dopamine [Intropin], etc.), corticosteroids, and ventilation equipment. (10) Tetanus prophylaxis is indicated. (11) Corticosteroids are the drugs of choice if antivenin is not available until 24 hours after the snake bite but are not recommended for concomitant administration. (12) Consider use of broad-spectrum antibiotic. (13) Do not pack bitten extremity in ice.

Contraindications: Hypersensitivity to horse serum unless only treatment available for life-threatening situation. Several techniques including preload of antihistamines and/or desensitization may be considered (see literature).

Incompatible with: Specific information not available. Do not mix with any other drug in syringe or solution due to specific use.

Side effects: Acute anaphylaxis with urticaria, respiratory distress, and vascular collapse. Serum sickness may occur. Usually appears in 7 to 12 days. Local pain, local erythema, and urticaria without systemic reaction can occur.

Antidote: Discontinue the drug and notify the physician of all side effects. Treat anaphylaxis immediately. Epinephrine (Adrenalin) and diphenhydramine (Benadryl), oxygen, vasopressors (dopamine), corticosteroids, and ventilation equipment must always be available. Resuscitate as necessary.

ANTIVENIN *(LATRODECTUS MACTANS)*

(Black widow spider antivenin)

Usual dose: Testing for sensitivity to horse serum is required before use (see precautions).

Entire contents of one vial of antivenin (2.5 ml) is recommended for adults and children. One vial is usually enough, but a second dose may be necessary in rare instances.

Dilution: Each single dose (6,000 antivenin units) must be initially diluted with 2.5 ml of sterile water for injection (supplied). Keep needle in rubber stopper of antivenin and shake vial to completely dissolve contents. Must be further diluted in 10 to 50 ml normal saline for IV injection.

Rate of administration: A single dose over a minimum of 15 minutes.

Actions: Prepared from the blood serum of horses immunized against the venom of the black widow spider. One unit will neutralize one average mouse lethal dose of black widow spider venom when both are injected simultaneously under laboratory conditions.

Indications and uses: Treatment of patients with symptoms due to black widow spider bites *(Latrodectus mactans)*.

Precautions: (1) Read drug literature supplied with antivenin completely before use. Essential to evaluate symptoms and individual status of each patient. (2) Determine patient response to any previous injections of serum of any type and history of any allergic type reactions. (3) Hospitalize patient if possible. (4) Test every patient for sensitivity to horse serum without exception (1 ml vial of 1:10 dilution horse serum supplied). Skin test and conjuctival test are recommended for maximum safety.

Skin test: Inject 0.02 ml of 1:10 horse serum into (not under) skin (intracutaneous). A like injection of normal saline can be used as a control. Compare in 20 minutes. An urticarial wheal surrounded by a zone of erythema is a positive reaction.

Conjunctival test: Instill 1 drop of 1:10 horse serum into conjunctival sac for adults (1 drop 1:100 di-

lution for children). Itching, redness, burning, and/
or lacrimation within 30 minutes is a positive reaction. A drop of normal saline in the opposite eye
is used as a control and should be asymptomatic.
Reverse adverse effects of positive reaction with 1
drop of epinephrine ophthalmic solution.

Other testing methods may be used. Use at least
two. (5) A systemic reaction may occur even when both
sensitivity tests are negative. (6) Supportive therapy
is indicated. 10 ml of 10% calcium gluconate IV may
control muscle pain. Morphine may be needed. Barbiturates or diazepam may be used for restlessness.
Prolonged warm baths are helpful; corticosteroids
have been used. (7) Observe patient constantly for respiratory paralysis. Can occur from toxin alone, and
narcotics and sedatives may precipitate respiratory
depression. (8) Muscle relaxants may be the initial
treatment of choice in healthy individuals between 16
and 60. Antivenin use may be deferred while patient
is observed. (9) May be given IM. IV route is preferred
in severe cases or if patient is in shock or under 12
years of age.

Contraindications: Hypersensitivity to horse serum unless only treatment available for a life-threatening situation. Several techniques including preload of antihistamine and/or desensitization may be considered
(see literature).

Incompatible with: Specific information not available.
Do not mix with any other drug in syringe or solution
due to specific use.

Side effects: Acute anaphylaxis with urticaria, respiratory distress, and vascular collapse. Serum sickness
may occur. Usually appears in 7 to 12 days. Local pain,
local erythema, and urticaria without systemic reaction can occur.

Antidote: Discontinue the drug and notify the physician
of all side effects. Treat anaphylaxis immediately. Epinephrine (Adrenalin), diphenhydramine (Benadryl),
oxygen, vasopressors (dopamine), corticosteroids, and
ventilation equipment must always be available. Resuscitate as necessary.

ANTIVENIN *(MICRURUS FULVIUS)*

(North American coral snake antivenin)

Usual dose: Testing for sensitivity to horse serum is required before use (see precautions).

Entire contents of 3 to 5 vials (30 to 50 ml) are recommended depending on the nature and severity of envenomation. Up to 10 vials may be required if the snake's entire venom load was delivered by the bite.

Dilution: Each single vial must be diluted with 10 ml of sterile water for injection (supplied). Start an IV infusion of 250 to 500 ml normal saline. May be administered through the tubing of the free-flowing IV or added to the infusion solution after the initial 2 ml is given without adverse reaction.

Rate of administration: Inject the first 1 to 2 ml over a minimum of 3 to 5 minutes. If no adverse reaction, give remaining initial dose at maximum rate of administration based on severity of envenomation and fluid tolerance appropriate for patient's body weight and condition.

Actions: Prepared from the blood serum of horses immunized against the venom of specific coral snakes. Will neutralize the venom of *Micrurus fulvius fulvius* (Eastern coral snake) and *M. fulvius tenere* (Texas coral snake). Response should be rapid and dramatic.

Indications and uses: Treatment of patients with symptoms due to the venom of *M. fulvius fulvius* (eastern coral snake) and *M. fulvius tenere* (Texas coral snake). Not effective for *M. euryxanthus* (Arizona or Sonoran coral snake).

Precautions: (1) Read drug literature supplied with antivenin completely before use. Essential to evaluate symptoms and individual status of each patient. (2) Determine patient response to any previous injections of serum of any type and history of any allergic type reactions. (3) Hospitalize patient if possible. (4) Test every patient for sensitivity to horse serum without exception (1 ml vial of 1:10 dilution horse serum supplied). Scratch test and conjunctival test recommended for maximum safety.

Scratch test: Place 1 drop of 1:100 solution on the skin. Make a ¼ inch scratch through this drop. Establish a normal saline control in the same manner on a like skin surface. Compare in 20 minutes. An urticarial wheal surrounded by a zone of erythema is a positive reaction.

Conjunctival test: Instill 1 drop of 1:10 horse serum into conjunctival sac for adults (1 drop of 1:100 dilution for children). Itching, redness, burning, and/or lacrimation within 30 minutes is a positive reaction. A drop of normal saline in the opposite eye is used as a control and should be asymptomatic. Reverse adverse effects of positive reaction with 1 drop of epinephrine ophthalmic solution. Other testing methods may be used. Use at least two. (5) A systemic reaction may occur even when both sensitivity tests are negative. (6) Observe patient constantly. Additional antivenin may be needed. Paralysis can occur within 2 to 2½ hours. Local tissue reaction does not reflect the amount of envenomation. Observe signs and symptoms to assess amount of toxin injected. Symptoms may begin in 1 hour or be delayed up to 18 hours. (7) Supportive therapy is indicated. Respiratory depressants (narcotics, sedatives, etc.) are contraindicated or used with extreme caution. Keep equipment for artificial ventilation immediately available. (8) Tetanus prophylaxis is indicated.

Contraindications: Hypersensitivity to horse serum unless only treatment available for a life-threatening situation. Several techniques including preload of antihistamines and/or desensitization may be considered (see literature).

Incompatible with: Specific information not available. Do not mix with any other drug in syringe or solution due to specific use.

Side effects: Acute anaphylaxis with urticaria, respiratory distress, and vascular collapse. Serum sickness may occur. Usually appears in 7 to 12 days. Local pain, local erythema, and urticaria without systemic reaction can occur.

Antidote: Discontinue the drug and notify the physician

of all side effects. Treat anaphylaxis immediately. Epinephrine (Adrenalin) and diphenhydramine (Benadryl), oxygen, vasopressors (dopamine), corticosteroids, and ventilation equipment must always be available. Resuscitate as necessary.

ARGININE HYDROCHLORIDE

(R-Gene 10)

Usual dose: 300 ml as a single test dose under specific clinical conditions and procedures.

Pediatric dose: 5 ml/kg of body weight.

Dilution: Available as 10% solution in 500 ml bottles ready for use as an IV infusion.

Rate of administration: A single dose evenly distributed over 30 minutes. Recommended dose must be infused in 30 minutes to ensure accurate test results.

Actions: A diagnostic aid, it is an IV stimulant to the pituitary that often induces a pronounced rise in plasma level of human growth hormone (HGH) in normal individuals. This rise does not occur if pituitary function is diminished or absent.

Indications and uses: IV stimulant to pituitary as a diagnostic aid. May be useful in panhypopituitarism, pituitary dwarfism, chromophobe adenoma, postsurgical craniopharyngiomia, hypophysectomy, pituitary trauma, acromegaly, gigantism, and problems of growth or stature.

Precautions: (1) Inspect each bottle. Discard if not clear or vacuum is not present. (2) Specific test procedure must be observed. Schedule in morning. Patient must be fasting overnight and have had a normal night's rest. Maintain bed rest and calming atmosphere from 30 minutes before infusion to completion of test process. Draw blood samples from opposite arm of infusion 30 minutes before, at time infusion is begun, and every 30 minutes times five. Technician should promptly centrifuge and store all samples at 6.7° C (20° F) until processed. (3) False positive or negative results occur 30% of time. Cross-check or confirm result with insulin hypoglycemia test and a second arginine test. Allow 1 day between each test. (4) Confirm serum electrolyte balance before administration, high chloride content. (5) Use caution in renal impairment, high nitrogen content. (6) False positive results will be obtained during pregnancy or with oral contraceptives.

Contraindications: Individuals with known severe allergic tendencies.

Incompatible with: Specific information not available. Should be considered incompatible with any other drug due to specific use.

Side effects: Usually due to rate or hypertonicity of solution. Flushing, headache, local venous irritation, nausea, numbness, rash, vomiting.

Antidote: Slow infusion to reduce side effects, but must be infused in 30 minutes for accurate results. Notify physician of all side effects. Discontinue drug and treat allergic reaction with diphenhydramine (Benadryl) or epinephrine. Resuscitate as necessary.

(Calcium ascorbate, Calscorbate, Cenolate, Cevalin, Cevita, sodium ascorbate, vitamin C)

Usual dose: 200 mg to 2 Gm/24 hr. Up to 6 Gm/24 hr has been given without toxicity.

Infant dose: 100 to 300 mg/24 hr is the curative dose recommended.

Dilution: May be given undiluted or may be administered diluted in IV infusion solutions. Soluble in the more commonly used solutions, such as 5% dextrose in water or saline, normal saline, lactated Ringer's injection, Ringer's injection, or sodium lactate injection.

Rate of administration: 100 mg or fraction thereof over 1 minute by direct IV administration.

Actions: This water-soluble vitamin is necessary to the formation of collagen in all fibrous tissue, carbohydrate metabolism, connective tissue repair, maintenance of intracellular stability of blood vessels, and many other body functions. Not stored in the body. Daily requirements must be met. Completely utilized, excess is excreted unchanged in the urine. Crosses placental barrier. Excreted in breast milk.

Indications and uses: (1) Preoperative and postoperative maintenance of optimum health; (2) prolonged IV therapy; (3) increased vitamin requirements or replacement therapy in severe burns, extensive injuries, and severe infections; (4) prematurity, (5) deficient intestinal absorption of water-soluble vitamins; (6) prolonged or wasting diseases; (7) hemovascular disorders and delayed fracture and wound healing require increased intake; (8) specific for the treatment of scurvy.

Precautions: (1) Vitamin C is better absorbed and utilized by IM injection. (2) Increased urinary excretion is diagnostic for vitamin C saturation. (3) Slight coloration does not affect the medication. Protect from freezing and from light. (4) Potentiates barbiturates, ferrous iron absorption, salicylates, and sulfonamides. (5) Antagonizes anticoagulants. (6) Use caution in pregnancy; high dosage may adversely affect fetus. (7) 2 Gm/day will lower urine pH and will cause reabsorp-

tion of acidic drugs and crystallization with sulfonamides. (8) Use caution in cardiac patients. Sodium
or calcium content may antagonize other drugs or
overall condition.

Contraindications: There are no absolute contraindications.

Incompatible with: Aminophylline, bleomycin (Blenoxane), chloramphenicol (Chloromycetin), chlordiazepoxide (Librium), chlorothiazide (Diuril), conjugated
estrogens (Premarin), dextran, erythromycin (Erythrocin), hydrocortisone, nafcillin (Unipen), phytonadione (Aquamephyton), sodium bicarbonate, sulfisoxazole, triflupromazine (Vesprin), vitamin B_{12} (Redisol, etc.), warfarin (Coumadin).

Side effects: Occur only with too-rapid injection: temporary dizziness or faintness. Diarrhea and or renal
calculi may occur with large doses.

Antidote: Discontinue administration temporarily. Re-
sume administration at a decreased rate. If side effects
persist, discontinue drug and notify the physician.

(Elspar)

Usual dose: *Skin test:* Required before initial dose and anytime 7 days or more occur between doses. Give 0.1 ml containing 2.0 IU intradermally and observe for 1 hour for the appearance of a wheal or erythema.

Direct IV: Very specific amount to be given on a specific day or days in a specific regime of other chemotherapeutic agents; i.e., 1,000 IU/kg of body weight/24 hr for 10 successive days beginning on day 22 of regime with specific prednisone and vincristine doses. When used as a single agent, the usual dose for adults and children is 200 IU/kg/24 hr for 28 days.

Desensitization process for administration: Extensive process. See drug literature.

Dilution: *Specific techniques required: see precautions.* Initially dilute each 10 ml vial (10,000 IU) with 5 ml of sterile water or sodium chloride for injection. 2,000 IU/ml.

Skin test: Withdraw 0.1 ml from the above solution and further dilute with 9.9 ml of sodium chloride for injection (20 IU/ml). 0.1 of this solution equals 2 IU.

Direct IV: Use 2,000 IU/ml solution. Must be further diluted by administering through Y tube or three-way stopcock of a free-flowing infusion of 5% dextrose in water or normal saline.

Rate of administration: *Direct IV:* Each dose evenly distributed over at least 30 minutes.

Actions: An enzyme derived from *Escherichia coli* that rapidly depletes asparagine from cells. Some malignant cells have a metabolic defect that makes them dependent on exogenous asparagine for survival, but they are unable to synthesize asparagine as normal cells do.

Indications and uses: Induces remissions in acute lymphocytic leukemia. Primarily used in specific combinations with other chemotherapeutic agents.

Precautions: (1) Follow guidelines for handling cytotoxic agents recommended by the National Study Commission on Cytotoxic Exposure (see Appendix, p. 528). (2) A lethal drug; administer in the hospital by or under the direction of the physician specialist. Toxicity and short-term effectiveness limit use. More toxic in adults than in children. (3) Appropriate treatment for anaphylaxis must always be available. (4) Rarely used as a single agent; not recommended for maintenance therapy. (5) Impairs liver function and may increase toxicity of other drugs. (6) Increases toxicity of vincristine and prednisone if given before or concurrently. (7) Inhibits methotrexate. (8) Allopurinol, increased fluid intake, and alkalinization of the urine may be required to reduce uric acid levels. (9) Frequent blood counts, bone marrow evaluation, serum amylase, blood sugar, and evaluation of liver and kidney function are necessary. (10) Will produce teratogenic effects on the fetus. Has a mutagenic potential. (11) Nausea and vomiting can be severe. Prophylactic administration of antiemetics is recommended to increase patient comfort. (12) Predisposition to infection is probable. (13) Refrigerate before and after dilution. Discard after 8 hours or anytime solution is cloudy. Use only clear solutions. (14) May contain fiberlike particles; use of 5.0 μm filter recommended. (15) Do not administer any vaccine or chloroquine to patients receiving antineoplastic drugs.

Contraindications: Hypersensitivity to asparaginase, pancreatitis, or past history of pancreatitis.

Incompatible with: Specific information not available. Consider incompatible with any other drug in syringe or solution due to toxicity and specific use.

Side effects: Occur frequently even with the initial dose and may cause death. Allergic reactions including anaphylaxis (even if skin test is negative and/or allergic symptoms have not occurred with previous doses), agitation, azotemia, bone marrow depression, coma, confusion, depression, fatigue, hallucinations, hyperglycemia, hyperthermia (fatal), hypofibrinogenemia and depression of other clotting factors, nausea and vomiting, fulminating pancreatitis (fatal).

Antidote: Notify physician of all side effects. Asparaginase may have to be discontinued until recovery or permanently discontinued. Symptomatic and supportive treatment is indicated. Treat anaphylaxis with epinephrine, corticosteroids, oxygen, and antihistamines. There is no specific antidote.

Usual dose: 0.4 to 0.6 mg bolus repeated every 3 to 5 minutes. Up to a total dose of 2 mg can be used to achieve a desired pulse rate above 60. Subsequent doses of 0.3 to 1.0 mg may be given at 4- to 6-hour intervals. 1.0 mg bolus recommended in asystole with specific protocol. 0.4 to 0.6 mg every 3 to 4 hours for smooth muscle relaxation. Up to 2 mg may be given in a single dose when used as an antidote for acute poisoning.

Dilution: May be given undiluted, but many prefer to dilute desired dose in at least 10 ml of sterile water for injection. Do not add to IV solutions. Inject through Y tube or three-way stopcock of infusion set.

Rate of administration: 0.6 mg or fraction thereof over 1 minute.

Actions: Atropine is an anticholinergic drug and a potent belladonna alkaloid. It produces local, central, and peripheral effects on the body. The main therapeutic uses of atropine are peripheral, affecting smooth muscle, cardiac muscle, and gland cells. This drug can interfere with vagal stimuli. It is widely distributed in all body fluids. Excretion is through all body fluids, but chiefly urine and bile.

Indications and uses: (1) Treatment of sinus bradycardia, syncope from Stokes-Adams syndrome, and high-degree atrioventricular block with profound bradycardia; (2) suppression of salivary, gastric, pancreatic, and respiratory secretions; (3) to relieve pylorospasm, hypertonicity of the small intestine, and hypermotility of the colon; (4) to relieve biliary and ureteral colic; (5) antidote for specific poisons such as organophosphorous insecticides, nerve gases, and mushroom poisoning *(Amanita muscaria);* (6) used in combination with many other drugs to produce a desired effect.

Precautions: (1) Use caution in prostatic hypertrophy, chronic lung disease, infants and small children, the elderly and debilitated, in urinary retention, and during cyclopropane anesthesia. (2) Potentiated by antidepressants (amitriptyline [Elavil], etc.), antihistamines, isoniazid, MAO inhibitors (pargyline [Eutonyl], etc.), and phenothiazines (prochlorperazine [Compazine], etc.). (3) Antagonistic to many drugs, such as acetylcholine, echothiophate (Phospholine), edrophonium (Tensilon), methacholine (Mecholyl), morphine, and pyridostigmine (Mestilon). (4) Use caution with cholinergics, digitalis, digoxin, diphenhydramine, levodopa, and neostigmine. May cause adverse effects.

Contraindications: Hypersensitivity to atropine; acute glaucoma; asthma; pyloric stenosis.

Incompatible with: Amobarbital (Amytal), ampicillin (Omnipen), chloramphenicol (Chloromycetin), chlortetracycline (Aureomycin), cimetidine (Tagamet), epinephrine (Adrenalin), heparin, isoproterenol (Isuprel), levarterenol (Levophed), metaraminol (Aramine), methicillin (Staphcillin), methohexital (Brevital), nitrofurantoin (Ivadantin), pentobarbital (Nembutal), promazine (Sparine), sodium bicarbonate, sodium iodide, thiopental (Pentothal), warfarin (Coumadin).

Side effects: *Average dose:* anhidrosis, blurred vision, respiratory failure, dilation of the pupils, dryness of the mouth, flushing, postural hypotension, bradycardia (temporary), and urinary retention may occur. *Overdose:* coma, death, delirium, elevated blood pressure, fever, paralytic ileus, rash, respiratory failure, stupor, tachycardia.

Antidote: Physostigmine salicylate (Antilirium) reverses most cardiovascular and CNS effects. Pilocarpine, 10 mg (H), until the mouth is moist. Sustain physiological functions at a normal level. Use diazepam (Valium), short-acting barbiturates (amobarbital), chloral hydrate, or paraldehyde to relieve excitement. Neostigmine methylsulfate (Prostigmin) is an alternate antidote.

AZATHIOPRINE SODIUM

(Imuran)

Usual dose: 3 to 5 mg/kg of body weight/24 hr. Begin treatment within 24 hours of renal homotransplantation. Some authorities recommend doses of 1 to 5 mg/kg for several days previous to transplant. Maintenance dose is 1 to 2 mg/kg/24 hr. Individualized adjustment is imperative and may be required on a daily basis.

Dilution: Each 100 mg should be diluted initially with 10 ml of sterile water for injection. Swirl the vial gently until completely in solution. May be further diluted in a minimum of 50 ml of sterile saline or glucose in saline and given as an infusion. Mixing with alkaline solutions may result in conversion to 6-mercaptopurine.

Rate of administration: A single dose properly diluted over at least 30 minutes.

Actions: An immunosuppressive drug. It is a derivative of the antineoplastic preparation mercaptopurine. Maximum response occurs if administered when antibody response begins. Has a selective action but achieves good response in many situations. Metabolized readily with small amounts excreted in the urine.

Indications and uses: Adjunct to prevent rejection in renal homotransplantation.

Precautions: (1) Oral dosage is preferred; begin as soon as feasible. (2) Diluted IV solution must be used within 24 hours. (3) Monitor bone marrow function, red and white blood cell counts, platelet count, and BUN frequently. Drug should be withdrawn or dosage reduced at first sign of abnormally large fall in the leukocyte count or other evidence of persistent bone marrow depression. (4) May increase possibility of malignant tumor growth. (5) Potentiated by allopurinol (Zyloprim). Reduce dose to one third or one fourth of usual. (6) Use caution with other myelosuppressive drugs or radiation therapy. (7) Reduce dosage in impaired kidney function (especially immediately after transplant or with cadaveric kidneys) and in persistent negative nitrogen balance. (8) Observe constantly for signs of infection. (9) Safety for use in pregnancy, lactation, and men and women capable of conception not established. (10) Toxic hepatitis or biliary stasis may necessitate discontinuing drug.

Contraindications: Anuria, known hypersensitivity, severe rejection.

Incompatible with: Sufficient information not available. Administer separately.

Side effects: Alopecia, anemia, anorexia, arthralgia, bleeding, diarrhea, fever, jaundice, leukopenia, nausea, oral lesions, pancreatitis, skin rash, thrombocytopenia, vomiting.

Antidote: Notify the physician of all side effects. Most can be treated symptomatically. Drug may be decreased or discontinued or other immunosuppressive agents utilized. Hematopoietic depression may require temporary or permanent withholding of treatment.

(Azlin)

Usual dose: 200 to 300 mg/kg of body weight/day equally divided in 4 to 6 doses (3 Gm every 4 hr equals 18 Gm/24 hr). Do not exceed 24 Gm/24 hr.

Pediatric dose: *Infants 1 month to children 12 years:* 75 mg/kg of body weight every 4 hours (450 mg/kg/24 hr). Limited data available on use in children.

Dilution: Each 1 Gm or fraction thereof should be diluted with at least 10 ml of sterile water, 5% dextrose, or 0.9% sodium chloride for injection. Shake vigrously to dissolve. Must be further diluted to desired volume (50 to 100 ml) with 5% dextrose in H_2O, 0.45 normal saline, or other compatible infusion solution (see literature) and given as an intermittent infusion. For direct IV administration dilute to a 10% solution.

Rate of administration: *Direct IV:* A single dose properly diluted over 3 to 5 minutes. *Intermittent infusion:* A single dose properly diluted over 30 minutes. Discontinue primary IV infusion during administration. Pediatric dose must be given over 30 minutes.

Actions: An extended-spectrum penicillin. Bactericidal against a variety of gram-negative and gram-positive bacteria including aerobic and anaerobic strains. Especially effective against *Pseudomonas*. Well distributed in all body fluids, tissue, bone, and through inflamed meninges. Onset of action is prompt. Crosses placental barrier. Some excretion in urine and breast milk.

Indications and uses: (1) Serious infections of the lower respiratory tract, urinary tract, and skin and skin structure, bone and joint infections, and bacterial septicemia caused by susceptible organisms. (2) Acute pulmonary exacerbation of cystic fibrosis in children.

Precautions: Stable at room temperature for only 24 hours. (2) Warm to 37° C (98.6° F) in a water bath for 20 minutes if precipitation occurs on refrigeration. Shake vigorously. (3) Slightly darkened color does not affect potency. (4) Frequently used concurrently with aminoglycosides (gentamycin [Garamycin]), etc., but must be administered in separate infusions. Inactivated by tetracyclines. (5) Sensitivity studies are indicated to determine the susceptibility of the causative organism to azlocillin. (6) Oral probenecid is indicated to achieve higher and more prolonged blood levels. (7) Watch for early symptoms of allergic reaction. (8) Avoid prolonged use of drug; superinfection caused by overgrowth of nonsusceptible organisms may result. (9) Periodic evaluation of renal, hepatic, and hematopoietic systems and serum potassium is recommended in prolonged therapy. (10) Electrolyte imbalance and cardiac irregularities resulting from high sodium content are very possible. Contains 2.17 mEq of sodium/Gm. (11) Confirm patency of vein; avoid extravasation or intraarterial injection. Slow infusion rate for pain along venipuncture site. (12) Usual duration of therapy is 7 to 10 days. Continue at least 2 days after symptoms of infection disappear. (13) Reduce dose only in severe renal impairment with creatinine clearance temporarily below 30 ml/min. May be given to patients undergoing hemodialysis and peritoneal dialysis (see literature for dose). (14) Test for syphilis also before treating gonorrhea.

Contraindications: History of sensitivity to multiple allergens, penicillin sensitivity.

Incompatible with: Aminoglycosides (amikacin, colistimethate, gentamicin, kanamycin, streptomycin, tobramycin), amphotericin B (Fungizone), chloramphenicol, lincomycin, oxytetracycline, polymyxin B, promethazine (Phenergan), tetracycline (Achromycin), vitamin B with C.

Side effects: Anaphylaxis; bleeding; convulsions; decreased hemoglobin or hematocrit; decreased uric acid level; diarrhea; eosinophilia; elevated SGOT, SGPT, and BUN; fever; hypokalemia; interstitial nephritis; leukopenia; nausea; neuromuscular excitability; neutropenia; pruritus; pseudoproteinuria; skin rash; taste sensation (abnormal); thrombocytopenia; thrombophlebitis; urticaria; vomiting.

Antidote: Notify the physician immediately of any adverse symptoms. For severe symptoms, discontinue the drug, treat allergic reaction (antihistamines, epinephrine, and corticosteroids), and resuscitate as necessary. Hemodialysis or peritoneal dialysis is effective in overdose.

BENZQUINAMIDE HYDROCHLORIDE

pH 3.0 to 4.0

(Emete-Con)

Usual dose: 25 mg (0.2 to 0.4 mg/kg of body weight) as initial dose one time only. If additional doses are indicated, give IM.

Dilution: Each 50 mg must be diluted with 2.2 ml of sterile water for injection (25 mg/ml). May be administered direct, IV through Y tube or three-way stopcock of infusion tubing. Further dilution is not recommended.

Rate of administration: A single dose over a minimum of 30 to 60 seconds.

Actions: Chemically unrelated to phenothiazines and other antiemetics. Exhibits antiemetic, antihistaminic, mild anticholinergic, and sedative actions. Mechanism of action unknown. Effective within minutes and lasts about 1 hour. Metabolized in the liver. Some excretion in the urine.

Indications and uses: Prevention and treatment of nausea and vomiting during anesthesia and surgery.

Precautions: (1) Prophylactic use restricted to specific situations under direction of the anesthesiologist. (2) Monitor blood pressure closely. (3) Markedly reduce dose of benzquinamide in patients receiving pressor agents (epinephrine, etc.). (4) Sudden hypertension, PVCs and PACs (transient) may result with IV injection. Limit use to patients who do not have cardiovascular disease and are not receiving preanesthetic or concomitant cardiovascular drugs. (5) Antiemetic action may mask signs of drug overdose or may obscure diagnosis of conditions such as intestinal obstruction or brain tumor. (6) Safety for use in pregnancy and children is not established. (7) Discard diluted solution after 14 days at room temperature.

Contraindications: Cardiovascular disease, hypersensitivity to benzquinamide hydrochloride.

Incompatible with: Chlordiazepoxide (Librium), diazepam (Valium), pentobarbital (Nembutal), phenobarbital (Luminal), secobarbital (Seconal), sodium chloride, thiopental (Pentothal).

49

Side effects: Allergic reactions, atrial fibrillation, blurred vision, diaphoresis, dizziness, dry mouth, excitement, fever, flushing, hiccups, hypertension, hypotension, nervousness, premature atrial contractions, premature ventricular contractions, salivation, tremors, weakness.

Antidote: Notify the physician of side effects. Depending on severity physician may discontinue the drug. For overdose treatment will be symptomatic and supportive. Atropine may be helpful. Resuscitate as necessary.

BENZTROPINE MESYLATE

(Cogentin mesylate)

Usual dose: 0.5 to 2 mg. May be increased gradually to 4 to 6 mg/24 hr if required.

Dilution: 1 ml of prepared solution equals 1 mg. May be given undiluted.

Rate of administration: 1 mg or fraction thereof over 1 minute.

Actions: Anticholinergic and antihistaminic agent. Effectively relieves tremor, rigidity, drooling, dysphagia, gait disturbances, pain caused by muscle spasm, and other annoying symptoms of parkinsonism. Provides excellent relief in combination with levodopa. Onset of action is prompt by IV or IM route. primarily excreted in the urine.

Indications and uses: Parkinsonism—drug induced (especially phenothiazines and reserpine), postencephalitic, idiopathic, or arteriosclerotic.

Precautions: (1) IV route seldom used, except in acute drug reactions or psychotic patients. (2) IM and oral routes are satisfactory. (3) Has a potent cumulative action; the patient must be under close observation. (4) Observe carefully in patients with hypotension, narrow angle glaucoma, myasthenia gravis, tachycardia, and prostatic hypertrophy, in children over 3 years, and in the elderly. Dosage adjustment is required if an inability to move particular muscle groups persists. (6) Treatment of drug-induced parkinsonism can precipitate toxic psychosis. (7) Side effects may be potentiated by alcohol, barbiturates, phenothiazines, and tricyclic antidepressants. (8) May reduce amount of levodopa absorbed in the GI tract. (9) Do not discontinue other antiparkinsonian drugs abruptly; reduce gradually. (10) May inhibit lactation.

Contraindications: Known hypersensitivity, pregnancy, children under 3 years. Ineffective in tardive dyskinesia.

Incompatible with: No specific incompatibilities are known.

Side effects: *Average dose:* allergic reactions including skin rash, blurred vision, constipation, depression, dizziness, dry mouth, listlessness, nausea, nervousness, numbness of the fingers, vomiting. *Overdose:* anhidrosis, circulatory collapse, coma, dilation of the pupils, dry mucous membranes, flushed skin, hyperpyrexia, incipient glaucoma, paralytic ileus, respiratory depression, tachycardia, urinary retention.

Antidote: Notify the physician of all side effects. Symptoms of an average dose may be relieved by reducing the dose or discontinuing for a day or so and then resuming at a lesser dose. Treat overdose symptomatically, including respiratory support. Physostigmine salicylate (Antilirium) will reverse symptoms of anticholinergic intoxication. Diazepam (Valium) reduces CNS excitation. Resuscitate as necessary.

Usual dose: 2 ml/24 hr. However, up to 20 ml may be added to 1 liter of IV infusion solution.

Dilution: May be given undiluted, but it is preferable to administer Berocca-C diluted in IV fluids. Soluble in all commonly used solutions, including amino acids, glucose solutions, normal saline, or electrolyte replacement fluids.

Rate of administration: 2 ml or fraction thereof over 5 minutes, direct IV administration.

Actions: Provides five B-complex vitamins and 100 mg (500 mg) of vitamin C essential for maintaining health. Water soluble and readily absorbable. Provides daily requirements or corrects an existing deficiency.

Indications and uses: (1) Preoperative and postoperative maintenance of optimum health (2) prolonged IV therapy; (3) increased vitamin requirements in fever, severe burns, increased metabolism, hyperthyroidism, and pregnancy; (4) deficient intestinal absorption of water-soluble vitamins; (5) prolonged or wasting diseases.

Precautions: (1) 2 ml undiluted is the maximum dose that may be given by direct IV route. (2) Previous injections of thiamine hydrochloride can cause sensitivity, and anaphylactic shock may result, especially with too-rapid injection (3) Darkening of the solution is acceptable. It results from a specific, more soluble form of riboflavin. (4) Causes an increased prothrombin time, which can result in hemorrhage with anticoagulants.

Contraindications: Sensitivity to thiamine hydrochloride.

Incompatible with : Amikacin (Amikin), aminophylline, bleomycin, chloramphenicol, chlorothiazide (Diuril), erythromycin (Erythrocin), hydrocortisone (Solu-Cortef), magnesium sulfate, methicillin (Staphcillin), methylprednisolone (Solu-Medrol), nafcillin (Unipen), phenytoin (Dilantin), procaine, prochlorperazine (Compazine), sodium bicarbonate, tetracycline, vancomycin (Vancocin), warfarin (Coumadin).

When combining Berocca-C with other drugs in IV solutions, check the incompatibilities of each drug.

Side effects: Rare when administered as recommended: anaphylactic shock, feeling of warmth, and flushing.

Antidote: Discontinue administration immediately and notify the physician. Treat anaphylaxis or resuscitate as necessary.

Usual dose: 2 ml/24 hr. May be increased to 5 ml/24 hour if indicated.

Pediatric dose: Proportionately less according to age.

Dilution: May be given undiluted. Dilution with 5 to 10 ml of sterile water or normal saline for injection is preferable to avoid discomfort during administration.

Rate of administration: 2 ml or fraction thereof undiluted medication (or its equivalent) over 5 minutes.

Actions: Provides five B-complex vitamins and 75 mg of ascorbic acid. These are water-soluble, readily absorbable vitamins that are essential for maintaining health. Provides daily requirements or corrects an existing deficiency.

Indications and uses: (1) Preoperative and postoperative maintenance of optimum health; (2) prolonged IV therapy; (3) increased vitamin requirements in fever, severe burns, increased metabolism, hyperthyroidism, and pregnancy; (4) deficient intestinal absorption of water-soluble vitamins; (5) prolonged or wasting diseases.

Precautions: (1) Must be refrigerated. (2) Do not use if any precipitate is present. (3) IM route is preferred. (4) If added to IV solutions, must be protected from light. (5) Previous injections of thiamine hydrochloride can cause sensitivity, and anaphylactic shock may result, especially with too-rapid injection. (6) Causes an increased prothrombin time, which can result in hemorrhage with anticoagulants.

Contraindications: Sensitivity to thiamine hydrochloride.

Incompatible with: Aminophylline, ampicillin (Polycillin-N), cephalothin (Keflin), chloramphenicol (Chloromycetin), chlorpromazine (Thorazine), clindamycin (Cleocin), cyanocobalamin (Redisol), erythromycin (Erythrocin), folic acid, heparin, hydrocortisone (Solu-Cortef), hydrocortisone phosphate, kanamycin (Kantrex), levarterenol (Levophed), magnesium sulfate, methicillin (Staphcillin), methylprednisolone (Solu-Medrol), nafcillin (Unipen), nitrofurantoin (Ivadantin), oxacillin (Prostaphlin), oxytetracycline (Terramycin), penicillin G sodium or potassium, phenobarbital (Luminal), phenytoin (Dilantin), prochlorperazine (Compazine), promazine (Sparine), sodium bicarbonate, tetracycline (Achromycin), thiopental (Pentothal), vancomycin (Vancocin), warfarin (Coumadin).

Side effects: Rare when administered as recommended: anaphylactic shock, feeling of warmth, flushing.

Antidote: Discontinue administration immediately and notify the physician. Treat anaphylaxis or resuscitate as necessary.

BIPERIDEN LACTATE

(Akineton)

Usual dose: 2 mg. Repeat every 30 minutes until symptoms are relieved. Do not exceed four doses of 2 mg in 24 hours.

Dilution: May be given undiluted.

Rate of administration: 2 mg or fraction thereof over 1 minute.

Actions: An anticholinergic agent with atropine-like effects. Inhibits the parasympathetic nervous system. Effectively relieves tremor, rigidity, drooling, dysphagia, gait disturbances, and pain caused by muscle spasm. Primarily excreted in the urine.

Indications and uses: (1) Control of drug-induced extrapyramidal disorders (reserpine, phenothiazines); (2) parkinsonism/postencephalitic, arteriosclerotic, and idiopathic.

Precautions: (1) IV route seldom used except in acute drug reactions or psychotic patients; use IM route for children. (2) Has a potent cumulative action; the patient must be under close observation. (3) Use caution in hypotension, hypertension, and tachycardia; cardiac, liver, and kidney disorders; narrow angle glaucoma; myasthenia gravis; obstructive disease of the gastrointestinal or genitourinary tracts; prostatic hypertrophy; pregnancy and lactation; and in the elderly. (4) Treatment of drug-induced parkinsonism can precipitate toxic psychosis. (5) Side effects may be potentiated by alcohol, barbiturates, phenothiazines, and tricyclic antidepressants. (6) May reduce the amount of levodopa absorbed in the GI tract. (7) Potentiated by isoniazid, MAO inhibitors (pargyline [Eutonyl], etc.).

Contraindications: Known hypersensitivity.

Incompatible with: No specific information available. Consider atropine similarities.

Side effects: *Average doses:* allergic reactions including skin rash, blurred vision, constipation, depression, dizziness, dry mouth, listlessness, nausea, nervousness, numbness of the fingers, vomiting. *Overdose:* anhidrosis, circulatory collapse, coma, dilation of the

57

pupils, dry mucous membranes, flushed skin, hyper-pyrexia, incipient glaucoma, paralytic ileus, respiratory depression, tachycardia, urinary retention.

Antidote: Notify the physician of all side effects. Symptoms of an average dose may be relieved by reducing the dose or discontinuing for a day or so and then resuming at a lesser dose. Treat overdose symptomatically, including respiratory support. Physostigmine salicylate (Antilirium) will reverse symptoms of anticholinergic intoxication. Diazepam (Valium) reduces CNS excitation. Resuscitate as necessary.

(Blenoxane)

Usual dose: 0.25 to 0.5 unit/kg of body weight/24 hr (10 to 20 units/M²), once or twice weekly. The first two doses in lymphoma patients should not exceed 2 units to rule out hypersensitivity.

Hodgkin's disease: dosage as above. After a 50% response a maintenance dose of 1 unit/24 hr or 5 units weekly is recommended.

Dilution: *Specific techniques required, see precautions.* Each 15 units or fraction thereof must be diluted with 5 ml or more of sterile water for injection, 5% dextrose, or sodium chloride for injection. Further dilution with 50 to 100 ml of same solution is recommended. May be given through Y tube or three-way stopcock of infusion set.

Rate of administration: Each 15 units or fraction thereof over 10 minutes.

Actions: An antibiotic antineoplastic agent, cell cycle phase nonspecific, that seems to act by splitting and fragmentation of double-stranded DNA, leading to chromosomal damage. It localizes in tumors. Improvement is usually noted within 2 weeks. Well distributed in skin, lungs, kidneys, peritoneum, and lymphatics. About 40% excreted in the urine.

Indications and uses: (1) Testicular carcinoma; may induce complete remission with vinblastine and cisplatin. (2) A palliative treatment, adjunct to surgery or radiation, in patients not responsive to other chemotherapeutic agents or those with squamous cell carcinoma of the skin, head, esophagus, neck, genitourinary tract including the cervix, vulva, scrotum, and penis, in Hodgkin's disease, and other lymphomas.

Precautions: (1) Follow guidelines for handling cytotoxic agents recommended by the National Study Commission on Cytotoxic Exposure (see Appendix, p. 528). (2) Usually administered in the hospital by or under the direction of the physician specialist. (3) Determine patency of vein; avoid extravasation. (4) Obtain a baseline chest x-ray film, and recheck every 1 to 2 weeks to detect pulmonary changes. (5) Monitor renal, hepatic, and central nervous systems and skin for symptoms of toxicity. (6) Dosage is based on average weight in the presence of edema or ascites. (7) Safety for use in pregnancy or lactation is not established. (8) Do not administer vaccines or chloroquine to patients receiving antineoplastic drugs. (9) May be used with other antineoplastic drugs to achieve tumor remission. (10) May cause severe anaphylaxis with lymphomas; use a test dose. (11) Pulmonary toxicity increases markedly with advancing age or larger doses; will occur at lower doses when bleomycin is used in combination with other antineoplastic agents. To identify subclinical pulmonary toxicity, monitor pulmonary diffusion capacity for carbon monoxide monthly. Should remain 30% to 35% above pretreatment value. Most toxic when total cumulative dose exceeds 350 to 450 units. (12) May decrease gastrointestinal absorption of digoxin and hydantoins (phenytoin, etc.). (13) Maintain adequate hydration. (14) Prophylactic antiemetics may reduce nausea and vomiting and increase patient comfort. (15) Observe closely for all signs of infection. (16) Aspirin and diphenhydramine (Benadryl) may be used prophylactically to reduce the incidence of fever and anaphylaxis.

Contraindications: Known hypersensitivity to bleomycin, elderly patients with pulmonary disease.

Incompatible with: Specific information not available; to be considered incompatible with any other drug in syringe or solution due to toxicity and specific use.

Side effects: *Minor:* alopecia, anorexia, chills, dyspnea, fever, hypotension, nausea, phlebitis (infrequent), rales, tenderness of the skin, tumor site pain, vomiting, weight loss. *Major:* anaphylaxis (up to 6 hours after test dose), pneumonitis, pulmonary fibrosis, skin toxicity (including nodules on hands, desquamation of skin, hyperpigmentation, and gangrene).

Antidote: Notify the physician of all side effects. Minor side effects will be treated symptomatically. Discontinue the drug immediately and notify the physician of any symptom of major side effects. Provide immediate treatment (epinephrine [Adrenalin] and diphenhydramine hydrochloride [Benadryl] for anaphylaxis, antibiotics and steroids for pneumonitis) or supportive therapy as indicated.

BRETYLIUM TOSYLATE

pH 5 to 7

(Bretylol)

Usual dose: *Ventricular fibrillation:* 5 mg/kg of body weight. Increase to 10 mg/kg and repeat at 15- to 30-minute intervals if arrhythmia persists. Do not exceed total dose of 30 mg/kg/24 hr.

Other ventricular arrhythmias: 5 to 10 mg/kg by IV infusion. Repeat in 1 to 2 hours if arrhythmia persists.

Maintenance dosage: 5 to 10 mg/kg by infusion every 6 hours or a continuous infusion at 1 to 2 mg/min. Replace with oral antiarrhythmic therapy in 3 to 5 days.

Dilution: May be given undiluted in ventricular fibrillation. For other ventricular arrhythmias, each dose must be diluted with 50 ml or more of 5% dextrose in water or normal saline to be given as an intermittent infusion. Larger amounts may be further diluted in any amount of the above solutions and given as a continuous infusion (1 Gm in 1,000 ml equals 1 mg/ml).

Rate of administration: *Ventricular fibrillation:* a single dose over 15 to 30 seconds.

Intermittent infusion: a single dose over a minimum of 10 to 30 minutes.

Continuous infusion: 1 to 2 mg of diluted solution/min. Use an infusion pump or microdrip (60 gtt/ml). Adjust as indicated by progress in patient's condition.

Actions: A quaternary ammonium compound with antiarrhythmic effects. It increases the ventricular fibrillation threshold, suppresses ventricular arrhythmias and aberrant impulses, and increases the refractory period without increasing heart rate. Probably effective through its adrenergic blocking action. Antifibrillatory effects occur within minutes; suppression of premature beats requires constant plasma levels. Half-life ranges from 4 to 17 hours. Excreted in the urine.

Indications and uses: Prophylaxis and treatment of ventricular fibrillation and treatment of life-threatening ventricular arrhythmias that have failed to respond to adequate doses of lidocaine or procainamide.

Precautions: (1) Monitor the patient's EKG and BP continuously. (2) Keep patient in supine position; postural hypotension is almost always present. Tolerance to hypotensive effect may develop after several days. (3) Correct dehydration or hypovolemia. (4) May aggravate digitalis toxicity; use with caution if patient is receiving digitalis. (5) May cause severe hypotension if fixed cardiac output is present (aortic stenosis, pulmonary hypertension). (6) Used during pregnancy or in children only in life-threatening situations. (7) Use caution if renal function is impaired. (8) Will potentiate catecholamines (dopamine [Intropin], etc.); use diluted solution and monitor BP closely when indicated. (9) Reduce dose under EKG monitoring after 3 to 5 days, then discontinue.

Contraindications: None when used as indicated.

Incompatible with: Specific information not available. Is physically compatible with calcium chloride, dopamine, lidocaine, nitroglycerin, potassium chloride, procainamide, and verapamil; however, therapeutic rates of administration may differ.

Side effects: Anginal attacks, bradycardia, dizziness, hypotension and postural hypotension, increased frequency of PVCs, light-headedness, nausea and vomiting, substernal pressure, syncope, transitory hypertension, vertigo.

Antidote: Notify the physician of all side effects. Nausea and vomiting may subside with reduction in rate of administration. Use dopamine to correct hypotension. Resuscitate as necessary.

(Dimetane-Ten)

Usual dose: 10 mg initially. 5 to 20 mg may be given. Repeat every 3 to 12 hours as indicated. Do not exceed 40 mg/24 hr.

Pediatric dose: Under 12 years, 0.5 mg/kg of body weight/24 hr divided into 3 or 4 doses.

Dilution: May be given undiluted, but further dilution of each ml with 10 ml normal saline for injection is preferred to reduce incidence of side effects. May be added to normal saline or 5% dextrose in water and given as an infusion.

Rate of administration: A single dose over 1 minute. A single dose in an IV infusion may be given at the desired or ordered rate.

Actions: An antihistamine with anticholinergic and sedative effects. Acts by blocking the effects of histamine at various receptor sites. Either eliminates allergic reaction or greatly modifies it. Readily absorbed, widely distributed, and excreted in changed form in the urine.

Indications and uses: (1) Prevention or reduction of allergic reactions to blood or plasma, (2) treatment of anaphylactic reactions, (3) treatment of other allergic conditions if IV route is indicated.

Precautions: (1) IM or subcutaneous use is generally preferred after an initial IV dose. (2) Often used in conjunction with epinephrine. (3) Use caution in patients with a history of bronchial asthma, cardiovascular disease, renal disease, diabetes, hypertension, hyperthyroidism, increased intravascular pressure, and the elderly. (4) Potentiates CNS depressants (alcohol, analgesics, antianxiety agents, hypnotics, sedatives, and tranquilizers). Reduced dosage of CNS depressant is indicated. (5) Keep patient in recumbent position. (6) Protect from light to prevent discoloration in ampoule. (7) If necessary, warm to dissolve any crystals that may have formed.

Contraindications: Hypersensitivity to antihistamines; pregnancy; lactation; newborn or premature infants;

patients taking MAO inhibitors (pargyline [Eutonyl], etc.); lower respiratory diseases.

Incompatible with: Aminophylline, insulin, iodipamide meglumine (Cholografin), pentobarbital (Nembutal).

Side effects: Anaphylaxis, confusion, convulsions, death, dizziness, dryness of mouth, nose and throat, hallucinations, headache, hypertension, hypotension, hysteria, nausea, palpitations, paresthesias, sedation, tachycardia, thickening of bronchial secretions, urinary retention, vomiting, wheezing.

Antidote: Notify the physician of all side effects. Most will subside after the drug is discontinued or will respond to symptomatic treatment. Anticonvulsant barbiturates or analeptics (doxapram [Dopram], etc.) may increase toxicity. Resuscitate as necessary.

BUMETANIDE

(Bumex)

Usual dose: 0.5 to 1.0 mg. May be repeated at 2- to 3-hour intervals. Do not exceed 10 mg/24 hr.

Dilution: May be given undiluted. Not usually added to IV solutions but compatible with 5% dextrose in water, 0.9% sodium chloride, and lactated Ringer's infusion solutions. Usually given through Y tube or three-way stopcock of infusion set.

Rate of administration: A single dose direct IV over 1 to 2 minutes.

Actions: A sulfonamide diuretic, antihypertensive, and antihypercalcemic agent related to the thiazides. A loop diuretic agent. Extremely potent and has a rapid onset of action. Effectiveness is noted within 5 minutes and may last for 4 hours. Apparently acts on the proximal and distal ends of the tubule and the ascending limb of the loop of Henle to excrete water, sodium, chlorides, and potassium. Will produce diuresis in alkalosis or acidosis. Rapidly absorbed and distributed, it is excreted unchanged in the urine.

Indications and uses: (1) Congestive heart failure, (2) acute pulmonary edema, (3) cirrhosis of the liver with ascites, (4) renal diseases including the nephrotic syndrome, (5) edema unresponsive to other diuretic agents, (6) diuresis in patients allergic to furosemide.

Precautions: (1) Can be used for patients allergic to furosemide. 1 mg to 40 mg ratio (bumetanide to furosemide) is used to determine dose. (2) Use only freshly prepared solutions for infusion. Discard after 24 hours. (3) Do not give concurrently with indomethacin (Indocin), probenecid, or lithium. (4) May precipitate excessive diuresis with water and electrolyte depletion. Routine checks on electrolyte panel, CO_2, and BUN are necessary during therapy. Potassium chloride replacement may be required. (5) May be used concurrently with aldosterone antagonists (spironolactone [Aldactone], etc.) for more effective diuresis and to prevent excessive potassium loss. (6) Potentiates antihypertensive drugs, salicylates, muscle relaxants (curare, tubocurarine, etc.), and hypotensive effect of other diuretics and MAO inhibitors (pargyline [Eutonyl], etc.). (7) May cause transient deafness in doses exceeding the usual or in conjunction with ototoxic drugs (dihydrostreptomycin, kanamycin, etc.). (8) May increase blood glucose and has precipitated diabetes mellitus; lowers serum calcium level, causing tetany, and rarely precipitates an acute attack of gout. (9) May cause cardiac arrhythmias with digitalis, ethacrynic acid (Edecrin), or any condition causing hypokalemia; increased toxicity with tetracycline.

Contraindications: Anuria, known hypersensitivity to bumetanide. Use caution and improve basic condition first in hepatic coma, electrolyte depletion, and advanced cirrhosis of the liver.

Incompatible with: Specific information not available. Note precautions.

Side effects: Usually occur in prolonged therapy, seriously ill patients, or following large doses. *Minor:* abdominal pain, arthritic pain, azotemia, dizziness, EKG changes, elevated serum creatinine, encephalopathy, headache, hyperglycemia, hyperuricemia, hypochloremia, hyponatremia, hypotension, impaired hearing, muscle cramps, nausea, pruritus, rash. *Major:* anaphylactic shock, blood volume reduction, circulatory collapse, dehydration, excessive diuresis, hypokalemia, metabolic acidosis, vascular thrombosis and embolism.

Antidote: If minor side effects are noted, discontinue the drug and notify the physician, who may treat the side effects symptomatically and continue the drug. If side effects are progressive or any major side effect occurs, discontinue the drug immediately and notify the physician. Treatment of major side effects is symptomatic and aggressive and includes fluid and electrolyte replacement. Resuscitate as necessary.

(Stadol)

Usual dose: 0.5 to 2 mg. Repeat every 3 to 4 hours as necessary.

Dilution: May be given undiluted.

Rate of administration: Each 2 mg or fraction thereof over 3 to 5 minutes. Frequently titrated according to symptom relief and respiratory rate.

Actions: A potent narcotic analgesic with some narcotic antagonist effects. Exact mechanism of action is unknown. Analgesia similar to morphine is produced. Does produce respiratory depression, but this does not increase markedly with larger doses. Pain relief is effected almost immediately, peaks at 30 minutes, and lasts about 3 hours. Causes some hemodynamic changes that increase the work load of the heart.

Indications and uses: (1) Relief of moderate to severe pain, (2) preoperative or prepartum medication.

Precautions: (1) Not used for narcotic-dependent patients because of antagonist activity. (2) Can produce dependency; monitor dosage carefully. (3) Oxygen and controlled respiratory equipment must be available. (4) Observe patient frequently and monitor vital signs. (5) Use in myocardial infarction, ventricular dysfunction, and coronary insufficiency only if the patient is hypersensitive to morphine or meperidine. (6) Use caution in respiratory depression or difficulty from any source, obstructive respiratory conditions, head injury, and impaired liver or kidney function. (7) Potentiated by barbiturates (secobarbital [Seconal]), phenothiazines (Compazine), cimetidine, droperidol, and other tranquilizers.

Contraindications: Hypersensitivity to butorphanol. Biliary surgery, labor, delivery, pregnancy, lactation, and children are probable contraindications

Incompatible with: Specific information not available.

Side effects: Anaphylaxis, clammy skin, confusion, diplopia, dizziness, dry mouth, floating feeling, flushing, hallucinations, headache, lethargy, light-headedness, nausea, respiratory depression, sedation, sensitivity to cold, sweating, unusual dreams, vertigo, vomiting, warmth.

Antidote: With increasing severity of any side effect or onset of symptoms of overdose, discontinue the drug and notify the physician. Naloxone hydrochloride (Narcan) will reverse respiratory depression. A patent airway, artificial ventilation, oxygen therapy, and other symptomatic treatment must be instituted promptly.

CAFFEINE AND SODIUM BENZOATE

Usual dose: 500 mg to 1 Gm. Maximum dose is 2.5 Gm/ 24 hr.

Dilution: May be given undiluted.

Rate of administration: 250 mg or fraction thereof over 1 minute.

Actions: A xanthine derivative and descending analeptic CNS stimulant. Small doses cause wakefulness and mental alertness. Larger doses stimulate the respiratory center and increase heart action. It is believed to constrict the intracranial blood vessels and lower intracranial pressure. Widely distributed throughout the body and excreted in the urine. Crosses the placental barrier. Excreted in breast milk.

Indications and uses: Rarely used. (1) To alleviate headaches after spinal cord puncture, (2) alcoholic stupor/ excitement, (3) barbiturate poisoning antidote, (4) narcotic poisoning antidote if levallorphan (Lorfan) or naloxone (Narcan) is not available.

Precautions: (2) Usually given IM; IV route is for emergencies only. (3) Most people have developed a tolerance level for caffeine because of daily ingestion of coffee or tea. (3) MAO inhibitors (isocarboxazid [Marplan], etc.) potentiate caffeine and can cause an acute hypertensive crisis. (4) May produce convulsions with overdose of propoxyphene (Darvon).

Contraindications: Acute myocardial infarction.

Incompatible with: Chlorpromazine (Thorazine).

Side effects: Generally only occur with very large doses: cardiac irregularities, diuresis, excessive irritability, hypertension (transient), insomnia, muscle twitching, nausea and vomiting, palpitations, and tachycardia.

Antidote: For major symptoms, discontinue drug and notify the physician. Short-acting sedatives (pentobarbital [Nembutal], etc.) will quiet CNS stimulation.

Usual dose: 5 to 10 ml (500 mg to 1 Gm) at intervals of 1 to 3 days. 5 ml (500 mg) every 10 minutes IV or into the ventricular cavity during cardiac resuscitation. 0.5 Gm for every 500 ml of whole blood if arrest occurs in a situation requiring copious blood replacement. *1 Gm (10 ml) contains 13.6 mEq (272 mg) of calcium.*

Infant dose: 0.2 to 0.3 ml/kg of body weight of a 10% solution for cardiac resuscitation.

Dilution: May be given undiluted, but preferably diluted with an equal amount of distilled water or normal saline for injection to make a 5% solution.

Rate of administration: 100 mg or fraction thereof of 10% solution over 1 minute. Total dose may be given over 30 to 60 seconds during cardiac resuscitation if necessary.

Actions: Calcium is a basic element very prevalent in the human body. It affects bones, nerves, muscles, glands, and cardiac and vascular tone, as well as normal coagulation of the blood. It is excreted in the urine and feces.

Indications and uses: Calcium preparations other than calcium chloride are preferred except in cardiac resuscitation. (1) Hypocalcemia tetany, (2) cardiac asystole or electromechanical dissociation, (3) sensitivity reactions, (4) insect bites or stings, (5) acute symptoms of lead colic, (6) antidote for magnesium sulfate.

Precautions: (1) Three times more potent than calcium gluconate. (2) For IV use only; however, vein irritation may occur. Necrosis and sloughing will occur with IM or subcutaneous injection. (3) Solution should be warmed to body temperature. (4) Will increase digitalis toxicity. Use with extreme care in patients receiving digitalis. (5) Can reduce neuromuscular paralysis and respiratory depression produced by antibiotics such as kanamycin (Kantrex). (6) Inhibits tetracycline absorption. (7) Vitamin D aids absorption. (8) Keep patient recumbent after injection to prevent postural hypotension.

Contraindications: Ventricular fibrillation.

Incompatible with: Amphotericin B (Fungizone), cephalothin (Keflin), chlorpheniramine (Chlortrimeton), chlortetracycline (Aureomycin), digitalis (Digitoxin, etc.), epinephrine (Adrenalin), methicillin (Staphcillin), nitrofurantoin (Ivadantin), oxytetracycline (Terramycin), sodium bicarbonate, tetracycline (Achromycin), warfarin (Coumadin). Calcium salts are not generally mixed with carbonates, phosphates, sulfates, or tartrates.

Side effects: Rare when given as recommended: bradycardia, calcium taste, cardiac arrest, depression, heat waves, prolonged state of cardiac contraction, tingling sensation.

Antidote: If side effects occur, discontinue the drug and notify the physician. Resuscitate as necessary. Disodium edetate may be used with extreme caution as a calcium-chelating agent if overdosage is critical.

CALCIUM DISODIUM EDETATE   pH 6.5 to 7.5

(Calcium Disodium Versenate)

Usual dose: 1 Gm (5 ml) twice in 24 hours for 3 to 5 days. Give second dose after 6 hours. Repeat after several days' rest if indicated. Do not exceed 50 mg/kg of body weight/24 hr.

Pediatric dose: Should not exceed 70 mg/kg of body weight/24 hr in two equal doses. *Do not exceed recommended dosage.*

Dilution: Each dose must be diluted in 250 to 500 ml of 5% dextrose in water or isotonic saline for IV infusion.

Rate of administration: Each dose must be given over at least 1 hour, 2 hours in the symptomatic patient. Physician will order a specific rate.

Actions: A chelating agent that helps to remove metals, especially lead, from the body. Forms stable compounds, which are then excreted in the urine.

Indications and uses: (1) Acute and chronic lead poisoning, (2) heavy metal poisoning, (3) removal of radioactive and nuclear fission products.

Precautions: (1) Establish urine flow before drug is administered. (2) Monitor vital signs, EKG, and urine output. (3) Daily urine specimens are recommended to determine status of renal function. (4) Obtain specific fluid orders from the physician. Increased fluid intake is desirable except in the presence of cerebral edema. (5) IM injection is preferred in presence of increased intracranial pressure. (6) May produce toxic and fatal effects. (7) Use with caution in active or healed tuberculosis and mild renal disease. (8) Do not confuse with disodium edetate (Endrate), which does not chelate lead but actually removes calcium from the body and can be very dangerous. (9) Not effective in mercury poisoning. (10) Usually given IM in children concurrently with dimercaprol (BAL).

Contraindications: Anuria, severe renal disease.

Incompatible with: Must be diluted in specific intravenous solutions. *Do not mix with any other IV medication.*

Side effects: Acute renal tubular necrosis, hematuria, hypotension, leg and other muscle cramps, malaise, weakness.

Antidote: Notify the physician of any side effects. Most will be treated symptomatically. Evidence of increasing renal damage will require temporary discontinuation of the drug.

CALCIUM GLUCEPTATE
INJECTION   pH 6.0 to 7.0

Usual dose: 5 to 20 ml (5 ml is equal in calcium content [0.09 Gm] to 10 ml of 10% calcium gluconate). May be repeated if indicated.

Newborn exchange transfusion: The average dose is 0.5 ml after each 100 ml of blood exchanged.

Dilution: May be given undiluted.

Rate of administration: 1 ml or fraction thereof over 1 minute.

Actions: Calcium is a basic element very prevalent in the human body. It affects bones, nerves, muscles, glands, and cardiac and vascular tone, as well as normal coagulation of the blood. It is excreted in the urine and feces.

Indications and uses: (1) Hypocalcemia caused by neonatal tetany, parathyroid deficiency tetany, vitamin D deficiency tetany, alkalosis; (2) prevention of hypocalcemia during exchange transfusions.

Precautions: (1) IV use is preferred in adults and mandatory for infants and young children. Necrosis and sloughing can occur with IM or subcutaneous injection. (2) Will increase digitalis toxicity. Use with extreme care in patients receiving digitalis. (3) Solution should be warmed to body temperature. (4) Keep patient lying down after injection to prevent postural hypotension.

Contraindications: IM use is contraindicated in infants and small children.

Incompatible with: Cefamandole (Mandol, cefazolin (Kefzol), cephalothin (Keflin), magnesium sulfate, prednisolone sodium phosphate (Hydeltrasol), prochlorperazine (Compazine), tetracyclines. Calcium salts are not generally mixed with carbonates, phosphates, sulfates, or tartrates.

Side effects: Usually occur only with rapid administration and may include tingling sensations, calcium taste, and heat waves.

Antidote: Decrease rate of administration. If side effects persist, discontinue the drug and notify the physician. Further dilution and a decrease in the rate of administration may be necessary.

CALCIUM GLUCONATE
INJECTION

(Kalcinate)

Usual dose: 10 ml/24 hr, every other day, or every third day. 10 ml of 10% solution equals 0.09 Gm of calcium. Up to 30 ml may be given if indicated. Up to 60 ml may be given in an IV infusion.

2 to 4 ml into the ventricular cavity or IV during cardiac resuscitation.

Pediatric dose: 2 to 5 ml/24 hr, every other day, or every third day.

Dilution: May be given undiluted or may be further diluted in 1,000 ml of normal saline solution for infusion.

Rate of administration: Undiluted, each 0.5 ml or fraction thereof over 1 minute. Diluted in 1,000 ml of normal saline, it may be given over 12 to 24 hours.

Actions: Calcium is a basic element very prevalent in the human body. It affects bones, nerves, glands, and cardiac and vascular tone, as well as normal coagulation of the blood. It is excreted in the urine and feces.

Indications and uses: (1) Calcium deficiency caused by hypoparathyroidism, osteomalacia, vitamin D deficiency, preeclampsia, uremia; (2) cardiac resuscitation; (3) sensitivity reactions; (4) uterine inertia; (5) insect bites or stings; (6) antidote for magnesium sulfate; (7) acute symptoms of lead colic; (8) may be given after blood transfusions to maintain calcium-potassium ratio.

Precautions: (1) Has only one third the potency of calcium chloride. (2) IV use is preferred in adults and mandatory for infants and young children. Necrosis and sloughing can occur with IM or subcutaneous injection. (3) Solution should be warmed to body temperature. (4) Will increase digitalis toxicity. Use with extreme care in patients receiving digitalis. (5) Vitamin D aids absorption. (6) Inhibits tetracycline absorption. (7) Vasodilation may cause mild hypotension.

Contraindications: IM use in infants and small children.

Incompatible with: Amphotericin B (Fungizone), cefamandole (Mandol), cefazolin (Ancef), cephalothin

(Keflin), chlortetracycline (Aureomycin), digitalis (digitoxin, etc.), epinephrine (Adrenalin), hydrocortisone phosphate, kanamycin (Kantrex), magnesium sulfate, methylprednisolone (Solu-Cortef), oxytetracycline (Terramycin), potassium phosphate, prochlorperazine (Compazine), promethazine (Phenergan), sodium bicarbonate, streptomycin, tetracycline. Calcium salts are not generally mixed with carbonates, phosphates, sulfates, or tartrates.

Side effects: Rare when given as recommended: bradycardia, calcium taste, cardiac arrest, depression of neuromuscular function, flushing, heat waves, prolonged state of cardiac contraction, tingling sensation.

Antidote: If side effects occur, discontinue the drug and notify the physician. Disodium edetate may be used with extreme caution as a calcium-chelating agent if overdosage is critical.

(Geopen, Pyopen)

Usual dose: 1 to 10 Gm every 4 to 6 hours (200 to 500 mg/kg of body weight/24 hr), depending on the severity of the infection. Not to exceed 40 Gm/24 hr; normal renal function is necessary for this dosage.

Pediatric dose: 50 to 500 mg/kg of body weight/24 hr in divided doses ever 4 to 6 hours, depending on the severity of the infection. Not to exceed 500 mg/kg/24 hr or 40 Gm/24 hr, whichever is less.

Newborn dose: 100 mg/kg of body weight initially, then 75 mg/kg of body weight every 8 hours.

Dilution: Each 1 Gm or fraction thereof is diluted with 2 to 2.6 ml of sterile water for injection. Further dilution of each gram with an additional 10 to 20 ml of sterile water for injection is required for direct IV administration. May be added to large volumes of standard IV fluids for infusion including 50 or 100 ml additive bottles.

Rate of administration: 1 Gm or fraction thereof over 5 minutes when given directly IV. Large doses may be given over 4 to 24 hours in an IV infusion. Administer newborn dose over 15 minutes.

Actions: An extended-spectrum penicillin. Bactericidal for *Pseudomonas*, indole-positive *Proteus* strains, *Haemophilus influenzae, Escherichia coli*, and other gram-negative organisms. Not active against penicillinase-producing organisms. Excreted in the urine. Excreted in breast milk.

Indications and uses: Urinary tract infections, severe systemic infections and septicemia, acute and chronic respiratory infections, and soft tissue infections. Useful in treating infections in acute leukemia or in patients receiving immunosuppressive or oncolytic drugs.

Precautions: (1) Administer within 24 hours of preparation. (2) Sensitivity studies are indicated to determine the susceptibility of the causative organism to carbenicillin. (3) Oral probenecid is advised to achieve higher and more prolonged blood levels. (4) Reduce daily dose commensurate with amount of renal impairment. Intervals between injections should also be increased. (5) Watch for early symptoms of allergic reaction. (6) Avoid prolonged use of drug; superinfection caused by overgrowth of nonsusceptible organisms may result. (7) Periodic evaluation of renal, hepatic, and hematopoietic systems is recommended in prolonged therapy. (8) Electrolyte imbalance and cardiac irregularities resulting from high sodium content are very possible. (9) Confirm patency of vein; avoid extravasation or intraarterial injection. Slow infusion rate for pain along venipuncture site. (10) Gentamicin used concurrently in severe infection. May not be combined in the same IV solution. (11) Tetracyclines inhibit bactericidal action.

Contraindications: History of sensitivity to multiple allergens, known penicillin sensitivity, pregnancy.

Incompatible with: Aminoglycosides (amikacin, colistimethate, gentamicin, kanamycin, streptomycin, tobramycin), amphotericin B (Fungizone), chloramphenicol, lincomycin, oxytetracycline, polymyxin B, promethazine (Phenergan), tetracycline (Achromycin), vitamin B with C.

Side effects: Abnormal clotting time or prothrombin time, anaphylaxis, anemia, convulsions, elevated temperature, elevated SGOT and SGPT, eosinophilia, hematuria, itching, nausea, neuromuscular irritability, thrombophlebitis, unpleasant taste in the mouth, urticaria.

Antidote: Notify the physician immediately of any adverse symptoms. For severe symptoms, discontinue the drug, treat allergic reaction (antihistamines, epinephrine, and corticosteroids), and resuscitate as necessary.

CARMUSTINE (BCNU)

pH 5.6 to 6.0

(BiCNU)

Usual dose: Initial dose is 200 mg/M^2. May be given as a single dose, or one half of the calculated dose may be given initially and repeated the next day. Repeat every 6 weeks if bone marrow has sufficiently recovered. Repeat doses adjusted according to hematological response of previous dose.

Dilution: *Specific techniques required, see precautions.* Initially dilute 100 mg vial with supplied sterile diluent (3 ml of absolute ethanol). Further dilute with 27 ml of sterile water for injection. Each ml will contain 3.3 mg of carmustine. Withdraw desired dose and further dilute in 100 to 500 ml of 5% dextrose or sodium chloride for injection and give as an infusion.

Rate of administration: Each single dose must be given as an infusion over a minimum of 1 hour. Reduce rate for pain or burning at injection site, flushing of the skin, or suffusion of the conjunctiva. Usually given over 1 to 2 hours.

Actions: An alkylating agent of the nitrogen mustard group with antitumor activity, cell cycle phase nonspecific. Degraded to metabolites within 15 minutes of administration. Concurrent concentration is higher in cerebrospinal fluid than in plasma. Excreted in changed form in urine. Small amounts are excreted as respiratory CO_2.

Indications and uses: Suppress or retard neoplastic growth of brain tumors; multiple myeloma; gastrointestinal, breast, bronchogenic, and renal carcinomas; meningeal leukemia; Hodgkin's disease; and some non-Hodgkin's lymphomas.

Precautions: (1) Follow guidelines for handling cytotoxic agents recommended by the National Study Commission on Cytotoxic Exposure (see Appendix, p. 528). (2) Usually administered in the hostpital by or under the direction of the physician specialist. (3) Adjust dose downward for platelet count below 75,000, leukocytes below 3,000, and when used with other myelosuppressive drugs. (4) Delayed toxicity is probable in 4 to 6 weeks; wait at least 6 weeks between doses.

81

Frequent leukocyte and platelet counts are indicated. (5) Store in refrigerator (2° to 8° C [36° to 46° F]) in all forms. Stable up to 48 hours after dilution. Temperatures above 27° C (80° F) will cause liquefication of the drug powder; discard immediately. (6) Often used with other antineoplastic drugs in reduced doses to achieve tumor remission. (7) Will produce teratogenic effects on the fetus. Has a mutagenic potential. (8) Nausea and vomiting can be severe. Prophylactic administration of antiemetics is recommended. (9) Do not administer vaccine or chloroquine to patients receiving antineoplastic drugs. (10) Avoid contact of carmustine solution with the skin. (11) Potentiates or is potentiated by hepatotoxic or nephrotoxic medications and radiation therapy. (12) Observe for any signs of infection. (13) Maintain hydration.

Contraindications: Hypersensitivity to carmustine, previous chemotherapy, or other causes that result in insufficient circulating platelets, leukocytes, or erythrocytes.

Incompatible with: Consider incompatible with any other drug in syringe or solution due to toxicity and specific use.

Side effects: Most are dose related and can be reversed. Bone marrow toxicity most pronounced at 4 to 6 weeks, can be severe and cumulative with repeated dosage. Anemia, elevated liver function test results, flushing of skin and suffusion of conjunctivia (from too-rapid infusion rate), hyperpigmentation of skin (from actual contact with solution), nausea and vomiting, renal abnormalities.

Antidote: Notify physician of all side effects. Most will decrease in severity with reduced dosage, increased time span between doses, or symptomatic treatment. May reduce therapeutic effectiveness. Hematopoietic depression may require withholding carmustine until recovery occurs. There is no specific antidote. Supportive therapy as indicated will help sustain the patient in toxicity.

CEFAMANDOLE NAFATE

(Mandol)

Usual dose: 500 mg to 2 Gm every 4 to 8 hours depending on severity of infection. Do not exceed 12 Gm/24 hr.

Perioperative prophylaxis: 1 or 2 Gm 30 minutes to 1 hour before incision. Follow with 1 to 2 Gm every 6 hours for 24 to 48 hours.

Pediatric dose: 50 to 150 mg/kg of body weight/24 hr in equally divided doses every 4 to 8 hours. Do not exceed maximum adult dose.

Perioperative prophylaxis: 50 to 100 mg/kg/24 hr in equally divided doses. Give first dose 30 minutes to 1 hour before incision and every 6 hours for up to 72 hours.

Dilution: *Direct IV:* each 1 Gm or fraction thereof must be diluted with at least 10 ml of sterile water for injection.

Intermittent infusion: further dilute in 100 ml of dextrose in water or normal saline for infusion and give through Y tube, three-way stopcock, or additive infusion set.

Continuous infusion: may be further diluted in up to 1,000 ml of compatible infusion solutions (see literature).

Rate of administration: Each 1 Gm or fraction thereof over 3 to 5 minutes or longer as indicated by amount of solution and condition of the patient. Discontinue IV infusion solution during administration of cefamandole by intermittent infusion. Rate of continuous infusion should be by physician order.

Actions: A semisynthetic cephalosporin antibiotic that is bactericidal to many gram-positive and gram-negative organisms. Absorbed by most body fluids. Excreted rapidly in the urine.

Indications and uses: (1) Treatment of serious infections of the respiratory tract, genitourinary tract, bones, joints, soft tissue, and skin, septicemia, and peritonitis. Effective only if the causative organism is susceptible. (2) Preoperative, intraoperative, and postoperative prophylaxis.

83

Precautions: (1) Sensitivity studies are indicated to determine the susceptibility of the causative organism to cefamandole. (2) Watch for early symptoms of allergic reaction. (3) Reduce total daily dose if renal function is impaired. (4) Avoid prolonged use of drug; superinfection caused by overgrowth of nonsusceptible organisms may result. (5) Administer within 24 hours of preparatoin or up to 96 hours if refrigerated. (6) Use extreme caution in the penicillin-sensitive patient; cross-sensitivity may occur. (7) Adverse interaction may occur with promethazine (Phenergan), procainamide (Pronestyl), quinidine, muscle relaxants, potent diuretics, and aminoglycosides. Will produce symptoms of acute alcohol intolerance with alcohol. (8) Frequently used concomitantly with aminoglycosides in severe infections, but these drugs must never be mixed in the same infusion or given concurrently. Nephrotoxicity is markedly increased when both drugs are utilized. (9) Use only if absolutely necessary in pregnancy. (10) Probenecid inhibits excretion and may require reduction in dosage. (11) Forms carbon dioxide after initial dilution; use caution when drawing from vial, and do not store in syringe. (12) Avoid concurrent administration of bacteriostatic agents.

Contraindications: Known cephalosporin sensitivity, infants under 1 month of age.

Incompatible with: Amikacin (Amikin), calcium, carbenicillin (Geopen, cimetidine (Tagamet), gentamicin (Garamycin), kanamycin (Kantrex), lidocaine (Xylocaine), magnesium, tobramycin (Nebcin).

Side effects: Allergic reactions including anaphylaxis; anorexia; false positive reaction for urine glucose except with Test-Tape or Keto-Diastix; leukopenia; local site pain; nausea and vomiting; neutropenia; oral thrush; phlebitis, positive direct Coomb's test; transient elevation of SGOT, SGPT, BUN, alkaline phosphatase, proteinuria; and thrombophlebitis.

Antidote: Notify physician of any side effects. Discontinue the drug if indicated. Treat allergic reaction as indicated and resuscitate as necessary.

CEFAZOLIN SODIUM

pH 4.8 to 5.5

(Ancef, Kefzol)

Usual dose: 250 mg to 1 Gm every 6 to 8 hours. Not to exceed 6 Gm/24 hr, depending on severity of infection. *Perioperative prophylaxis:* 0.5 to 1 Gm 30 minutes to 1 hour before incision. May be repeated in 2 hours in the OR and every 6 to 8 hours for up to 5 days.

Pediatric dose: 25 to 50 mg/kg of body weight/24 hr in three or four equally divided doses. May be increased to 100 mg/kg/24 hr in severe infections. Do not exceed adult dose.

Dilution: Each 1 Gm or fraction thereof must be diluted with at least 10 ml of sterile water for injection. To reduce the incidence of thrombophlebitis, may be further diluted in 50 ml of 5% dextrose in water, normal saline for injection, or other compatible infusion solutions (see literature). May be administered through Y tube, three-way stopcock, additive infusion set, or as a continuous infusion.

Rate of administration: Each 1 Gm or fraction thereof over 5 minutes or longer as indicated by amount of solution and condition of patient.

Actions: A semisynthetic cephalosporin antibiotic that is bactericidal through inhibition of cell wall synthesis to many organisms, including staphylococci and streptococci. A number of organisms are resistant to this cephalosporin. Absorbed by most body fluids. Excreted rapidly in the urine.

Indications and uses: (1) Treatment of serious infections of the bone, joints, skin, soft tissue, bloodstream, cardiovascular system, respiratory tract, and genitourinary tract. Effective only if the causative organism is susceptible. (2) Preoperative, intraoperative, and postoperative prophylaxis.

Precautions: (1) Sensitivity studies are indicated to determine the susceptibility of the causative organisms to cefazolin. (2) Watch for early symptoms of allergic reaction. (3) Reduce total daily dose if renal function is impaired. (4) Avoid prolonged use of drug; superinfection caused by overgrowth of nonsusceptible organisms may result. (5) Administer within 24 hours

85

of preparation, or up to 96 hours if under refrigeration (5° C [41° F]). (6) Continuous IV infusion is not recommended; markedly increases incidence of phlebitis. (7) Use extreme caution in the penicillin-sensitive patient; cross-sensitivity may occur. (8) Adverse interaction may occur with promethazine (Phenergan), procainamide (Pronestyl), quinidine, muscle relaxants, aminoglycosides (gentamicin, etc.), and potent diuretics. (9) Use only if absolutely necessary in pregnancy. (10) Higher blood levels are obtained with probenecid. (11) Avoid concurrent administration of bacteriostatic agents.

Contraindications: Known cephalosporin sensitivity, infants under 1 month of age.

Incompatible with: Amobarbital (Amytal), calcium gluceptate, calcium gluconate, colistimethate (Coly-Mycin M), erythromycin, kanamycin (Kantrex), oxytetracycline, pentobarbital (Nembutal), polymyxin B, tetracycline.

Side effects: Allergic reactions including anaphylaxis; anorexia; false positive reaction for urine glucose except with Tes-Tape or Keto-Diastix; leukopenia; local site pain; nausea and vomiting; neutropenia; oral thrush; phlebitis; positive direct and indirect Coombs' test; transient elevation of SGOT, SGPT, BUN, and alkaline phosphatase.

Antidote: Notify the physician of any side effects. Discontinue the drug if indicated, treat allergic reaction as indicated, and resuscitate as necessary.

CEFOPERAZONE

(Cefobid)

Usual dose: 2 to 4 Gm/24 hr in equally divided doses every 12 hours. Total daily dose and frequency may be increased in severe infections.

Dilution: Each 1 Gm must be diluted with 5 ml of sterile water. Difficult to put into solution. Shake vigorously to ensure solution, then allow to sit and examine for clarity. Each 1 Gm may be further diluted with 20 to 40 ml of 5% dextrose in water, normal saline, or other compatible solutions (see literature) to a maximum dilution of 50 mg/ml for intermittent infusion or diluted to 2 to 25 mg/ml and given as a continuous infusion.

Rate of administration: *Direct IV:* a single dose equally distributed over 3 to 5 minutes. May be given through Y tube or three-way stopcock of infusion set.
Intermittent IV; a single does over 15 to 30 minutes. Discontinue primary infusion during administration.
Continous infusion: 500 to 1,000 ml over 6 to 24 hours, depending on total dose and concentration.

Actions: A broad-spectrum cephalosporin antibiotic similar to cefamandole. Bactericidal to many gram-negative and gram-positive organisms. Effective against organisms resistant to other second- and third-generation cephalosporins. Absorbed by most body fluids including inflamed meninges and bone tissue. Excreted in bile. Crosses placental barrier. Excreted in breast milk.

Indications and uses: Treatment of serious respiratory tract, intraabdominal, skin and skin structure, and gynecological infections and bacterial septicemia. Most effective against specific organisms (see literature).

Precautions: (1) Sensitivity studies are indicated to determine the susceptibility of the causitive organism to cefoperazone. (2) Watch for early symptoms of allergic reaction. (3) Reduce total daily dose if renal function is impaired. Calculated according to degree of impairment. (4) Avoid prolonged use of drug; superinfection caused by overgrowth of nonsusceptible organisms may result. (5) Administer within 24 hours of preparation. Selected solutions may be preserved 5 days with refrigeration. (6) Use extreme caution in the penicillin-sensitive patient; cross-sensitivity may occur. (7) Adverse interaction may occur with promethazine (Phenergan), procainamide (Pronestyl), quinidine, muscle relaxants, potent diuretics, and aminoglycosides. Will produce symptoms of acute alcohol intolerance with alcohol. (8) Frequently used concomitantly with aminoglycosides in severe infections, but these drugs must never be mixed in the same infusion or given concurrently. Nephrotoxicity is markedly increased when both drugs are utilized. (9) Use only if absolutely necessary in pregnancy. (10) Use caution in patients with liver impairment. (11) Probenecid inhibits excretion and may require reduction in dosage. (12) Avoid concurrent administration of bacteriostatic agents. (13) May cause thrombophlebitis. Use small needles and large veins and rotate infusion sites. (14) Electrolyte imbalance and cardiac irregularities resulting from high sodium content are very possible. Contains 1.5 mEq of sodium/Gm.

Contraindications: Known sensitivity to cephalosporins or related antibiotics (penicillins). Not recommended for use in children.

Incompatible with: Specific information not available. Any other bacteriostatic agent and all aminoglycosides (kanamycin [Kantrex], etc.).

Side effects: Full scope of allergic reactions including anaphylaxis. Abnormal bleeding; decreased hemoglobin or decreased hematocrit; decreased prothrombin time; decreased platelet functions; diarrhea; dyspnea; eosinophilia; elevation of SGOT, SGPT, total bilirubin, alkaline phosphatase, LDH, and BUN (transient); false positive reaction for urine glucose except with Tes-Tape or Keto-Diastix; fever; leukopenia; local site pain; pseudomembranous colitis; thrombocytopenia; thrombophlebitis; transient neutropenia; vaginitis; vomiting.

Antidote: Notify the physician of any side effects. Discontinue the drug if indicated. Treat allergic reaction as indicated and resuscitate as necessary. Hemodialysis may be useful in overdose. Vitamin K, fresh frozen plasma, packed red cells, or platelet concentrates may be indicated in abnormal bleeding tendencies confirmed by lab evaluations.

CEFOTAXIME
(Claforan)

Usual dose: Depends on seriousness of infection. 1 to 2 Gm every 4 to 6 or 8 hours. Usually 1 Gm every 6 to 8 hours. Maximum daily dose is 12 Gm. Higher doses are often reduced with positive clinical response.

Perioperative prophylaxis: 1 Gm 30 to 90 minutes prior to incision, then 1 Gm 30 to 120 minutes later. May be repeated in a lengthy operation. In cesarean section give initial dose after cord is clamped then 1 Gm at 6 and 12 hours post operatively.

Pediatric dose: *Newborn to 1 week:* 50 mg/kg of body weight every 12 hours.

1 to 4 weeks: 50 mg/kg every 8 hours.

1 month to 12 years: less than 50 kg, 50 to 180 mg/kg/ 24 hr in 4 to 6 divided doses.

Dilution: Each single dose must be diluted with 10 ml of sterile water, 5% dextrose in water, 0.9% sodium chloride, or other compatible infusion solution for injection (see literature). May be further diluted with compatible solutions and given as an intermittent infusion or added to larger volumes and given as a continuous infusion.

Rate of administration: *Direct IV:* a single dose equally distributed over 3 to 5 minutes. May be given through Y tube or three-way stopcock of infusion set.

Intermittent IV: a single dose over 30 minutes. Discontinue primary infusion during administration.

Continuous infusion: 500 to 1,000 ml over 6 to 24 hours, depending on total dose and concentration.

Actions: A broad-spectrum cephalosporin antibiotic similar to cefamandole. Bactericidal to many gram-negative and gram-positive organisms. Effective against many otherwise resistant organisms. Absorbed by most body fluids including inflamed meninges. Some metabolites are formed. Excreted in the urine. Crosses placental barrier. Excreted in breast milk.

Indications and uses: (1) Treatment of serious lower respiratory tract, urinary tract, skin and skin structure, intraabdominal, bone and joint, CNS, and gynecological infections and bacteremia/septicemia. Most effective against specific organisms (see literature). (2) Perioperative prophylaxis.

Precautions: (1) Sensitivity studies are indicated to determine the susceptibility of the causative organism to cefotaxime. (2) Watch for early symptoms of allergic reaction. (3) Reduce total daily dose if renal function is impaired. Calculated according to degree of impairment. (4) Avoid prolonged use of drug; superinfection caused by overgrowth of nonsusceptible organisms may result. (5) Administer within 24 hours of preparation or up to 5 days if refrigerated. (6) Use extreme caution in the penicillin-sensitive patient; cross-sensitivity may occur. (7) Adverse interaction may occur with promethazine (Phenergan), procainamide (Pronestyl), quinidine, muscle relaxants, potent diuretics, and aminoglycosides. (8) Frequently used concomitantly with aminoglycosides in severe infections, but these drugs must never be mixed in the same infusion or given concurrently. Nephrotoxicity is markedly increased when both drugs are utilized. (9) Use only if absolutely necessary in pregnancy. (10) Probenecid inhibits excretion and may require reduction in dosage. (11) Avoid concurrent administration of bacteriostatic agents. (12) May cause thrombophlebitis. Use small needles and large veins and rotate infusion sites. (13) Electrolyte imbalance and cardiac irregularities resulting from high sodium content are very possible. Contains 2.2 mEq of sodium/Gm.

Contraindications: Known sensitivity to cephalosporins or related antibiotics (penicillins).

Incompatible with: Should be considered incompatible in syringe or solution with any other bacteriostatic agent. All aminoglycosides (kanamycin [Kantrex], etc.). All diluents with a pH of 7.5 or more and sodium bicarbonate.

Side effects: Full scope of allergic reactions including anaphylaxis. Decreased hemoglobin or decreased hematocrit; decreased prothrombin time; decreased platelet functions; diarrhea; dyspnea; elevation of SGOT, SGPT, total bilirubin, alkaline phosphatase, LDH, and BUN (transient); eosinophilia; false positive reaction for urine glucose except with Tes-Tape or

Keto-Diastix; fever; leukopenia; local site pain; nausea; oral thrush; positive direct Coombs' test; pseudomembranous colitis; thrombocytopenia; thrombophlebitis; transient neutropenia; vaginitis; vomiting.

Antidote: Notify the physician of any side effects. Discontinue the drug if indicated. Treat allergic reaction as indicated and resuscitate as necessary. Hemodialysis may be useful in overdose.

(Mefoxin)

Usual dose: 1 to 2 Gm every 6 to 8 hours depending on severity of the infection.

> *Perioperative prophylaxis:* 2 Gm 30 minutes to 1 hour before incision. Follow with 2 Gm every 6 hours for 24 to 72 hours.

Dilution: Each 1 Gm or fraction thereof must be diluted with at least 10 ml of sterile water, 5% dextrose in water, or normal saline for injection. A single dose may be further diluted in 50 to 1,000 ml of most common infusion solutions (see literature) and given through a Y tube, three-way stopcock, or additive infusion set or as a continuous infusion.

Rate of administration: Each 1 Gm or fraction thereof over 3 to 5 minutes or longer as indicated by amount of solution and condition of the patient. Discontinue IV infusion solution during administration of cefoxitin by intermittent infusion. Rate of continuous infusion should be by physician's order.

Actions: A semisynthetic cephalosporin antibiotic that is bactericidal to many gram-positive and gram-negative organisms. Absorbed by most body fluids. Excreted rapidly in the urine.

Indications and uses: (1) Treatment of serious respiratory, genitourinary, intraabdominal, gynecological, bone and joint, skin and structure infections, and septicemia. Effective only if the causative organism is susceptible. (2) Preoperative, intraoperative, and postoperative prophylaxis.

Precautions: (1) Sensitivity studies are indicated to determine the susceptibility of the causative organism to cefoxitin. (2) Watch for early symptoms of allergic reaction. (3) Reduce total daily dose if renal function is impaired. (4) Avoid prolonged use of drug; superinfection caused by overgrowth of nonsusceptible organisms may result. (5) Administer within 24 hours of preparation or up to 48 hours if refrigerated. (6) Use extreme caution in the penicillin-sensitive patient; cross-sensitivity may occur. (7) Adverse interaction may occur with promethazine (Phenergan), procainamide (Pronestyl), quinidine, muscle relaxants, potent diuretics, and aminoglycosides. (8) Frequently used concomitantly with aminoglycosides in severe infections, but these drugs must never be mixed in the same infusion or given concurrently. Nephrotoxicity is markedly increased when both drugs are utilized. (9) Use only if absolutely necessary in pregnancy. (10) Probenecid inhibits excretion and may require reduction in dosage. (11) Use of scalp vein needles may reduce incidence of phlebitis.

Contraindications: Known cephalosporin sensitivity; safety for infants and children is not established.

Incompatible with: Amikacin (Amikin), carbenicillin (Geopen), gentamicin (Garamycin), kanamycin (Kantrex), tobramycin (Nebcin).

Side effects: Allergic reactions including anaphylaxis; anorexia; false positive reaction for urine glucose except with Tes-Tape or Keto Diastix; leukopenia; local site pain; nausea and vomiting; neutropenia; oral thrush; phlebitis; positive direct Coombs' test; transient elevation of SGOT, SGPT, BUN, alkaline phosphatase; proteinuria; and thrombophlebitis.

Antidote: Notify physician of any side effects. Discontinue the drug if indicated. Treat allergic reaction as indicated, and resuscitate as necessary.

CEFTIZOXIME

(Cefizox)

Usual dose: Dependent on seriousness of infection. Range is 500 mg to 4 Gm every 8 to 12 hours. Higher doses are often reduced with positive clinical response.

Dilution: Each 1 Gm must be diluted with 10 ml of sterile water. Shake well. May be further diluted with 50 to 100 ml of sodium chloride or other compatible solutions and given as an intermittent infusion. Not given as a continuous infusion.

Rate of administration: *Direct IV:* a single dose equally distributed over 3 to 5 minutes. May be given through Y tube or three-way stopcock of infusion set.
Intermittent IV: a single dose over 30 minutes.

Actions: A broad-spectrum cephalosporin antibiotic similar to cefamandole. Bactericidal to many gram-negative and gram-positive organisms. Effective against many otherwise resistant organisms. Absorbed by most body fluids including inflamed meninges and bone tissue. Excreted in the urine. Crosses placental barrier. Excreted in breast milk.

Indications and uses: Treatment of serious lower respiratory tract, urinary tract, intraabdominal, skin and skin structure, and bone and joint infections, septicemia, and gonorrhea. Most effective against specific organisms (see literature).

Precautions: (1) Sensitivity studies are indicated to determine the susceptibility of the causative organism to ceftizoxime. (2) Watch for early symptoms of allergic reaction. (3) Reduce total daily dose if renal function is impaired. Calculated according to degree of impairment. (4) Avoid prolonged use of drug; superinfection caused by overgrowth of nonsusceptible organisms may result. (5) Administer within 8 hours of preparation or up to 48 hours if refrigerated. (6) Use extreme caution in the penicillin-sensitive patient; cross-sensitivity may occur. (7) Adverse interaction may occur with promethazine (Phenergan), procainamide (Pronestyl), quinidine, muscle relaxants, potent diuretics, and aminoglycosides. (8) Frequently used concomitantly with aminoglycosides in severe infections, but these drugs must never be mixed in the same infusion or given concurrently. Nephrotoxicity is markedly increased when both drugs are utilized. (9) Use only if absolutely necessary in pregnancy. (10) Probenecid inhibits excretion and may require reduction in dosage. (11) Avoid concurrent administration of bacteriostatic agents. (12) May cause thrombophlebitis. Use small needles and large veins and rotate infusion sites. (13) Electrolyte imbalance and cardiac irregularities resulting from high sodium content are very possible. Contains 2.6 mEq of sodium/Gm.

Contraindications: Known sensitivity to cephalosporins or related antibiotics (penicillins). Not recommended for use in children.

Incompatible with: Should be considered incompatible in syringe or solution with any other bacteriostatic agent. All aminoglycosides (kanamycin [Kantrex], etc.).

Side effects: Full scope of allergic reactions including anaphylaxis. Decreased hemoglobin or decreased hematocrit; decreased platelet functions; decreased prothrombin time; diarrhea; dyspnea; elevation of SGOT, SGPT, total bilirubin, alkaline phosphatase, LDH, and BUN (transient); eosinophilia; false positive reaction for urine glucose except with Tes-Tape or Keto-Diastix; fever; leukopenia; local site pain; nausea; oral thrush; positive direct Coombs' test; thrombocytopenia; thrombophlebitis; vaginitis; vomiting.

Antidote: Notify the physician of any side effects. Discontinue the drug if indicated. Treat allergic reaction as indicated and resuscitate as necessary. Hemodialysis may be useful in overdose.

CEFUROXIME

(Zinacef)

Usual dose: Dependent on seriousness of infection. Range is from 750 mg to 3 Gm every 8 hours for 5 to 10 days. 1.5 Gm every 6 hours is used for life-threatening infections.

Perioperative prophylaxis: 1.5 Gm IV 30 minutes to 1 hour before incision, then 750 mg every 8 hours for 24 hours or 1.5 Gm every 12 hours to total dose of 6 Gm in open heart surgery.

Pediatric dose: Infants and children over 3 months of age: 50 to 100 mg/kg of body weight/24 hr in equally divided doses every 6 to 8 hours. Increase to 200 to 240 mg/kg/24 hr in bacterial meningitis.

Dilution: Each 750 mg must be diluted with 9 ml of sterile water, 5% dextrose in water, 0.9% sodium chloride, or other compatible infusion solution for injection (see literature). Shake well. May be further diluted with compatible solutions to 50 ml and given as an intermittent infusion or added to 500 to 1,000 ml and given as a continuous infusion.

Rate of administration: *Direct IV:* a single dose equally distributed over 3 to 5 minutes. May be given through Y tube or three-way stopcock of infusion set. *Intermittent IV:* a single dose over 30 minutes. Discontinue primary infusion during administration. *Continuous infusion:* 500 to 1,000 ml over 6 to 24 hours, depending on total dose and concentration.

Actions: A broad-spectrum cephalosporin antibiotic similar to cefamandole. Bactericidal to many gram-negative and gram-positive organisms. Effective against many otherwise resistant organisms. Absorbed by most body fluids including inflamed meninges and bone tissue. Excreted in the urine. Crosses placental barrier. Excreted in breast milk.

Indications and uses: (1) Treatment of serious lower respiratory tract, urinary tract, and skin and skin structure infections, septicemia, meningitis, and gonorrhea. Most effective agaist specific organisms (see literature). (2) Perioperative prophylaxis.

Precautions: (1) Sensitivity studies are indicated to determine the susceptibility of the causative organism to cefuroxime. (2) Watch for early symptoms of allergic reaction. (3) Reduce total daily dose if renal function is impaired. Calculated according to degree of impairment. (4) Avoid prolonged use of drug; superinfection caused by overgrowth of nonsusceptible organisms may result. (5) Administer within 24 hours of preparation or up to 48 hours if refrigerated. (6) Use extreme caution in the penicillin-sensitive patient; cross-sensitivity may occur. (7) Adverse interaction may occur with promethazine (Phenergan), procainamide (Pronestyl), quinidine, muscle relaxants, potent diuretics, and aminoglycosides. (8) Frequently used concomitantly with aminoglycosides in severe infections, but these drugs must never be mixed in the same infusion or given concurrently. Nephrotoxicity is markedly increased when both drugs are utilized. (9) Use only if absolutely necessary in pregnancy. (10) Probenecid inhibits excretion and may require reduction in dosage. (11) Avoid concurrent administration of bacteriostatic agents. (12) May cause thrombophlebitis. Use small needles and large veins and rotate infusion sites. (13) Electrolyte imbalance and cardiac irregularities resulting from high sodium content are very possible. Contains 2.4 mEq of sodium/Gm.

Contraindications: Known sensitivity to cephalosporins or related antibiotics (penicillins). Infants under 3 months of age.

Incompatible with: Should be considered incompatible in syringe or solution with any other bacteriostatic agent. All aminoglycosides (kanamycin [Kantrex], etc.).

Side effects: Full scope of allergic reactions including anaphylaxis. Decreased hemoglobin or decreased hematocrit; decreased platelet functions; decreased prothrombin time; diarrhea; dyspnea; elevation of SGOT, SGPT, total bilirubin, alkaline phosphatase, LDH, and BUN (transient); eosinophilia; false positive reaction for urine glucose except with Tes-Tape or Keto-Diastix; fever; leukopenia; local site pain; nausea; oral thrush; positive direct Coombs' test; pseudomembranous colitis; transient neutropenia; thrombocytopenia; thrombophlebitis; vaginitis; vomiting.

Antidote: Notify physician of any side effects. Discontinue the drug if indicated. Treat allergic reaction as indicated and resuscitate as necessary. Hemodialysis may be useful in overdose.

CEPHALOTHIN SODIUM

pH 6.0 to 8.5

(Keflin)

Usual dose: 1 to 2 Gm every 4 to 6 hours. Not to exceed 12 Gm/24 hr, depending on severity of infection.

Perioperative prophylaxis: 1 to 2 Gm 30 minutes to 1 hour before incision. May be repeated in OR and every 6 hours for 24 hours.

Pediatric dose: 80 to 160 mg/kg of body weight/24 hr in equally divided doses. *Do not exceed adult dose.*

Perioperative prophylaxis: 20 to 30 mg/kg. Give first dose 30 minutes to 1 hour before incision. May be repeated in OR and every 6 hours for 24 hours.

Dilution: Each 1 Gm or fraction thereof must be diluted with at least 10 ml of sterile water for injection. To reduce incidence of thrombophlebitis, may be further diluted in 50 ml or more of 5% dextrose in water, normal saline, or other compatible infusion solutions (see literature). May be administered through Y tube, three-way stopcock, or additive infusion set.

Rate of administration: 1 Gm over 3 to 5 minutes or longer as indicated by amount of solution and condition of patient. Discontinue IV infusion solution during administration of cephalothin. May be given as a continuous infusion.

Actions: A broad-spectrum cephalosporin antibiotic. Bactericidal against many gram-positive and gram-negative organisms. Absorbed by all body fluids except bile and spinal fluid. Excreted rapidly in urine.

Indications and uses: (1) Treatment of severe infections of bone, joint, skin, soft tissue, bloodstream, cardiovascular system, respiratory tract, genitourinary tract, and gastrointestinal tract, peritonitis, septic abortion, and staphylococcal and pneumococcal meningitis. (2) Preoperative, intraoperative, and postoperative prophylaxis.

Precautions: (1) Sensitivity studies are necessary to determine the susceptibility of the causative organism to cephalothin. (2) Watch for early symptoms of allergic reaction. (3) Reduce total daily dose if renal function is impaired. (4) Avoid prolonged use of drug; superinfection caused by overgrowth of nonsusceptible organisms may result. (5) *Pseudomonas* is almost always resistant to cephalothin. (6) Administer within 24 hours of preparation. Warm to body temperature if precipitate forms on refrigeration. Agitate to dissolve. (7) Sometimes given to the penicillin-sensitive patient. Use extreme caution; cross-sensitivity is common (see contraindications). (8) Rotation of vein sites is recommended at least every 3 days. Use larger veins when possible. (9) Adverse interaction may occur with promethazine (Phenergan), procainamide (Pronestyl), quinidine, muscle relaxants, aminoglycosides, and potent diuretics. (10) Use only if absolutely necessary in pregnancy. (11) Higher blood levels obtained with probenecid.

Incompatible with: Alkaline earth metals, amikacin (Amikin), aminophylline, amobarbital (Amytal), calcium chloride, calcium gluceptate, calcium gluconate, chlorpromazine (Thorazine), chlortetracycline (Aureomycin), cimetidine (Tagamet), colistimethate (Coly-Mycin M), diphenhydramine (Benadryl), dopamine (Intropin), doxorubicin (Adriamycin), epinephrine (Adrenalin), ergonovine (Ergotrate), erythromycin (Iloytcin, Erythrocin), gentamicin (Garamycin), heparin, kanamycin (Kantrex), levarterenol (Levophed), metaraminol (Aramine), methylprednisolone (Solu-Medrol), nitrofurantoin (Ivadantin), oxytetracycline (Terramycin), penicillin G potassium or sodium, pentobarbital (Nembutal), phenobarbital (Luminal), phenytoin (Dilantin), phytonadione (Aquamephyton), polymyxin B sulfate (Aerosporin), prochlorperazine (Compazine), succinylcholine (Anectine), sulfisoxazole (Gantrisin), tetracycline, thiopental (Pentothal), warfarin (Coumadin).

Contraindications: Known penicillin or cephalothin sensitivity; pregnancy.

Side effects: Allergic reactions including anaphylaxis, false positive reaction for urine glucose except with Tes-Tape and Keto-Diastix; local site pain; neutropenia and hemolytic anemia; positive direct Coombs' test; redness; thrombophlebitis.

Antidote: Notify the physician immediately of any adverse symptoms. Discontinue the drug if indicated. Treat allergic reaction as indicated and resuscitate as necessary.

CEPHAPIRIN SODIUM

(Cefadyl)

Usual dose: 500 mg to 1 Gm every 4 to 6 hours. 8 to 12 Gm/24 hr has been given in severe infections.

Perioperative prophylaxis: 1 to 2 Gm 30 minutes to 1 hour before incision. May be repeated in OR and every 6 hours for 24 hours or up to 5 days in specific situations.

Pediatric dose: 40 to 80 mg/kg of body weight/24 hr in four equally divided doses. *Do not exceed adult dose.*

Dilution: Each 1 Gm or fraction thereof must be diluted with at least 10 ml of sterile water for injection. To reduce incidence of thrombophlebitis, may be further diluted in 50 ml of 5% dextrose in water, normal saline for injection, or other compatible infusion solutions (see literature). May be administered through Y tube, three-way stopcock, or additive infusion set.

Rate of administration: Each 1 Gm or fraction thereof over 5 minutes or longer as indicated by amount of solution and condition of patient. Discontinue IV infusion solution during administration of cephapirin.

Actions: A semisynthetic cephalosporin antibiotic that is bactericidal through inhibition of cell wall synthesis to many organisms, including staphylococci and streptococci. A number of organisms are resistant to this cephalosporin. Absorbed by most body fluids and excreted in the urine.

Indications and uses: (1) Treatment of moderate to severe infections of the skin, soft tissue, respiratory tract, and genitourinary tract. Effective only if the causative organism is susceptible. (2) Preoperative, perioperative, and postoperative prophylaxis.

Precautions: (1) Sensitivity studies are necessary to determine the susceptibility of the causative organism to cephapirin. (2) Watch for early symptoms of allergic reaction. (3) Reduce total daily dose if renal function is impaired. (4) Avoid prolonged use of drug; superinfection caused by overgrowth of nonsusceptible organisms may result. (5) Administer within 24 hours of preparation. (6) Use extreme caution in the penicillin-sensitive patient; cross-sensitivity can occur. (7)

Use only if absolutely necessary in pregnancy. (8) Adverse interaction may occur with promethazine (Phenergan), procainamide (Pronestyl), quinidine, muscle relaxants, aminoglycosides, and potent diuretics. (9) Higher blood levels are obtained with probenecid. (10) Avoid concurrent administration of bacteriostatic agents.

Contraindications: Known cephalosporin sensitivity; infants under 3 months of age.

Incompatible with: Amikacin (Amikin), chlortetracycline (Aureomycin), epinephrine (Adrenalin), kanamycin (Kantrex), levarterenol (Levophed), mannitol, oxytetracycline (Terramycin), phenytoin (Dilantin), tetracycline (Achromycin), thiopental (Pentothal).

Side effects: Allergic reactions including anaphylaxis; anemia; false positive reaction for urine glucose except with Tes-Tape or Keto-Diastix; leukopenia; local site pain; neutropenia; phlebitis; positive direct and indirect Coombs' test; transient elevation of SGOT, SGPT, BUN, and alkaline phosphatase.

Antidote: Notify the physician of any side effects. Discontinue the drug if indicated, treat allergic reaction as indicated, and resuscitate as necessary.

(Velosef)

Usual dose: 500 mg to 1 Gm every 4 to 6 hours. Not to exceed 8 Gm/24 hr, depending on severity of infection. *Perioperative prophylaxis:* 1 Gm 30 to 90 minutes before incision. Repeat every 6 hours for 24 hours.

Pediatric dose: 50 to 100 mg/kg of body weight/24 hr in equally divided doses every 6 hours. Up to 300 mg/kg/24 hr has been used in severe infections. Do not exceed adult dose.

Dilution: Each 500 mg or fraction thereof must be diluted with at least 5 ml of sterile water for injection. To reduce incidence of thrombophlebitis or for doses of 2 Gm or over, further dilute each 500 mg in 10 to 20 ml of 5% dextrose in water, normal saline for injection, or other compatible infusion solutions. May be administered through Y tube, three-way stopcock, or additive infusion set.

Rate of administration: Each 1 Gm or fraction thereof over 3 to 5 minutes or longer as indicated by amount of solution and condition of patient.

Actions: A semisynthetic cephalosporin antibiotic that is bactericidal through inhibition of cell wall synthesis to many organisms, including staphylococci and streptococci. A number of organisms including *Pseudomonas* are resistant to this cephalosporin. Readily absorbed by most body fluids and rapidly excreted in the urine.

Indications and uses: (1) Treatment of serious infections of the bone, joint, skin, soft tissue, gastrointestinal tract, respiratory tract, genitourinary tract, and bloodstream, peritonitis, and meningococcal meningitis. Effective only if the causative organism is susceptible. (2) Preoperative, perioperative, and postoperative prophylaxis.

Precautions: (1) Sensitivity studies are indicated to determine the susceptibility of the causative organism to cephradine. (2) Watch for early symptoms of allergic reaction. (3) Reduce total daily dose if renal function is impaired. (4) Avoid prolonged use of drug; superinfection caused by overgrowth of nonsusceptible organisms may result. (5) Administer within 2 hours of preparation. Stable for 10 hours in compatible infusion fluids or 24 hours if refrigerated. Protect solution from direct sunlight. (6) Continuous IV infusion may increase incidence of phlebitis. Rotation of vein sites is recommended at least every 3 days. Use larger veins when possible. (7) Use extreme caution in the penicillin-sensitive patient; cross-sensitivity may occur. (8) Use only if absolutely necessary in pregnancy. (9) Probenecid inhibits excretion; may require reduction of dosage. (10) Adverse interaction may occur with promethazine (Phenergan), procainamide (Pronestyl), quinidine, muscle relaxants, aminoglycosides, and potent diuretics. (11) Avoid concurrent administration of bacteriostatic agents.

Contraindications: Known cephalosporin sensitivity; infants under 1 month of age.

Incompatible with: Do not mix in syringe or solution with any other antibiotic. Calcium salts, epinephrine (Adrenalin), lidocaine (Xylocaine), tetracyclines.

Side effects: Allergic reactions including anaphylaxis; diarrhea; dizziness; dyspnea; edema; false positive reaction for urine glucose except with Tes-Tape, Clinistix, and Diastix; headache; joint pains; monilial overgrowth; nausea; paresthesia; thrombophlebitis; transient leukopenia and neutropenia; transient elevated SGOT, SGPT, total bilirubin, alkaline phosphatase, LDH, BUN, and serum creatinine; vaginitis; vomiting.

Antidote: Notify the physician of any side effects. Discontinue the drug if indicated, treat allergic reaction as indicated, and resuscitate as necessary.

CHLORAMPHENICOL SODIUM SUCCINATE

(Chloromycetin, Mychel-S)

Usual dose: Adults and children: 50 mg/kg of body weight/24 hr in equally divided doses every 6 hours. Exceptional cases may require up to 100 mg/kg/24 hr, but this dose must be reduced as soon as possible.

Infant dose: (Includes young children) 25 mg/kg of body weight/24 hr divided in 2 to 4 equal doses.

Dilution: Each 1 Gm should be diluted with 10 ml of sterile water or 5% dextrose in water for injection to prepare a 10% solution. May be further diluted in 50 to 100 ml of 5% dextrose in water for infusion. Give through Y tube, three-way stopcock, or additive infusion set.

Rate of administration: 1 Gm or fraction thereof over at least 1 minute. Diluted in 50 to 100 ml, give as an infusion over 30 to 60 minutes.

Actions: Effective against many life-threatening organisms; bacteriostatic and bactericidal. Acts by inhibiting protein synthesis. Quickly absorbed, well distributed in therapeutic doses throughout the body, especially in the liver and kidneys. Lowest concentrations are found in the brain and spinal fluid. Excreted in urine, bile, and feces. Crosses the placental barrier. Excreted in breast milk.

Indications and uses: Only in serious infections in which potentially less dangerous drugs are ineffective or contraindicated; acute *Salmonella typhi* infections, meningeal infections, bacteremia, Rocky Mountain spotted fever, lymphogranuloma psittacosis, and others. Cystic fibrosis regimes.

Precautions: (1) *This is a lethal drug.* (2) Observe baseline blood studies at least every 2 to 3 days during therapy and discontinue drug if indicated. Desired blood level range is 5 to 20 µg/ml. (3) Potentiates oral anticoagulants, oral antidiabetics, hydantoins (phenytoin [Dilantin], etc.), and cyclophosphamide. (4) This drug causes bone marrow depression. Avoid concurrent therapy with other similar acting drugs. (5) Has a cumulative potency effect in impaired or immature

107

liver and kidney metabolic functions. (6) Superinfection caused by overgrowth of nonsusceptible organisms, including fungi, is possible. (7) Avoid repeated courses of the drug. (8) For IV use only; not effective IM. (9) Sensitivity studies are mandatory to determine the susceptibility of the causative organism not only to chloramphenicol but to other less dangerous drugs. (10) Use caution in infants and children; causes gray syndrome. (11) Inhibits iron dextran and penicillins.

Contraindications: Known chloramphenicol sensitivity, pregnancy, labor, delivery, and lactation.

Incompatible with: Ampicillin (Polycillin), amobarbital (Amytal), ascorbic acid, carbenicillin (Geopen), chlorpromazine (Thorazine), digitoxin (Crystodigin), erythromycins (Ilotycin, Erythrocin), hydrocortisone phosphate, hydroxyzine (Vistaril), nitrofurantoin (Ivadantin), oxacillin (Prostaphlin), pentobarbital (Nembutal), phenytoin (Dilantin), polymyxin B (Aerosporin), procaine (Novocain), prochlorperazine (Compazine), promazine (Sparine), promethazine (Phenergan), solutions with a pH below 5.5 or above 7.0, sulfisoxazole (Gantrisin), tetracyclines (Aureomycin, Achromycin, Terramycin), thiopental (Pentothal), tripelennamine hydrochloride (Pyribenzamine), vancomycin (Vancocin), warfarin (Coumadin).

Side effects: Anaphylaxis, aplastic anemia, bone marrow depression, confusion, depression, diarrhea, fever, granulocytopenia, gray syndrome of newborns and infants, headache, hypoplastic anemia, leukemia, nausea, optic and peripheral neuritis, paroxysmal nocturnal hemoglobinuria, rashes, stomatitis, thrombocytopenia, vomiting, and many others. *May be fatal.*

Antidote: Notify the physician immediately of any adverse symptoms. Discontinue the drug if indicated, treat allergic reaction as indicated, and resuscitate as necessary.

CHLORDIAZEPOXIDE HYDROCHLORIDE

(Librium)

Usual dose: 50 to 100 mg initially. Repeat 25 to 100 mg in 2 to 4 hours if indicated or 25 to 50 mg three or four times in 24 hours. Maximum dose is 300 mg in a 6- to 24-hour period.

Dilution: Each 100 mg ampoule of sterile powder should be diluted with 5 ml of normal saline or sterile water for injection. Agitate gently to dissolve completely. *Do not use diluent provided; for IM use only.* May not be mixed with infusion fluids. Give through Y tube or three-way stopcock of infusion set. Observe closely for occurrence of fine white precipitate.

Rate of administration: 100 mg or fraction thereof over a minimum of 1 minute.

Actions: A CNS depressant that produces a calming effect. Also relaxes skeletal muscles. Wide margin of safety between therapeutic and toxic doses. Response is extremely rapid by IV route. Slowly metabolized and excreted very slowly in the urine.

Indications and uses: (1) Acute or severe agitation, (2) tremor, (3) anxiety, (4) acute alcoholism withdrawal.

Precautions: (1) Use only freshly prepared solutions; discard unused portion. (2) Bed rest is required for a minimum of 3 hours after IV injection. (3) Withdrawal symptoms are possible after long-term use. (4) Potentiated by narcotics, phenothiazines (prochlorperazine [Compazine], etc.), barbiturates, MAO inhibitors (pargyline [Eutonyl], etc.), alcohol and other CNS depressants, cimetidine (Tagamet), digoxins, and phenytoin (Dilantin). Concomitant use is not recommended, or reduce dose by one third. (5) Reduce dosage for the elderly, debilitated, children over 12 years of age, and patients with impaired renal or hepatic function. (6) May potentiate oral anticoagulants. (7) Use caution in depressed patients; may develop suicidal tendencies. (8) Keep resuscitation equipment available.

Contraindications: Known hypersensitivity to chlordiazepoxide; children under 12 years; known psychoses;

pregnancy or childbirth; shock or comatose states; untreated narrow angle glaucoma.

Incompatible with: Ascorbic acid, heparin, pentobarbital (Nembutal), phenytoin (Dilantin), promethazine (Phenergan), secobarbital (Seconal).

Side effects: *Average dose:* blood dyscrasias, constipation, EEG changes, hiccups, hypotension, menstrual irregularities, nausea, skin eruptions, syncope, tachycardia, urinary retention, urticaria. *Overdose:* may be caused by too-rapid injection. Apnea, ataxia, bradycardia, cardiovascular collapse, confusion, coma, diminished reflexes, drowsiness, edema, hypotension (severe), paradoxical reactions, somnolence.

Antidote: Notify the physician of all side effects. Reduction of dosage may be required. Discontinue the drug for paradoxical reactions including hyperexcitability, hallucinations, and acute rage. Do not treat with barbiturates or CNS stimulants. For overdose, symptomatic and supportive treatment is indicated. Treat hypotension with dopamine (Intropin). Resuscitate as necessary.

(Diuril)

Usual dose: 0.5 to 1.0 Gm once or twice every 24 hours as indicated. Sometimes given every second or third day.

Dilution: Each 0.5 Gm must be diluted with at least 18 ml of sterile water for injection. May be further diluted in dextrose or sodium chloride IV solutions.

Rate of administration: 0.5 Gm or fraction thereof over 5 minutes.

Actions: A nonmercurial diuretic and antihypertensive drug with carbonic anhydrase inhibitor as well as thiazide effects. Related to the sulfonamides. Effectiveness is noted within 15 to 30 minutes. Apparently acts in the renal tubules to excrete sodium, chlorides, potassium, water, and in high doses, some bicarbonate. Potassium excretion is usually not excessive, and rigid low salt intake is never indicated. Rapidly absorbed and excreted unchanged in the urine.

Indications and uses: (1) Edema of any etiology, (2) toxemia of pregnancy, (3) antidiuretic in diabetes insipidus.

Precautions: (1) Use of oral form is preferred. (2) Discard reconstituted solution after 24 hours. (3) Do not give simultaneously with whole blood or its derivatives. (4) Determine absolute patency of vein. Avoid extravasation. For IV use only. (5) May precipitate excessive diuresis with water and electrolyte depletion. Routine checks on electrolyte panel, CO_2, and BUN are necessary during therapy. Potassium chloride replacement may be required. (6) Has antihypertensive actions. Reduced dosage of both agents is required when used concurrently with other antihypertensive drugs. (7) Monitor blood pressure frequently. (8) Hypotensive effect is increased by alcohol, barbiturates, and narcotics. (9) Discontinue 48 hours previous to elective surgery. (10) Use caution in impaired liver or renal function and bronchial asthma. (11) May cause excessive potassium depletion with corticosteroids, cardiac arrhythmias with digitalis, changes in insulin requirements in diabetes, and exacerbation of symptoms of gout or lupus erythematosus. (12) Potentiates lithium, salicylates, muscle relaxants (tubocurarine, etc.), hypotensive effect of other diuretics, and MAO inhibitors (pargyline [Eutonyl], etc.). (13) Inhibits oral anticoagulants and pressor amines (norepinephrine, etc.). (14) May alter laboratory test results, especially K, BUN, uric acid, glucose, and PBI.

Contraindications: Anuria, increasing azotemia and oliguria; known sulfonamide sensitivity; not recommended for children; pregnancy and lactation except in preeclampsia.

Incompatible with: Amikacin (Amikin), ascorbic acid, chlorpromazine (Thorazine), codeine, digitoxin (Crystodigin), insulin (aqueous), levarterenol (Levophed), levorphanol (Levo-Dromoran), methadone, morphine, polymyxin B (Aerosporin), procaine (Novocain), prochlorperazine (Compazine), promazine (Sparine), promethazine (Phenergan), protein hydrolysate, streptomycin, tetracycline, triflupromazine (Vesprin), vancomycin (Vancocin), vitamin B with C, warfarin (Coumadin).

Side effects: *Minor:* diarrhea, dizziness, fatigue, hyperuricemia, muscle cramps, nausea, paresthesias, photosensitivity, purpura, rash, urticaria, vertigo, vomiting, weakness. *Major:* anaphylaxis, blood volume reduction, circulatory collapse, dehydration, excessive diuresis, hematuria, hypokalemia, metabolic acidosis, vascular thrombosis or embolism.

Antidote: If minor side effects are noted, discontinue the drug and notify the physician, who may treat the side effects and continue the drug. If side effects are progressive or any major side effect occurs, discontinue the drug immediately and notify the physician. Treatment of major side effects is symptomatic and aggressive. Resuscitate as necessary.

CHLORPHENIRAMINE MALEATE   pH 4.0 to 5.2

(Chlor-Pro, Chlor-Trimeton)

Usual dose: 10 mg initially. 10 mg may be repeated as necessary (prior to administration of each unit of blood), but do not exceed 40 mg/24 hr. In anaphylactic reactions 20 mg may be given initially.

Pediatric dose: 0.35 mg/kg of body weight/24 hr (10 mg/ M^2/24 hr) in divided doses every 6 hours.

Dilution: May be given undiluted.

Rate of administration: 10 mg or fraction thereof over 1 minute. Extend injection time when possible.

Actions: An antihistamine, acts by blocking the effects of histamine at various receptor sites. Either eliminates an allergic reaction or greatly modifies it. Readily absorbed, widely distributed, and excreted in changed form in the urine.

Indications and uses: (1) Prophylaxis of allergic (not pyrogenic) transfusion reactions, (2) treatment of anaphylactic reactions, (3) treatment of other allergic reactions if IV route is indicated.

Precautions: (1) IM or subcutaneous use is indicated in all situations except the above specific indications. (2) Note label; only the 10 mg/ml chlorpheniramine may be used IV. (3) Do not add to unit of blood. Give direct IV only. (4) Protect from light to prevent discoloration. (5) Use with caution for severely asthmatic patients. (6) Increases effectiveness of epinephrine and is often used in conjunction with it. (7) Antagonizes heparin. (8) Reduce dosage for the elderly and debilitated.

Contraindications: Antihistamine hypersensitivity, lactation, pregnancy, severe cardiac conditions.

Incompatible with: Calcium chloride, iodipamide meglumine (Cholografin), kanamycin (Kantrex), levarterenol (Levophed), pentobarbital (Nembutal).

Side effects: Occur infrequently. *Minor:* drowsiness, headache, nervousness, polyuria, transitory stinging at injection site. *Major:* acute CNS excitement, convulsions, diaphoresis, pallor, transitory hypotension, weak pulse, death.

Antidote: For major side effects, discontinue the drug and notify the physician. The side effects will usually subside within an hour or may be treated symptomatically. Anticonvulsant barbiturates or analeptics (doxapram [Dopram], etc.) will increase toxicity. Resuscitate as necessary.

CHLORPROMAZINE HYDROCHLORIDE

pH 4.0 to 4.3

(Chlorazine, Ormazine, Promaz, Psychozine, Thorazine)

Usual dose: *Nausea and vomiting:* 2 mg. May repeat at 2-minute intervals as indicated. Do not exceed 25 mg. *Tetanus:* 25 to 50 mg three to four times daily.

Pediatric dose: *Nausea and vomiting:* 1 mg. May repeat at 2-minute intervals as indicated. Maximum is usually 12 mg. Not commonly used for children.
   Tetanus: 0.5 mg/kg of body weight every 6 to 8 hours. Do not exceed 40 mg for up to 23 kg and 75 mg for up to 50 kg.

Dilution: Each 25 mg (1 ml) must be diluted with 24 ml of normal saline for injection. 1 ml will equal 1 mg. May be further diluted in 500 ml of normal saline and given as an infusion.

Rate of administration: Direct IV administration; each 1 mg or fraction thereof over 1 to 2 minutes.

Actions: A phenothiazine derivative with effects on the central, autonomic, and peripheral nervous systems. Decreases anxiety and tension, relaxes muscle, produces sedation, and tranquilizes. Has an antiemetic effect and some antihistamine action and potentiates CNS depressants. Onset of action is prompt and of short duration in small IV doses. Excretion is slow through the kidneys.

Indications and uses: (1) Treatment of acute nausea, vomiting, hiccups, restlessness, or retching; primarily used during operative procedures; (2) tetanus; (3) treatment of drug-induced hypertension (methylergonovine [Methergine], etc.), lysergic acid (LSD) intoxication, and amphetamine overdose (IM injection is preferred).

Precautions: (1) IV use is limited to above specific indications. (2) Sensitive to light. Slightly yellow color does not alter potency. Discard if markedly discolored. (3) Handle carefully; may cause contact dermatitis. (4) Keep patient in supine position. Monitor blood pressure and pulse before administration and between doses. (5) Use caution in cardiovascular, liver, chronic respiratory, and acute respiratory diseases of children. (6) Cough reflex is often depressed. (7) May discolor urine pink to reddish brown. (8) Photosensitivity of skin is possible. (9) May mask diagnosis of brain tumor, drug intoxication, and intestinal obstruction. (10) Potentiates CNS depressants, such as narcotics, alcohol, anesthetics, barbiturates, MAO inhibitors (pargyline [Eutonyl], etc.), and anticholinergics, antihistamines, antihypertensives, hypnotics, muscle relaxants, and rauwolfia alkaloids. Reduce dosage of any medication potentiated by phenothiazines by one fourth to one half. (11) May reduce anticonvulsant activity of barbiturates and other anticonvulsants. (12) Contraindicated with quinidine, dipyrone, epinephrine, thiazide diuretics, and orphenadrine. (13) Capable of innumerable other interactions.

Contraindications: Bone marrow depression; comatose or severely depressed states; hypersensitivity to phenothiazines; lactation; pregnancy.

Incompatible with: Ampicillin, aminophylline, amphotericin B (Fungizone), atropine, caffeine and sodium benzoate, cephalothin (Keflin), chloramphenicol (Chloromycetin), chlorothiazide (Diuril), dimenhydrinate (Dramamine), epinephrine (Adrenalin), folic acid, hydrocortisone (Solu-Cortef), kanamycin (Kantrex), magnesium sulfate, methicillin (Staphcillin), methohexital (Brevital), methylprednisolone (Solu-Medrol), paraldehyde, penicillin G potassium, pentobarbital (Nembutal), phenobarbital (Luminal), secobarbital (Seconal), sodium bicarbonate, tetracycline (Achromycin), thiopental (Pentothal).

Side effects: Usually transient if drug is discontinued, but may require treatment if severe. Anaphylaxis, cardiac arrest, distorted Q and T waves, excitement, extrapyramidal symptoms (such as abnormal positioning, extreme restlessness, pseudoparkinsonism, weakness of extremities), fever, hypersensitivity reactions, hypertension, hypotension, tachycardia, and many others.

Antidote: Discontinue the drug at onset of any side effect and notify the physician. Counteract hypotension with dopamine (Intropin) or phenylephrine (Neo-Synephrine) and extrapyramidal symptoms with benztropine (Cogentin) or diphenhydramine (Benadryl). Epinephrine is contraindicated for hypotension; further hypotension will occur. Avoid analeptics such as caffeine sodium benzoate in treating respiratory depression and unconsciousness; they may cause convulsions. Resuscitate as necessary.

(Tagamet)

Usual dose: 300 mg every 6 hours. Increase frequency of dose, not amount, if necessary for pain relief. Do not exceed 2,400 mg/24 hr.

Hemorrhagic gastritis: If above dosage method is not effective, try a continuous infusion of 2 mg/kg of body weight/hr. May be increased to 4 mg/kg/hr if necessary.

Pediatric dose: 5 to 10 mg/kg of body weight every 6 hours. (note contraindications)

Dilution: *Direct IV:* Each 300 mg must be diluted with 20 ml of normal saline for injection.

Intermittent infusion: Each 300 mg may be diluted in 100 ml of 5% dextrose in water or other compatible infusion solution and given piggyback. Do not add to continuous IV fluids except in hemorrhagic gastritis, then dilute an easily calculated amount in 1,000 ml of most common IV solutions (2,000 mg in 1,000 ml equals 2 mg/ml).

Rate of administration: *Direct IV:* Each 300 mg or fraction thereof over 2 minutes.

Intermittent infusion: Each 300 mg dose over 15 to 20 minutes.

IV infusion: Use rate to administer calculated dose/kg of body weight/hr.

Actions: A histamine H_2 antagonist, it inhibits both daytime and nocturnal basal gastric acid secretion. It also inhibits gastric acid secretion stimulated by food, histamine, pentagastrin, caffeine, and insulin. Onset of action is prompt and effective for 4 to 5 hours. Excreted in the urine. Crosses placental barrier. Excreted in breast milk.

Indications and uses: Duodenal ulcers, pathological hypersecretory conditions. Adjunctive to specific therapy in hemorrhagic gastritis, pancreatic insufficiency, electrolyte imbalance from prolonged nasogastric suctioning, and prophylactically in situations where "stress ulcers" are frequent (extensive burns, severe trauma, some neurological procedures).

Precautions: (1) IV bolus administration has precipitated rare instances of cardiac arrhythmias, hypotension, and death. (2) Use antacids concomitantly to relieve pain. (3) May potentiate warfarin-type anticoagulants; monitor prothrombin times. (4) Gastric malignancy may be present even though patient is asymptomatic. (5) Increase intervals between injections to achieve pain relief with least frequent dosage in impaired renal function. (6) Stable at room temperature for 48 hours after dilution. (7) Gastric pain and ulceration may recur after medication is stopped. (8) Usually discontinued after 4 to 8 weeks; effects maintained with oral dosage. (9) Potentiates effects of benzodiazepines (diazepam [Valium], etc.), beta blockers (propranolol [Inderal], etc., hydantoins (phenytoin [Dilantin], etc.), lidocaine, and theophyllines (aminophylline, etc.). (10) May inhibit digoxin absorbtion. (11) Clinical effect (inhibition of nocturnal gastric secretion) is reversed by cigarette smoking.

Contraindications: No known contraindications but pregnancy, lactation, and children under 16 should be considered.

Incompatible with: Aminophylline, amphotericin B, barbiturates, cefamandole (Mandol), cefazolin (Ancef), cephalothin (Keflin).

Side effects: *Average dose:* bradycardia, confusion, diarrhea, delirium, dizziness, elevated SGOT, fever, galactorrhea, hallucinations, impotence, interstitial nephritis, muscular pain, rash. *Overdose:* cardiac arrhythmias, death, hypotension, respiratory failure, tachycardia.

Antidote: Notify physician of all side effects. May be treated symptomatically or may respond to decrease in frequency of dosage. Resuscitate as necessary for overdosage. Physostigmine may be useful to reverse CNS toxicity.

CISPLATIN

pH 3.5 to 5.5

(Platinol)

Usual dose: *Metastatic testicular tumors:* 20 mg/M² daily for 5 days every 3 weeks for 3 courses. Bleomycin and vinblastine are also indicated.

Metastatic ovarian tumors: 50 mg/M² once every 3 weeks, sequentially with doxorubicin.

As a single agent: 100 mg/M² once every 4 weeks.

Dilution: *Specific techniques required, see precautions.* Initially dilute each 10 mg vial with 10 ml of sterile water for injection. Withdraw desired dose. Each one half of a single dose should be diluted in 1 liter of 5% dextrose in 0.2% or 0.45% saline containing 37.5 Gm of mannitol. Will decompose if adequate chloride ion is not available.

Rate of administration: Each 1 liter of infusion solution over 3 to 4 hours. Give total dose (2 liters) over 6 to 8 hours.

Actions: A heavy metal complex (platinum and chloride atoms). Has properties similar to alkylating agents and is cell cycle nonspecific. Concentrates in liver, kidneys, and large and small intestines. Little is absorbed into the CNS. Only one fourth to one half of the drug is excreted in the urine by the end of 5 days.

Indications and uses: Suppress or retard neoplastic growth of metastatic tumors of the testes, ovaries, bladder, head and neck, thyroid, cervix, and endometrium; neuroblastoma; and osteogenic sarcoma. Most commonly used in specific combinations with other chemotherapeutic drugs.

Precautions: (1) Follow guidelines for handling cytotoxic agents recommended by the National Study Commission on Cytotoxic Exposure (see Appendix, p. 528). (2) Usually administered in the hospital by or under the direction of the physician specialist. (3) Hydrate patient with 1 to 2 liters of infusion fluid for 8 to 12 hours previous to injection. (4) Maintain adequate hydration and urinary output for 24 hours after each dose. (5) Frequent kidney function tests and blood counts are indicated. Repeat doses may not be given unless serum creatinine is below 1.5 mg/100 ml and/

or the BUN is below 25 mg/100 ml; platelets should be 100,000/mm^3 and leukocytes 4,000/mm^3; verify auditory acuity as within normal limits. (6) Refrigerate dry powder only. Reconstituted solutions must be kept at room temperature. Discard after 20 hours. (7) Do not use needles or intravenous tubing with aluminum parts to administer; a precipitate will form and potency will be decreased. (8) Will produce teratogenic effects on the fetus. Has a mutagenic potential. (9) Nausea and vomiting are frequently severe and prolonged (up to a week). Prophylactic administration of antiemetics is recommended. Metoclopramide (Reglan) and dexamethasone or droperidol are effective in most patients. (10) Ototoxicity is increased in children. (11) Allopurinol may be indicated to reduce uric acid levels. (12) May inhibit phenytoin (Dilantin). (13) Ototoxicity is potentiated with aminoglycosides (gentamicin, etc.) and ethacrynic acid (Edecrin).

Contraindications: Hypersensitivity to cisplatin or other platinum-containing compounds, myelosuppressed patients, preexisting impaired renal function or hearing deficit.

Incompatible with: Limited information available. Should be considered incompatible in syringe or solution with any other drug (except for mannitol) due to toxicity and specific use.

Side effects: Frequent; can occur with the initial dose and will become more severe with succeeding doses. Anaphylaxis (facial edema, hypotension, tachycardia, and wheezing within minutes of administration), hyperuricemia, myelosuppression, nausea and vomiting, nephrotoxicity (often noted in the second week after a dose), ototoxicity including tinnitus and hearing loss in the high-frequency range, and peripheral neuropathy (may be irreversible).

Antidote: Notify physician of all side effects. Cisplatin may have to be discontinued until recovery or permanently. Symptomatic and supportive treatment is indicated. Treat anaphylaxis with epinephrine, corticosteroids, oxygen, and antihistamines. There is no specific antidote.

CLINDAMYCIN PHOSPHATE

pH 6.0 to 6.3

(Cleocin phosphate)

Usual dose: 600 to 2,700 mg/24 hr in two, three, or four equally divided doses. Up to 4.8 Gm has been given in life-threatening infections.

Pediatric dose: Children over 1 month of age: 15 to 40 mg/kg of body weight/24 hr in three or four equally divided doses. A minimum dose of 300 mg/24 hr is recommended.

Dilution: Each 300 mg or fraction thereof must be diluted with a minimum of 50 ml of 5% dextrose in water, normal saline for injection, or other compatible infusion solution.

Rate of administration: Each 300 mg or fraction thereof over a minimum of 10 minutes. Do not give more than 1,200 mg in single 1-hour infusion.

Actions: A semisynthetic antibiotic that quickly converts to active clindamycin. It inhibits protein synthesis in the bacterial cell, producing irreversible changes in the protein-synthesizing ribosomes. Widely distributed in most body fluids, tissues, and bones. There is no clinically effective distribution to cerebrospinal fluid. Excreted in urine and feces in small amounts. Most excreted in inactive form in the urine. Crosses placental barrier. Excreted in breast milk.

Indications and uses: Treatment of serious infections caused by susceptible anaerobic bacteria or susceptible aerobic bacterial infections in penicillin-sensitive patients.

Precautions: (1) A highly toxic drug, to be used only when absolutely necessary and an alternate drug (e.g., erythromycin) is not acceptable. (2) Sensitivity studies are indicated to determine the susceptibility of the causative organism to clindamycin. (3) Avoid prolonged use of drug; superinfection caused by overgrowth of nonsusceptible organisms may result. (4) Capable of causing severe, even fatal, colitis; observe for symptoms of diarrhea. (5) Periodic blood cell counts and liver and kidney studies are indicated in prolonged therapy. (6) May potentiate other neuromuscular blocking agents (kanamycin, streptomycin, etc.). (7) Antagonized by erythromycin. (8) Use caution with a history of gastrointestinal, severe renal, or liver disease. (9) Should not be injected IV as a bolus.

Contraindications: Known hypersensitivity to clindamycin or lincomycin; pregnancy; newborns.

Incompatible with: Aminophylline, ampicillin, barbiturates, calcium gluconate, magnesium sulfate, phenytoin (Dilantin), Ringer's solution.

Side effects: Abdominal pain, allergic reactions, anaphylaxis, colitis, diarrhea, jaundice, nausea, thrombophlebitis, vomiting.

Antidote: Notify the physician of any side effects. Discontinue the drug if indicated (colitis, diarrhea, or allergic reactions, etc.), treat allergic reaction as indicated, and resuscitate as necessary. Treat colitis with fluid, electrolyte, and protein supplements, systemic corticosteroids, and corticoid retention enemas.

COLCHICINE

Usual dose: 2 mg (4 ml) as initial dose. Follow with 0.5 mg (1 ml) every 6 hours. Do not exceed 4 mg (8 ml) in 24 hours. Maintenance doses of 0.5 to 2 mg (1 to 4 ml)/24 hr may be given or divided into two doses every 24 hours.

Dilution: May be given undiluted or diluted with 0.9% sodium chloride without a bacteriostatic agent.

Rate of administration: Each 0.5 mg (1 ml) or fraction thereof over 1 minute.

Actions: An alkaloid. Its mode of action has not been determined, but it has a distinct antiinflammatory and analgesic effect. IV administration is preferred for rapid response and fewer gastrointestinal side effects. Readily absorbed into the liver, spleen, kidneys, and intestinal tract. Excreted in urine and feces.

Indications and uses: Specific for the treatment of acute gout.

Precautions: (1) Must be given IV. Will cause severe local reaction IM or subcutaneously. Maintain absolute patency of vein; severe irritation will occur with leakage along vein pathway. (2) Use only clear solutions. (3) Use with caution for the elderly and debilitated and in renal, gastrointestinal, or heart disease. (4) Reduce dosage if weakness, anorexia, nausea, vomiting, or diarrhea occurs. (5) Symptoms of overdosage do not occur right away. The patient must be continuously observed while hospitalized and well informed of all side effects when treated outside the hospital. (6) Thrombophlebitis can occur at the injection site. (7) Inhibited by acidifying agents, potentiated by alkalinizing agents.

Contraindications: *Absolute:* IM and subcutaneous use.

Incompatible with: Specific information not available. Interaction with other drugs does occur. Should be considered incompatible with any other drug in a syringe.

Side effects: Rare when recommended dose is not exceeded but may be latent. *Average doses:* abdominal pain, aplastic anemia, bone marrow depression, diarrhea, nausea, thrombocytopenia, thrombophlebitis at injection site, vomiting. *Overdose:* usual side effects plus ascending CNS paralysis; burning sensations in the throat, stomach, and skin; convulsions; delirium; electrolyte imbalance; hematuria; hemorrhagic gastroenteritis; muscular weakness; oliguria; respiratory depression; severe bloody diarrhea; shock; death.

Antidote: Discontinue the drug at initial onset of symptoms and notify the physician. For acute overdosage treatment is symptomatic and includes treatment of shock and electrolyte imbalance and respiratory assistance as necessary. Morphine and atropine may be used to relieve pain. Hemodialysis or peritoneal dialysis may promote elimination of the drug.

COLISTIMETHATE SODIUM

pH 7.0 to 8.0

(Coly-Mycin M)

Usual dose: Adults, children, and infants 2.5 to 5.0 mg/ kg of body weight/24 hr (150 mg/M^2/24 hr) equally divided into two to four doses and given every 6 to 12 hours. Normal renal funciton is necessary for this dosage.

Dilution: 150 mg vial is diluted with 2 ml of sterile water for injection. 1 ml equals 75 mg. Further dilute each single dose with 20 ml of sterile water for injection for direct IV administration. May be further diluted with 50 ml or more of 5% dextrose in water, isotonic saline, lactated Ringer's solution, or 10% invert sugar solution and given as an infusion through the Y tube, three-way stopcock, or additive infusion tubing.

Rate of administration: Direct IV administration. Each 75 mg or fraction thereof over 5 minutes. Initial dose should be direct IV. Second dose is sometimes given in 1 to 2 hours at 5 to 6 mg/hr.

Actions: A polypeptide antibiotic with neuromuscular blocking action. Bactericidal against specific gram-negative bacilli. Serum and urine levels remain adequate for up to 6 to 8 hours. Crosses the placental barrier. Excreted through the kidneys.

Indications and uses: Acute and chronic infections, especially of the urinary tract, due to gram-negative bacilli, such as *Pseudomonas aeruginosa, Aerobacter aerogenes, Escherichia coli, and Klebsiella pneumoniae.*

Precautions: (1) Read the label carefully. Only a specific powder can be diluted for intravenous use. (2) Sensitivity studies indicated to determine susceptibility of the causative organism to colistimethate. (3) Not effective against *Proteus* or *Neisseria.* (4) Reduce daily dose commensurate with amount of renal impairment. Intervals between injections should also be increased. (5) Watch for decrease in urine output and for rising BUN and serum creatinine. Dosage may require decreasing. (6) Be especially observant in infants, children, and the elderly. (7) Potentiated by anesthetics, other neuromuscular blocking antibiotics (kanamycin, streptomycin, etc.), anticholinesterases (endrophonium [Tensilon], etc.) and muscle relaxants (tubocurarine, etc.). *Apnea can occur.* (8) Avoid prolonged use of drug; superinfection caused by overgrowth of nonsusceptible organisms may result. (9) Motor coordination is impaired; supervise ambulation. (10) Store reconstituted drug in refrigerator for up to 7 days. Discard solutions diluted for infusion after 24 hours.

Contraindications: History of sensitivity to multiple allergens, known colistimethate sensitivity, pregnancy.

Incompatible with: Administer separately as recommended by manufacturer. Cefazolin (Kefzol), cephalothin (Keflin), chlortetracycline (Aureomycin), erythromycin (Erythrocin), hydrocortisone (Solu-Cortef), hydroxyzine (Vistaril), kanamycin (Kantrex).

Side effects: *Average dose:* circumoral paresthesia, dizziness, formication of extremities, numbness of extremities, pruritus, slurring of speech, tingling of extremities, vertigo. *Overdose:* anaphylaxis, apnea, decreased urine output, elevated BUN, elevated serum creatinine, muscle weakness, renal insufficiency.

Antidote: Side effects are expected with an average dose; notify the physician. Reduction of dose will usually alleviate symptoms. If any symptom of overdose occurs, discontinue the drug immediately and notify the physician. Nephrotoxicity is reversible. Maintain an adequate airway and artificial ventilation as indicated. Treat allergic reactoins symptomatically, that is, with antihistamines, pressor amines, corticosteroids.

CONJUGATED ESTROGENS

pH 6.8 to 7.4

(Premarin intravenous)

Usual dose: 25 mg in one injection. May be repeated in 6 to 12 hours if indicated.

Dilution: Withdraw all air from the vial of powder. Carefully withdraw contents from ampoule of sterile diluent provided. Direct flow of diluent gently against the side of the vial of powder. Mix solution by rotating the vial between the palms of the hands. Do not shake.

Rate of administration: 5 mg or fraction thereof over 1 minute. Must be given direct IV or through IV tubing close to needle site. Infusion solution must be compatible.

Actions: Produces a prompt increase in circulating prothrombin and accelerator globulin and decrease in antithrombin activities of the blood. The coagulability of the blood, especially in capillary beds, is enhanced. Promptly corrects bleeding due to estrogen deficiency. It is probably excreted in the urine.

Indications and uses: Dysfunctional uterine bleeding due to hormonal imbalance in the absence of organic pathology.

Precautions: (1) IV infusion is not recommended. (2) Must be refrigerated before and after reconstitution. Most frequently used promptly, but it is stable, if protected from light, for up to 60 days. (3) Do not use if discolored or precipitate is present. (4) Even though bleeding is controlled, the etiology of the bleeding must be determined and definitive therapy instituted. (5) Follow immediately with oral estrogens as recommended for dysfunctional uterine bleeding. (6) Potentiates oral antidiabetics and oxytocin injections. (7) May increase blood glucose levels. (8) Use with caution in epilepsy, migraine, asthma, or cardiac or renal disease, induces salt and water retention. (9) Estrogens are carcinogenic; use only for specific indications.

Contraindications: Pregnancy, thrombophlebitis, or thromboembolic disorders. Other specific contraindications for estrogens must be considered.

Incompatible with: Ascorbic acid, lactated Ringer's injection, Ringer's injection, sodium lactate injection (⅙ molar lactate), any solution with an acid pH.

Side effects: Rare when used as directed: flushing, nausea, vomiting.

Antidote: No toxicity has been reported throughout years of clinical use.

CORTICOTROPIN INJECTION

pH 3.0 to 7.0

(ACTH, Acthar)

Usual dose: 10 to 25 units/24 hr. Up to 80 units as a single injection has been used for diagnostic testing.

Dilution: Dilute lyophilized powder initially with 2 ml of water or sodium chloride for injection. Withdraw desired dose of corticotropin and further dilute in 500 ml of 5% glucose in water. An isotonic saline solution may be used unless salt is restricted.

Rate of administration: Given as a continuous IV infusion over an 8-hour period.

Actions: Synthesized anterior pituitary hormone, a polypeptide, not absorbed through the gastrointestinal tract. Given intravenously, it rapidly disappears from the bloodstream and little effect remains 6 hours after termination of the infusion. Effective only when the adrenal glands are normal and can respond to its stimulation. A normal increase in plasma corticol rules out primary adrenocortical failure. Prolonged therapy may be initiated if no acute response. Excreted in the urine. Excreted in breast milk.

Indications and uses: Diagnosis of adrenocortical function.

Precautions: (1) Skin test for allergy if a known sensitivity exists to polypeptides or to hogs. (2) Continuous observation for at least the first 30 minutes is mandatory. Observe frequently throughout administration. (3) Refrigerate remainder of medication after initial dilution. (4) Check blood pressure frequently; may cause elevated blood pressure and salt and water retention. (5) May increase insulin needs in diabetes. (6) Do not vaccinate for smallpox during therapy. (7) Use with caution in hypothyroidism and cirrhosis.

Contraindications: Do not use in ocular herpes simplex, acute psychoses, scleroderma, osteoporosis, systemic fungal infections, or recent surgery. *Relative contraindications:* active or latent peptic ulcer, congestive heart failure, diabetes mellitus, diverticulitis, hypertension, pregnancy (especially during the first trimester), protein sensitivity, psychotic tendencies, renal insufficiency, thromboembolic tendencies, and tuberculosis (active or healed).

Incompatible with: Aminophylline and sodium bicarbonate. Many drug interactions are possible with corticosteroids. Some drugs markedly potentiate their effects, and others necessitate increased doses.

Side effects: Do occur, but are usually reversible: alteration of glucose metabolism, including hyperglycemia; Cushing's syndrome (moon face, fat pads, etc.); electrolyte imbalance; increased blood pressure; increased intracranial pressure with papilledema; masking of infection; pancreatitis; perforation and hemorrhage from aggravation of peptic ulcer; protein catabolism with negative nitrogen balance; psychic disturbances, especially euphoria; suppression of growth; thromboembolism; and many others, including anaphylaxis.

Antidote: Notify the physician of any side effect so that it can be treated as necessary. Dosage may be reduced. Resuscitate as necessary for anaphylaxis and notify the physician. Keep epinephrine immediately available.

COSYNTROPIN

(Cortrosyn)

Usual dose: 250 μg (0.25 mg).

Pediatric dose: Same as adult dose for children over 2 years of age.

Dilution: Diluent provided (1.1 ml vial of 0.9% sodium chloride for injection). May be given direct IV after this initial dilution or further diluted in 5% dextrose or 0.9% saline solution and given as an infusion. (250 μg in 250 ml equals 1 μg/ml).

Rate of administration: *Direct IV:* A single dose over 2 minutes. *Infusion:* A single dose at 40 μg/hr over 6 hours.

Actions: A synthetic form of adrenocorticotropic hormone (ACTH). Stimulates the adrenal cortex to secrete cortisol, corticosterone, androgenic substances, and aldosterone. Does not increase cortisol secretion in patients with primary adrenocortical insufficiency. Peak serum concentrations occur 45 to 60 minutes after direct IV injection.

Indications and uses: Diagnostic aid for adrenocortical insufficiency.

Precautions: (1) Preferable to ACTH because it is less likely to cause allergic reactions. May be used in patients who have had an allergic reaction to ACTH. (2) Plasma cortisol may be falsely elevated for patients taking spironolactone when fluorometric procedure is used, patients receiving corticosteroids, and individuals with increased plasma bilirubin levels or free hemoglobin in the plasma. (3) Infusion method is used if greater stimulus is needed to effect results. (4) Use caution in pregnancy and lactation. (5) Stable after reconstitution for 24 hours at room temperature and 21 days if refrigerated. Infusion is stable 12 hours at room temperature.

Contraindications: Hypersensitivity to cosyntropin.

Incompatible with: Specific information not available. Should be considered incompatible with any other drug due to specific use.

Side effects: Bradycardia, dizziness, dyspnea, fainting, fever, irritability, rash, seizures, urticaria.

Antidote: Notify the physician of any side effect. Keep epinephrine and diphenhydramine available to treat anaphylaxis. Resuscitate as necessary.

CYCLOPHOSPHAMIDE

pH 5.05

(Cytoxan, Neosar)

Usual dose: Initial dose may be up to a maximum of 40 to 50 mg/kg of body weight, usually given in divided doses (10 to 20 mg/kg/24 hr) over 2 to 5 days. This dose is reduced by one third to one half if hematological disease is present or there has been extensive radiation therapy. Maintenance doses vary from 3 to 5 mg/kg twice weekly to 10 to 15 mg/kg every 7 to 10 days.

Dilution: *Specific techniques required, see precautions.* Each 100 mg must be diluted with 5 ml of sterile water or bacteriostatic water for injection (paraben-preserved only). Shake solution gently and allow to stand until clear. Additional diluent (up to 250 ml 5% glucose or normal saline) is recommended by some researchers to reduce side effects.

Rate of administration: Each 100 mg or fraction thereof may be given over 1 minute. Cyclophosphamide may be given IV through the lumen of the rubber tubing or three-way stopcock if the IV solution is glucose or saline.

Actions: An alkylating agent of the nitrogen mustard group with antitumor activity, cell cycle phase nonspecific and most effective in S phase. It is an inert compound but is activated in the body (probably in the liver) by an unknown action to produce regression in the size of malignant tumors, to relieve pain and fever, and to increase appetite, strength, and a sense of well-being. Well absorbed, this drug or its metabolites are excreted in the urine. Excreted in breast milk.

Indications and uses: To suppress or retard neoplastic growth. Good response has been experienced in hematopoietic malignancies, such as Hodgkin's disease and leukemia, and in solid malignancies of the breast and ovary.

Precautions: (1) Follow guidelines for handling cytotoxic agents recommended by the National Study Commission on Cytotoxic Exposure (see Appendix, p. 528). (2) Usually administered in the hospital by or under

134

the direction of the physician specialist. (3) Marked leukopenia will occur after the initial dose. Recovery should begin in 7 to 10 days. Maintenance doses are regulated by an acceptable leukocyte count (2,500 to 4,000 cells/mm³) and the absence of serious side effects. The maximum effective maintenance dose should be used. (4) Do not store cyclophosphamide in temperatures over 32.2° C (90° F). (5) Diluted solution is not stable and must be used within 24 hours. Stable up to 6 days if refrigerated. (6) Dosage based on average weight in presence of edema or ascites. (7) Use caution in leukopenia, thrombocytopenia, bone marrow infiltrated with malignant cells, recent x-ray therapy, and severe hepatic and renal disease. Observe for infection. (8) Wait 5 to 7 days after a major surgical procedure before beginning treatment. May interfere with normal wound healing. (9) Cyclophosphamide interacts with numerous drugs, including antidiabetics, barbiturates, chloramphenicol, corticosteroids, succinylcholine (Anectine), and other alkylating agents to produce potentially serious reactions. (10) Often used with other antineoplastic drugs in reduced doses to achieve tumor remission. (11) May produce teratogenic effects on the fetus. Has a mutagenic potential. (12) Potentiates anticoagulants. (13 Administer before 4 PM to decrease amount of drug remaining in bladder overnight. Encourage fluid intake and frequent voiding to prevent cystitis. (14) Do not administer any vaccine or chloroquine to patients receiving antineoplastic drugs. (15) Adjust dose for adrenalectomized patient. (16) Do not use heat to facilitate dilution.

Contraindications: None.

Incompatible with: Limited information available. Note precautions. Give separately.

Side effects: *Minor:* alopecia (regrowth may be slightly darker), amenorrhea, gonadal suppression, leukopenia (see precautions), mucosal ulcerations, nausea and vomiting, skin and fingernails become darker, susceptibility to infection. *Major:* bone marrow depression, pulmonary fibrosis, sterile hemorrhagic cystitis, which can be fatal.

Antidote: Minor side effects will be treated symptomatically if necessary. Discontinue the drug and notify the physician of hematuria immediately. There is no specific antidote. Supportive therapy as indicated will help sustain the patient in toxicity. Will respond to hemodialysis.

(Cytosine arabinoside, ARA-C, Cytosar-U)

Usual dose: Variable depending on specific regime or protocol.

IV injection: 2 mg/kg of body weight/24 hr for 5 to 10 days. Increase to 4 mg/kg/24 hr. Maintain treatment until therapeutic effect or toxicity occurs. Modify on a day-to-day basis for maximum individualized effectiveness.

IV infusion: 200 mg/M^2/24 hr for 5 days. Maintain treatment and modify dosage as above.

Dilution: *Specific techniques required, see precautions.* Each 100 mg must be initially diluted with 5 ml (500 mg with 10 ml) of sterile water for injection with preservative. Solution pH is about 5.0. May be given by direct IV administration as is or further diluted in 50 to 100 ml or more of normal saline or 5% dextrose in water and given as an infusion. Direct IV administration through a free-flowing IV tube is preferred.

Rate of administration: *IV injection:* each 100 mg or fraction thereof over 1 to 3 minutes.

IV infusion: single daily dose properly diluted over 1 to 24 hours, depending on amount of infusion solution and dosage regime.

Actions: An antimetabolite and pyrimidine antagonist that interferes with the synthesis of DNA and RNA. Cell cycle specific for S phase. Through various chemical processes this deprivation acts more quickly on rapidly growing cells and causes their death. Cytotoxic and cytostatic. A potent bone marrow depressant. Crosses the blood-brain barrier. Metabolized in the liver and excreted in the urine.

Indications and uses: Induction of remission in acute granulocytic leukemia of adults and other acute leukemias in adults and children.

Precautions: (1) Follow guidelines for handling cytotoxic agents recommended by the National Study Commission on Cytotoxic Exposure (see Appendix, p. 528). (2) Administered only to a hospitalized patient by or under the directon of the physician specialist. (3) Must be refrigerated until after dilution; then stable at

137

room temperature for 48 hours. (4) Use only clear solutions. (5) Leukocyte and platelet counts should be monitored daily. Discontinue therapy for platelet count under 50,000 or polymorphonuclear granulocytes under 1,000 cells/mm³. (6) Use caution with impaired liver function. (7) Monitor bone marrow, liver, and renal function at intervals during therapy. (8) Higher doses are tolerated by IV injection compared with IV infusion, but the incidence and intensity of nause and vomiting are increased. (9) May produce teratogenic effects on the fetus. (10) May be used with other antineoplastic drugs in reduced doses to achieve tumor remission. (11) Dosage based on average weight in presence of edema or ascites. (12) Potentiates anticoagulants. (13) Be alert for signs of bone marrow depression, bleeding, or infection. (14) Do not administer any vaccines or chloroquine to patients receiving antineoplastic drugs. (15) Monitor uric acid levels, maintain hydration; allopurinol may be indicated.

Contraindications: Hypersensitivity to cytarabine, preexisting drug-induced bone marrow depression.

Incompatible with: Specific information not available. Consider incompatible with any other drug due to toxicity and specific use.

Side effects: Anemia, bone marrow depression, diarrhea, esophagitis, fever, hepatic dysfunction, hyperuricemia, leukopenia, megaloblastosis, mucosal bleeding, nausea, rash, stomatitis, thrombocytopenia, thrombophlebitis, vomiting.

Antidote: Notify the physician of all side effects. Most will be treated symptomatically. Some toxicity is necessary to produce remission. Discontinue the drug for serious hematological depression. Drug must be restarted as soon as signs of bone marrow recovery occur or its effectiveness will be lost. There is no specific antidote; supportive therapy as indicated will help to sustain the patient in toxicity.

(DTIC-Dome, Imidazole carboxamide)

Usual dose: 2 to 4.5 mg/kg of body weight/24 hr for 10 days. May be repeated at 4-week intervals. May administer 250 mg/M² for 5 days. Repeat in 3 weeks. Has proved as effective in lesser doses as in larger doses. Individualized response determines dosage of succeeding treatments.

Dilution: *Specific techniques required, see precautions.* Each 100 mg vial is diluted with 9.9 ml (200 mg with 19.7 ml) of sterile water for injection (10 mg/ml). Additional diluent may be used. May be given through Y tube or three-way stopcock of infusion set. Administration through a free-flowing IV tubing is preferred. May be further diluted in 50 to 250 ml of 5% dextrose in water or normal saline for infusion.

Rate of administration: Total dose over 1 minute. If diluted with 50 to 250 ml, administer over 30 minutes.

Actions: An antineoplastic agent. Exact mechanism of action is not known; may inhibit DNA and RNA synthesis. It is an alkylating agent, cell cycle phase nonspecific. Probably localizes in the liver and is excreted in the urine through renal tubular secretion.

Indications and uses: Induction of remission of malignant melanoma with metastasis after surgical excision of the tumor, Hodgkin's disease, and soft tissue sarcomas.

Precautions: (1) Follow guidelines for handling cytotoxic agents recommended by the National Study Commission on Cytotoxic Exposure (see Appendix, p. 528). (2) Usually administered in the hospital by or under the direction of the physician specialist. (3) Determine absolute patency of vein; a stinging or burning sensation indicates extravasation; severe cellulitis and tissue necrosis will result. Discontinue injection, use another vein. (4) Diluted solution stable for 72 hours only if refrigerated at 4° C (39° F); discard in 6 to 8 hours if kept at room temperature. (5) Used with other antineoplastic drugs and radiation therapy in reduced doses to achieve tumor remission. (6) Monitor bone marrow function, WBC, RBC, and platelet count frequently. (7) Nausea and vomiting may be reduced by restricting oral intake of fluid and foods for 4 to 6 hours before administration. Use antiemetics. (8) Dosage based on average weight in presence of edema or ascites. (9) Safety for use in pregnancy or lactation and in men and women capable of conception not established. (10) Do not administer any vaccines or chloroquine to patients receiving antineoplastic drugs. (11) Use caution in impaired liver and renal function. (12) Inhibited by phenobarbital and phenytoin (Dilantin). Potentiates allopurinol. (13) Be alert for signs of bone marrow depression, bleeding, or infection.

Contraindications: Known hypersensitivity to dacarbazine.

Incompatible with: Limited information available; hydrocortisone sodium succinate, hydrocortisone sodium phosphate, and lidocaine. Should be considered incompatible in syringe or solution with any other drug due to toxicity and specific use.

Side effects: Leukopenia and thrombocytopenia may be serious enough to cause death. Alopecia, anaphylaxis, anorexia, facial flushing, facial paresthesias, fever, hepatotoxicity, malaise, myalgia, nausea, skin necrosis, vomiting.

Antidote: Notify physician of all side effects. Most will be treated symptomatically. Hematopoietic depression may require temporary or permanent withholding of treatment. There is no specific antidote. Supportive therapy as indicated will help sustain the patient in toxicity. For extravasation inject long-acting dexamethasone (Decadron-LA) or hyaluronidase (Wydase) throughout extravasated tissue. Use a 27- or 25-gauge needle. Apply heat.

DACTINOMYCIN

(Act, Actinomycin D, Cosmegen)

Usual dose: 0.5 mg/24 hr for up to 5 days. May be repeated after 3 weeks if all signs of toxicity have disappeared. Do not exceed 15 µg/kg of body weight/day in adults or children.

Pediatric dose: 0.015 mg (15 µg)/kg of body weight/24 hr for 5 days. May be repeated after 2 weeks if all signs of toxicity have disappeared.

Dilution: *Specific techniques required, see precautions.* Dilute each 0.5 mg vial with 1.1 ml of sterile water for injection without preservative (0.5 mg/ml). Use 2.2 ml to yield 0.25 mg/ml (vent vial to relieve pressure). May be given direct IV (see precautions), through the Y tube or three-way stopcock of a free-flowing infusion of compatible solutions, or further diluted in 50 ml 5% dextrose in water or normal saline for infusion.

Rate of administration: *Direct IV:* each 0.5 mg or fraction thereof over 1 minute.

IV infusion: A single dose over 10 to 15 minutes.

Actions: A highly toxic antibiotic antineoplastic agent, cell cycle phase nonspecific. Cytotoxic, it interferes with cell division by binding DNA to slow production of RNA. Found in high concentrations in the kidney, liver, and spleen.

Indications and uses: To suppress or retard neoplastic growth in (1) Wilms' tumor, (2) rhabdomyosarcoma, (3) carcinoma of the testis and uterus, (4) choriocarcinoma.

Precautions: (1) Follow guidelines for handling cytotoxic agents recommended by the National Study Commission on Cytotoxic Exposure (see Appendix, p. 528). (2) Usually administered in the hospital by or under the direction of the physician specialist. (3) Determine absolute patency of vein; a stinging or burning sensation indicates extravasation; severe cellulitis and tissue necrosis will result. Discontinue injection, use another vein. (4) Use sterile two-needle technique for direct IV administration: one needle to dilute and withdraw and one needle to inject into the vein (rinse with blood before removing). (5) Light sensitive in dry

141

form. (6) Discard any unused portion. (7) Used with other antineoplastic drugs in reduced doses to achieve tumor remission. (8) Reduce dose of dactinomycin and radiation therapy when used concurrently, if either has been used previously, or if previous chemotherapy has been employed. (9) X-ray therapy potentiates dactinomycin. (10) Dactinomycin alone may reactivate erythema from previous x-ray therapy. (11) May produce teratogenic effects on the fetus; use caution in men and women capable of conception. (12) Monitor renal, hepatic, and bone marrow function frequently. (13) Except for immediate nausea and vomiting, side effects may not appear for 2 to 4 days. Always observe closely. Use prophylactic antiemetics. (14) Do not administer any vaccines or chloroquine to patients receiving antineoplastic drugs. (15) Inhibits action of penicillin. (16) Allopurinol, increased fluid intake, and alkalinization of the urine may be required to reduce uric acid levels.

Contraindications: Exposure to chickenpox, known sensitivity to dactinomycin, and infants under 6 months of age.

Incompatible with: Specific information not available. Should be considered incompatible in syringe or solution with any other drug.

Side effects: Abdominal pain, acne, alopecia, anaphylaxis, anemia, anorexia, cheilitis, diarrhea, dysphagia, erythema flare-up, esophagitis, fatigue, fever, gastrointestinal ulceration, hypocalcemia, lethargy, leukopenia, malaise, myalgia, nausea, pharyngitis, proctitis, skin eruptions, thrombocytopenia, ulcerative stomatitis, vomiting.

Antidote: Any side effect can result in death. Notify the physician of all side effects. Most will be treated symptomatically. Hematopoietic depression may require withholding dactinomycin until recovery occurs. There is no specific antidote. Supportive therapy as indicated will help sustain the patient in toxicity. For extravasation inject long-acting dexamethasone (Decadron-LA) or hyaluronidase (Wydase) throughout extravasted tissue. Use a 27- or 25-gauge needle. Apply heat.

(Dantrium Intravenous)

Usual dose: 1 mg/kg of body weight as an initial dose. Repeat as necessary until symptoms subside or a cumulative dose of 10 mg/kg is reached. Entire regime may be repeated if symptoms reappear. Dosage required depends on degree of susceptibility to malignant hyperthermia, length of time of exposure to triggering agent, and time lapse between onset of crisis and beginning of treatment.

Dilution: Each 20 mg must be diluted with 60 ml of sterile water for injection without a bacteriostatic agent. Shake until solution is clear. May be administered through Y tube or three-way stopcock of infusion tubing.

Rate of administration: Each single dose should be given by rapid continuous IV push. Follow immediately with subsequent doses as indicated.

Actions: A direct-acting skeletal muscle relaxant. Inhibits excitation-contraction coupling by interfering with the release of the calcium ion from the sarcoplasmic reticulum to reverse the physiological cause of malignant hyperthermia. Has no appreciable effect on cardiovascular or respiratory function. Onset of action is prompt and lasts about 5 hours. Metabolized in the liver and excreted in urine.

Indications and uses: To manage the fulminant hypermetabolism of skeletal muscle characteristic of malignant hyperthermia crisis (tachycardia, tachypnea, central venous desaturation, hypercapnia, metabolic acidosis, skeletal muscle rigidity, cyanosis, mottling of skin, fever, and increased use of anesthesia circuit CO_2 absorber).

Precautions: (1) Discontinue all anesthetic agents immediately when onset of malignant hyperthermia is recognized. (2) Monitor EKG, vital signs, electrolytes, and urine output continuously. Oxygen needs are increased; manage metabolic acidosis, institute cooling measures. (3) Confirm absolute patency of vein; avoid extravasation. (4) Protect diluted solution from direct light and discard after 6 hours. Store between 15° and

143

30° C (59° F and 86° F). (5) Oral dantrolene is indicated preoperatively in known susceptible patients and postoperatively for 1 to 3 days to follow emergency IV treatment. (6) Ability to bind to plasma proteins is inhibited by warfarin and clofibrate, increased by tolbutamide. (7) Use caution in pregnancy, lactation, and children under 5 years.

Contraindications: None when used as indicated.

Incompatible with: Specific information not available.

Side effects: None when used as short-term therapy for this specific indication.

Antidote: No specific antidote is available or needed when used correctly. Notify physician and initiate supportive measures (adequate airway and ventilation, monitor EKG) in overdosage. Large amounts of IV fluids may be needed to prevent crystalluria. Treat anaphylaxis and resuscitate as necessary.

DAUNORUBICIN HYDROCHLORIDE

(Cerubidine)

Usual dose: 60 mg/M²/24 hr for 3 days. Repeat every 3 to 4 weeks. Reduce dose to 45 mg/M²/24 hr for 3 days in combination with cytarabine 100 mg/M²/24 hr for 7 days. Repeat daunorubicin, 45 mg/M²/24 hr for only 2 days in subsequent courses every 3 to 4 weeks. Cytarabine 100 mg/M²/24 hr given daily for 5 days in subsequent courses. Normal liver and kidney function are required. When remission is complete, an individual maintenance program should be established.

Pediatric dose: 45 mg/M²/24 hr for 3 days. Repeat every 3 to 4 weeks.

Dilution: *Specific techniques required, see precautions.* Each 20 mg must be diluted with 4 ml of sterile water for injection (5 mg/ml). Agitate gently to dissolve completely. Further dilute each dose with 10 to 15 mg of normal saline. Do not add to IV solutions. Must be given through Y tube or three-way stopcock of a free-flowing infusion of 5% dextrose or normal saline.

Rate of administration: A single dose of properly diluted medication over 3 to 5 minutes.

Actions: A highly toxic antibiotic antineoplastic agent. Rapidly cleared from plasma, it inhibits synthesis of DNA. Cell cycle specific for S phase. Exact method of aciton is unknown, antimitotic, cytotoxic, and immunosuppressive. Slowly excreted in bile and urine.

Indications and uses: To induce remission of acute non-lymphocytic leukemia in adults.

Precautions: (1) Follow guidelines for handling cytotoxic agents recommended by the National Study Commission on Cytotoxic Exposure (see Appendix, p. 528). (2) Usually administered in the hospital by or under the direction of the physician specialist. (3) Determine absolute patency of vein; a stinging or burning sensation indicates extravasation; severe cellulitis and tissue necrosis will result. Discontinue injection, use another vein. (4) Diluted solution is stable 24 hours at room temperature, 48 hours if refrigerated; then discard. (5) Protect from sunlight. (6) Urine may be reddish in color (from dye, not hematuria). (7) Monitoring of white blood cells, red blood cells, platelet count, liver function, kidney function, EKG, chest x-ray, echocardiography, and systolic ejection fraction indicated before and during therapy. (8) May produce teratogenic effects on the fetus. (9) Observe closely for all signs of infection. (10) Use extreme caution in preexisting drug-induced bone marrow suppression, existing heart disease, previous treatment with doxorubicin (Adriamycin), or radiation therapy encompassing the heart. (11) May cause acute congestive heart failure with total cumulative doses over 550 mg/M^2 (400 mg/M^2 if previous treatment with doxorubicin or radiation therapy in area of heart). (12) Reduce dose up to one half if liver or renal function is impaired. (13) Prophylactic antiemetics may reduce nausea and vomiting and increase patient comfort. (13) Monitor uric acid levels, maintain hydration; allopurinol may be indicated. (14) Dosage is based on average weight if edema or ascites is present. (15) Do not administer any vaccines or chloroquine to patients receiving antineoplastic drugs.

Contraindications: Not absolute: preexisting bone marrow suppression, impaired cardiac function, preexisting infection (see Precautions).

Incompatible with: Should be considered incompatible with any other drug due to toxicity and specific use.

Side effects: Acute congestive heart failure, alopecia (reversible), bone marrow suppression (marked with average doses), chills, decrease in systolic ejection fraction, depressed QRS voltage, diarrhea, fever, gonadal suppression, mucositis, myocarditis, nausea, pericarditis, skin rash, and vomiting.

Antidote: Most side effects will be tolerated or treated symptomatically. Keep physician informed. Close monitoring of accumulated dosage, bone marrow, EKG, chest x-ray, echocardiography, and systolic ejection fraction may prevent most serious and potentially fatal side effects. There is no specific antidote. Supportive therapy as indicated will help sustain the patient in toxicity. For extravasation inject long-acting dexamethasone (Decadron-LA) or hyaluronidase (Wydase) throughout extravased tissue. Use a 27- or 25-gauge needle. Apply heat.

DEFEROXAMINE MESYLATE

(Desferal)

Usual dose: *Acute iron intoxication:* An initial dose of 1 Gm may be followed by doses of 500 mg every 4 hours as indicated by clinical response. *Do not exceed 6 Gm in 24 hours by way of any or all routes—IV, IM, or oral. Chronic iron overload:* 2 Gm with each unit of blood. Use a separate vein.

Dilution: Each 500 mg must be diluted in 2 ml of sterile water for injection. When completely dissolved, deferoxamine must be further diluted in an IV solution; normal saline, glucose in water, and Ringer's lactate solution are compatible.

Rate of administration: The fully diluted solution must not exceed a rate of 15 mg/kg of body weight/hr. Deferoxamine, 2 Gm in 1,000 ml of infusion fluid, equally distributed over 24 hours, constitutes a reasonably safe dose for anyone over 25 kg.

Actions: An iron-chelating agent, deferoxamine complexes with iron to form ferrioxamine, a stable chelate that prevents the iron from entering into further chemical reactions. Readily soluble in water, it passes easily through the kidney, giving the urine a characteristic reddish color. It will remove iron from ferritin and transferrin but not from hemoglobin.

Indications and uses: To facilitate the removal of iron in the treatment of acute iron intoxication or chronic overload from multiple transfusions.

Precautions: (1) Deferoxamine is adjunctive therapy. Standard measures for treating acute iron intoxication are also indicated: induction of emesis and/or gastric lavage; suction and maintenance of a clear airway; control of shock with IV fluids, blood, oxygen, and vasopressors; and correction of acidosis. (2) IM administration is the preferred route. IV administration should be used only in a state of cardiovascular shock or chronic iron overload. (3) For long-term therapy, check for cataract development. (4) Use care during early pregnancy or during childbearing years. (5) Under sterile conditions, deferoxamine diluted with sterile water may be stored at room temperature for 1 week.

Contraindications: Severe renal disease or anuria.

Incompatible with: Should be considered incompatible in syringe or solution with any other drug.

Side effects: Occur more frequently with too-rapid administration: abdominal discomfort; allergic type of reactions including anaphylaxis; blurring of vision; diarrhea; flushing of the skin; fever; hypotension; leg cramps; shock; tachycardia; urticaria.

Antidote: At first sign of side effects, decrease rate of administration. If side effects persist, discontinue drug and notify physician. Further dilution and decrease in rate of administration may be necessary. Resuscitate as indicated.

DESLANOSIDE INJECTION pH 5.9 to 6.5

(Cedilanid D)

Usual dose: 1.2 to 1.6 mg (6 to 8 ml) for digitalization. May be given as a single dose or equally divided over approximately 12 hours. Maintenance dose is usually about one fourth of the digitalizing dose. Give one half of the maintenance dose every 12 hours.

Pediatric dose: Total digitalizing dose for newborns is 0.022 mg/kg of body weight; for children 2 weeks to 3 years of age, 0.025 mg/kg; 3 years and over, 0.022 mg/kg. Give in divided doses every 3 to 4 hours or in a single dose if necessary.

Dilution: May be given undiluted or further diluted with 10 ml of sodium chloride injection (preferred). Do not mix with infusion fluids. Give through Y tube or three-way stopcock of IV infusion tubing.

Rate of administration: 0.2 mg (1 ml) or fraction thereof over 1 minute.

Actions: This is a rapid-acting derivative of lanatoside C. Effective within 5 to 15 minutes, it lasts 2 to 3 days. It increases the strength of myocardial contraction. It alters myocardial automaticity, conduction velocity, and refractory period. Results are a slower, stronger beat and increased cardiac output. Venous pressure falls, coronary circulation is increased, and heart size may become more normal. It is widely distributed throughout the body and excreted in the urine.

Indications and uses: (1) Congestive heart failure; (2) atrial fibrillation; (3) atrial flutter; (4) paroxysmal tachycardia; (5) cardiogenic shock; (6) ventricular arrhythmias with congestive heart failure; (7) preoperative, intraoperative, and postoperative need for digitalis because of stress on the heart.

Precautions: (1) IV administration is the preferred route. (2) Do not give digitalized patients calcium; death has occurred. (3) Potassium depletion makes the heart sensitive to digitalis intoxication. Check electrolytes during therapy. (4) Use with caution in patients with hypercalcemia or liver or kidney disease. (5) Reduce dose in impaired renal function and partially digitalized patients. (6) Potentiated by phenytoin sodium

(Dilantin), thyroid preparations, reserpine, quinidine, propranolol (Inderal), verapamil, mercurial and thiazide and loop diuretics, pressor agents (epinephrine), and others. (7) Inhibited by potassium salts, spironolactone (Aldactone), triamterene (Dyrenium), and others. (8) EKG monitoring is suggested.

Contraindications: Digitalis toxicity; ventricular tachycardia, or known sensitivity to deslanoside. *Relative contraindications:* myocardial infarction or angina pectoris without congestive heart failure.

Incompatible with: Acids, alkalies, calcium chloride, calcium disodium edetate, calcium gluceptate, calcium gluconate.

Side effects: Seldom last more than 3 days after drug is discontinued. Any form of digitalis may cause partial or AV block and almost any arrhythmia, including paroxysmal tachycardia, atrial tachycardia, fibrillation, or standstill. *First electrocardiographic signs of toxicity* are ST segment sagging, PR prolongation, and possible bigeminal rhythm. *Clinical signs of toxicity* are mostly gastrointestinal and visual: abdominal discomfort or pain, anorexia, blurred vision, confusion, diarrhea, disturbed colored (yellow) vision, headache, nausea, salivation, vomiting.

Antidote: Discontinue the drug at first sign of toxicity and notify the physician. Dosage may be decreased or discontinued. For severe toxicity use one or more of the following depending on symptoms: atropine, phenytoin (Dilantin), potassium salts (potassium chloride), procainamide (Pronestyl), or disodium edetate (EDTA disodium). Resuscitate as necessary. Treatment with Fab fragments is new and still investigational.

DEXAMETHASONE SODIUM PHOSPHATE

pH 7.0 to 8.5

(Ak-Dek, Betamethasone, Dalalone, Decadrol, Decadron phosphate, Decaject, Decameth, Delladec, Demasone, Dexacen-4, Dexasone, Dexon, Dexone, Dezone, Hexadrol phosphate, Savacort-D, Solurex, Wexaphos)

Usual dose: 0.5 to 9 mg daily, may be divided into 2 to 4 doses. Larger doses may be justified by patient condition. Repeat until adequate response, then decrease dose as indicated. Total dose usually does not exceed 80 mg/24 hr. Dosage must be individualized.
Unresponsive shock: 1.0 to 6 mg/kg of body weight (maximum 40 mg), as a single injection. Repeat every 2 to 6 hours while shock persists.

Dilution: May be given undiluted or added to IV glucose or saline solutions and given as an infusion.

Rate of administration: A single dose over 1 minute or less if necessary. As an IV infusion, give at prescribed rate.

Actions: An antiinflammatory glucocorticoid. A synthetic adrenocortical steroid with little sodium retention. Very soluble in water and seven times as potent as prednisolone and 20 to 30 times as potent as hydrocortisone. May be used in conjunction with other forms of therapy, such as epinephrine for acute allergic reactions or antibiotics for acute infections. Excreted in urine and breast milk.

Indications and uses: (1) Supplementary therapy for severe allergic reactions; (2) reduction of acute edematous states (cerebral edema); (3) shock unresponsive to conventional therapy; (4) acute life-threatening infections with massive antibiotic therapy; (5) acute exacerbations of disease for patients receiving steroid therapy; (6) viral hepatitis; (7) thyroid crisis; (8) diagnostic aid to distinguish adrenocortical hyperplasia or tumor; (9) adrenocortical insufficiency, total, relative, and operative; (10) chemotherapy; (11) antiemetic for cisplatin-induced vomiting; (12) betamethasone is used in respiratory distress syndrome of premature infants.

Precautions: (1) Use diluted solutions within 24 hours. (2) Sensitive to heat. (3) Protect from freezing. (4) May cause hypertension, but often effects diuresis rather than salt and water retention. (5) May mask signs of infection. (6) Inhibited by hydantoins (phenytoin [Dilantin], etc.), barbiturates (phenobarbital, etc.), ephedrine, and rifampin. (7) Withdrawal from therapy should be gradual to avoid precipitation of symptoms of adrenal insufficiency. The patient is observed, especially under stress, for up to 2 years. (8) Maintain on ulcer regime and antacids prophylactically. (9) May increase insulin needs in diabetes. (10) Salt and potassium replacement may be necessary. (11) Do not vaccinate against smallpox during therapy. (12) Use with caution in hypothyroidism and cirrhosis.

Contraindications: Tuberculosis (active or healed), ocular herpes simplex, or acute phychoses. *Relative contraindications:* active or latent peptic ulcer, acute or chronic infections (especially chickenpox and vaccinia), diabetes mellitus, diverticulitis, fresh intestinal anastomoses, myasthenia gravis, osteoporosis, pregnancy, psychotic tendencies, renal insufficiency, thromboembolic tendencies.

Incompatible with: Amikacin (Amikin), daunorubicin (Cerubidine), doxorubicin (Adriamycin), metaraminol (Aramine), prochlorperazine (Compazine), vancomycin (Vancocin). Limited information available. Give other drugs concurrently through a three-way stopcock.

Side effects: Do occur but are usually reversible: burning, Cushing's syndrome, electrolyte imbalance, embolism, euphoria, glycosuria, headache, hyperglycemia, hypersensitivity reactions (including anaphylaxis), hypertension, menstrual irregularities, peptic ulcer, perforation and hemorrhage, protein catabolism, sweating, thromboembolism, tingling, weakness, and many others.

Antidote: Notify the physician of any side effect. Will probably treat the side effect. Resuscitate as necessary for anaphylaxis and notify physician. Keep epinephrine immediately available.

DEXPANTHENOL

(Ilopan, Panol)

Usual dose: 2 ml (500 mg) every 6 hours until effective peristalsis returns. Treatment may be required for 72 hours or more.

Dilution: Each 2 ml (500 mg) or fraction thereof must be diluted in 500 ml or more of 5% dextrose in water or lactated Ringer's solution and given as an infusion.

Rate of administration: Each single dose properly diluted should be slowly and consistently infused over 3 to 6 hours.

Actions: A coenzyme precursor that helps to promote acetylcholine synthesis. Smooth muscle contraction is increased, promoting improved intestinal motility.

Indications and uses: (1) Paralytic ileus, (2) intestinal atony, (3) postoperative or postpartum retention of flatus or delay in resumption of intestinal motility, (4) prophylactic use immediately after major abdominal surgery.

Precautions: (1) IM route of administration is preferred; rarely given IV. (2) Allergic reactions of unknown cause have occurred when dexpanthenol is used concomitantly with antibiotics, narcotics, and barbiturates. (3) Must not be given within 12 hours of neostigmine (Prostigmin), other parasympathomimetics, or anticholinesterases or within 1 hour of succinylcholine (Anectine). (4) Hypokalemia will impede effect of dexpanthenol.

Contraindications: Hemophilia.

Incompatible with: Specific information not available. Note precautions.

Side effects: Rarely occur, but respiratory depression and allergic reactions are possible.

Antidote: Discontinue the drug and notify the physician of any symptoms of respiratory depression or allergic reaction. Treat anaphylaxis with epinephrine, antihistamines (diphenhydramine [Benadryl], etc.), vasopressors (dopamine [Intropin], etc.), aminophylline, and corticosteroids as indicated. Maintain a patent airway and resuscitate as necessary.

DEXTRAN, HIGH MOLECULAR WEIGHT

(Dextran 75, Dextran 70, Gentran 75, Macrodex)

Usual dose: Variable, depending on amount of fluid loss and resultant hemoconcentration. Initially 500 ml. Total dose should not exceed 20 ml/kg of body weight/24 hr for adults and children.

Dilution: Available as a 6% solution in 500 ml bottles properly diluted in normal saline or 5% dextrose in water and ready for use. Dextran 70 (Cutter) is available in a 250 ml bottle.

Rate of administration: Variable, depending on indication, present blood volume, and patient response. Initial 500 ml may be given at 20 to 40 ml/min. If additional high molecular weight dextran is required, reduce flow to lowest rate possible to maintain hemodynamic status desired.

Actions: Approximates colloidal properties of human albumin. Provides hemodynamically significant plasma volume expansion in excess of the amount infused for about 24 hours. Dilutes total serum proteins and hematocrit values. A glucose polymer, it is degraded to glucose and excreted in the urine.

Indications and uses: Treatment of shock or impending shock due to burns, hemorrhage, surgery, or trauma.

Precautions: (1) For IV use only. (2) Used when whole blood or blood products are not available. Not a substitute for whole blood or plasma proteins. (3) Monitor pulse, blood pressure, central venous pressure, and urine output every 5 to 15 minutes for the first hour and hourly thereafter while indicated. (4) Maintain hydration of patient with additional IV fluids; dextran promotes tissue dehydration. Avoid overhydration with dilution of electrolyte balance. (5) Change IV tubing or flush well with normal saline before infusing blood. Dextran will promote coagulation of blood in the tubing (glucose content). (6) Use caution in heart disease, renal shutdown, congestive heart failure, pulmonary edema. (7) May reduce coagulability of the circulating blood. Observe patient for increased bleeding; maintain hematocrit above 30%. (8) Draw blood for laboratory tests and type and cross-match before giving dextran, or notify laboratory of its use. May alter blood sugar and total bilirubin evaluation. (9) May produce elevated urine specific gravity (also symptom of dehydration) and increase SGOT and SGPT. (10) Crystallization of dextran can occur at low temperatures. Submerge in warm water and dissolve all crystals before administration. (11) Hemoglobin, hematocrit, electrolyte, and serum protein evaluations are necessary during therapy. (12) Use only clear solution. Store at constant temperature not above 25° C (76° F). Discard partially used solution; no preservative added.

Contraindications: Severe bleeding disorders, marked hemostatic defects (thrombocytopenia, hypofibrinogenemia, etc.) even if drug induced, known hypersensitivity to dextran, severe congestive cardiac failure, renal failure.

Incompatible with: Ascorbic acid, chlortetracycline (Aureomycin), phytonadione (Aquamephyton), promethazine (Phenergan). Do not add any drug to a bottle of dextran solution.

Side effects: Bleeding, dehydration, fever, hypotension, joint pain, nausea, overhydration, tightness of the chest, urticaria, vomiting, wheezing. Severe anaphylaxis and death have occurred.

Antidote: Notify the physician of any side effect. Discontinue the drug immediately at the first sign of an allergic reaction, provided other means of sustaining the circulation are available. Use epinephrine (Adrenalin) and/or antihistamines (diphenhydramine [Benadryl]), as indicated. Factor VIII infusion may reverse excessive bleeding. Resuscitate as necessary.

DEXTRAN 40, LOW MOLECULAR WEIGHT

(Gentran 40, L.M.D. 10%, Rheomacrodex)

Usual dose: 20 ml/kg of body weight total over first 24 hours; 10 ml/kg total over each succeeding 24 hours. Discontinue infusion after 5 days of therapy.

Prophylaxis: 10 mg/kg of body weight on day of surgery. 500 ml daily for 2 to 3 days, then 500 ml every 2 to 3 days up to 2 weeks.

As priming fluid: 10 to 20 ml/kg of body weight. Do not exceed this dose.

Dilution: Available as a 10% solution in 500 ml bottles properly diluted in normal saline or 5% dextrose in water and ready for use.

Rate of administration: Initial 500 ml may be given over 15 to 30 minutes. Remainder of any desired daily dose should be evenly distributed over 8 to 24 hours depending on use.

Actions: A low molecular weight, rapid but short-acting plasma volume expander. Increases plasma volume by once or twice its own volume. Helps to restore normal circulatory dynamics, increasing arterial and pulse pressure, central venous pressure, and cardiac output. Improves microcirculatory flow and prevents sludging in venous channels. Mobilizes water from body tissues and increases urine output. Each 1 Gm of dextran will hold 25 ml of water in the vascular space.

Indications and uses: (1) Adjunctive therapy in the treatment of shock caused by hemorrhage, burns, trauma, or surgery; (2) prophylaxis during surgical procedures with a high incidence of venous thrombosis and pulmonary embolism; (3) pump priming during extracorporeal circulation.

Precautions: (1) For IV use only. (2) Monitor pulse, blood pressure, central venous pressure, and urine output every 5 to 15 minutes for the first hour and hourly thereafter while indicated. Slow rate or discontinue dextran for rapid increase of central venous pressure (normal 7 to 14 mm H_2O pressure). If anuric or oliguric after 500 ml of dextran, discontinue the dextran. Mannitol may help increase urine flow. (3) Maintain hy-

157

dration of patient with additional IV fluids; dextran promotes tissue dehydration. Avoid overhydration with dilution of electrolyte balance. (4) Change IV tubing or flush well with normal saline before superimposing blood. Dextran will promote coagulation of blood in the tubing (glucose content). (5) Use caution in heart disease, renal shutdown, congestive heart failure, and pulmonary edema. (6) May reduce coagulability of the circulating blood slightly. Combined with increased volume, additional blood loss is possible. Maintain hematocrit above 30%. (7) Draw blood for laboratory tests and type and cross-match before giving dextran, or notify laboratory of its use. May alter blood sugar and total bilirubin evaluation. (8) May produce elevated urine specific gravity (also a symptom of dehydration) and increase SGOT and SGPT. (9) Crystallization can occur at low temperatures. Submerge in warm water and dissolve all crystals before administration. (10) Use only clear solution. Store at constant temperature not above (25° C) 76° F. Discard partially used solution; no preservative added.

Contraindications: Congestive heart failure, hypofibrinogenemia, known sensitivity to dextran, lactation and pregnancy unless needed as a lifesaving measure, renal disease with severe oliguria or anuria, thrombocytopenia.

Incompatible with: Ascorbic acid, chlortetracycline (Aureomycin), phytonadione (Aquamephyton), promethazine (Phenergan). Do not add any drug to a bottle of dextran solution.

Side effects: Bleeding, dehydration, fever, hypotension, joint pain, nausea, overhydration, tightness of chest, urticaria, vomiting, wheezing; severe anaphylaxis and death can occur.

Antidote: Notify the physician of any side effect. Discontinue the drug immediately at the first sign of an allergic reaction, provided other means of sustaining the circulation are available. Use epinephrine (Adrenalin) and/or antihistamines (diphenhydramine [Benadryl]) as indicated. Factor VIII infusion may reverse excessive bleeding. Resuscitate as necessary.

DEXTROSE

(Glucose)

Usual dose: Depends on use, age, weight, and clinical condition of the patient.

50 to 1,000 ml 2.5% and 5% dextrose may be repeated as indicated. Consider total amount of fluid.

5 ml of 10% dextrose. May repeat as necessary.

500 to 1,000 ml of 10% dextrose once or twice every 24 hours as indicated.

500 ml of 20% dextrose once or twice every 24 hours as indicated.

50 ml of 50% dextrose. May repeat if indicated.

500 to 1,500 ml/24 hr of 40% to 70% dextrose for nutrition.

Dilution: May be given undiluted in prepared solutions.

Rate of administration: 2.5% and 5% solution—rate depedent on amount.

10% solution—5 ml over 10 to 15 seconds.

10% solution—1,000 ml over at least 3 hours.

20% solution—500 ml over 30 to 60 minutes.

50% solution—10 ml over 1 minute.

500 ml of 40% to 70% solution over 4 to 12 hours, depending on body weight (0.5 to 0.8 Gm/kg/hr). Will cause glycosuria.

Actions: A monosaccharide, it provides glucose calories for metabolic needs. Its oxidation provides water to sustain volume. It lowers excess ketone production, protects body proteins, and prevents loss of electrolytes. Hypertonic solutions (20% to 50%) act as a diuretic and reduce CNS edema. Readily excreted by the kidneys, producing diuresis.

Indications and uses: (1) Cerebral and meningeal edema (eclampsia, acute glomerulonephritis, etc.) (50% solution); (2) shock (to sustain blood volume) (40% to 70% solution); (3) diuresis (20% to 50% solution); (4) hyperkalemia (20% solution); (5) hypoglycemia (insulin) in diabetic coma (50% solution); (6) adequate caloric intake (20% to 70% solution); (7) a sclerosing solution (50% solution, 3 to 20 ml).

Precautions: (1) Use caution in severe kidney damage. (2) Do not use as a diluent for blood; dextrose in any dilution causes clumping of red blood cells unless sodium chloride is added. (3) Dextrose solutions are excellent media for bacterial growth. Do not use unless the solution is entirely clear and the vial is sterile. (4) For concentrations over 20%, very large veins and slow administration are absolutely necessary. 50% dextrose can be used as a sclerosing agent and will cause thrombosis. (5) Insulin requirements may be increased. Monitor blood glucose. (6) Potassium and vitamins are readily depleted. Watch for any signs of beginning deficiency.

Contraindications: Delirium tremens with dehydration, intracranial or intraspinal hemorrhage.

Incompatible with: Cyanocobalamin (vitamin B_{12}), kanamycin (Kantrex), sodium bicarbonate, warfarin (Coumadin), whole blood.

Side effects: Rare in small doses administered slowly: acidosis, alkalosis, hyperglycemia (during infusion), hyperosmolar syndrome (mental confusion, loss of consciousness), hypoglycemia (after infusion), hypokalemia, hypovitaminosis, thrombosis.

Antidote: Discontinue the drug and notify the physician of the side effect. Symptomatic treatment is probable.

(Valium)

Usual dose: 2 to 10 mg (0.4 to 2.0 ml) every 3 to 4 hours. May be repeated in 1 hour. Maximum dose is 30 mg in 8 hours.

Cardioversion: 5 to 15 mg (1 to 3 ml) before procedure begins.

Endoscopy: Up to 20 mg before procedure begins if a narcotic is not used. Titrate to desired sedation.

Pediatric dose: *Tetanus in infants over 30 days:* 1 to 2 mg every 3 to 4 hours.

Tetanus in children 5 years or older: 5 to 10 mg every 3 to 4 hours.

Status epilepticus in infants over 30 days: 0.2 to 0.5 mg every 2 to 5 minutes to maximum 5 mg dose.

Status epilepticus in children 5 years or older: 0.5 to 1 mg every 2 to 5 minutes to maximum 10 mg dose.

Dilution: Do not dilute or mix with any other drug. *Do not add to any IV solution.*

Rate of administration: 5 mg (1 ml) or fraction thereof over 1 minute. Give total dose over a minimum of 3 minutes in infants and children.

Actions: Depresses the central, autonomic, and peripheral nervous systems in an undetermined manner. Exerts antianxiety, sedative/hypnotic, amnesic, anticonvulsant, skeletal muscle relaxant, and antitremor effects. Diminishes patient recall. Stays in the body in appreciable amounts for several days and is excreted very slowly in the urine.

Indications and uses: (1) Moderate to severe psychoneurotic reactions; (2) acute alcohol withdrawal; (3) acute stress reactions; (4) muscle spasm; (5) status epilepticus and severe recurrent convulsive seizures, including tetany; (6) preoperative medication, including endoscopic procedures; (7) cardioversion.

Precautions: (1) Should be given directly into the vein. Not soluble in any solution. Inject into IV tubing close to vein site only when direct IV injection is not feasible. Some precipitation or absorption into plastic tubing may take place. Consider heparin lock for frequent injection. Change site every 2 to 3 days. If dilution is imperative, add diluent solution to diazepam, not diazepam to diluent. Consult pharmacist. (2) To reduce incidence of thrombophlebitis, avoid smaller veins. Extravasation or arterial administration is hazardous. (3) Respiratory assistance must be available. (4) Bed rest is required for a minimum of 3 hours after IV injection. (5) Potentiates narcotics, phenothiazines (prochlorperazine [Compazine], etc.), barbiturates, and MAO inhibitors (pargyline [Eutonyl], etc.). Potentiated by cimetidine (Tagamet), alcohol, and other CNS depressants. (6) Reduce dosages for the elderly and debilitated and in those with impaired liver or renal function. (7) Withdrawal symptoms will occur for several weeks after extended or large doses. (8) Intended for short-term use only.

Contraindications: Acute narrow angle glaucoma; infants and children under 12 years, except in tetany and status epilepticus; manifestation of allergic reaction; known psychoses; pregnancy and childbirth; shock, coma, or acute alcoholic intoxication with depression of vital signs.

Incompatible with: Any other drug in syringe or solution. Precipitation will occur.

Side effects: *Minor:* ataxia, blurred vision, bradycardia, confusion, coughing, depressed respiration, depression, diminished reflexes, drowsiness, dyspnea, headache, hiccups, hyperexcited states, hyperventilation, laryngospasm, neutropenia, nystagmus, somnolence, syncope, venous thrombosis and phlebitis at injection site, vertigo. *Major:* apnea, cardiac arrest, cardiovascular collapse, coma.

Antidote: Notify the physician of minor symptoms. For major symptoms, discontinue drug, treat allergic reaction, or resuscitate as necessary and notify the physician. Caffeine and sodium benzoate effectively combats CNS depression of diazepam overdose. Use dopamine (Intropin), levarterenol (Levophed), or metaraminol (Aramine) for hypotension.

162

(Hyperstat IV)

Usual dose: 150 mg (10 ml) initially. 1 to 3 mg/kg of body weight may be used to calculate exact dose. May be repeated in 5 to 15 minutes if an adequate response is not obtained. This second injection may effect a greater response. Repeat as indicated at intervals of 4 to 24 hours to maintain desired blood pressure. For short-term use until a regime of oral antihypertensive medication is effective.

Pediatric dose: 1 to 3 mg/kg of body weight.

Dilution: Should be given undiluted.

Rate of administration: Rapidly as a single dose over 30 seconds or less. Not as effective when administered at a slower rate.

Actions: A potent, rapid-acting antihypertensive agent. Produces vasodilation by relaxing the smooth muscle of peripheral arterioles. Increases cardiac output while maintaining coronary and cerebral blood flow. Effects on renal blood flow are not significant. Effective in patients not responsive to other antihypertensive agents. Acts within 1 to 5 minutes. Usually no further decrease in blood pressure after 30 minutes, but a gradual increase over 2 to 12 hours. Crosses placental barrier, probably excreted in breast milk.

Indications and uses: Malignant hypertension.

Precautions: (1) Give only into a peripheral vein; avoid extravasation. (2) Maintain patient in recumbent position during injection and for at least 30 minutes after injection. (3) Check blood pressure every 5 minutes until stabilized and hourly thereafter. (4) Take blood pressure with patient in standing position before ambulation. (5) Use caution in diabetes; monitor blood glucose levels. May cause hyperglycemia. (6) Diuresis may be required to reverse sodium and water retention before diazoxide can be effective. (7) Use caution in impaired cerebral or cardiac circulation. (8) Potentiates coumarin and its derivatives; a reduced dose of anticoagulant may be required. (9) Potentiated by thiazides, side effects increased. (10) Inhibits phenytoin (Dilantin). (11) Profound hypotension will result if used with peripheral vasodilators (hydralazine [Apresoline], nitroprusside sodium [Nipride], etc.).

Contraindications: Compensatory hypertension (e.g., arteriovenous shunt or coarctation of the aorta); known sensitivity to thiazides; pregnancy; children; not effective in pheochromocytoma.

Incompatible with: Do not mix in syringe or solution with any other drug.

Side effects: Abdominal discomfort, cerebral ischemia, confusion, congestive heart failure, convulsions, edema, flushing, headache, hyperglycemia, hypotension (severe), ileus, light-headedness, myocardial ischemia, nausea, orthostatic hypotension, palpitations, paralysis, sensations of warmth, sensitivity reactions, sodium and water retention, supraventricular tachycardia, sweating, vomiting, weakness.

Antidote: Notify the physician of all side effects. Some will subside spontaneously, others will require symptomatic treatment. Treat sensitivity reaction as indicated and resuscitate as necessary. Treat undesirable hypotension with levarterenol (Levophed). If no response, diazoxide is probably not the cause of the hypotension; excessive hyperglycemia may be treated with insulin. Hemodialysis or peritoneal dialysis may be required in overdose.

DIETHYLSTILBESTROL
pH DIPHOSPHATE pH 9 to 10.5

(Stilphostrol)

Usual dose: 0.5 Gm/24 hr initially. Increase to 1 Gm/24 hr, beginning with second day, and give 1 Gm/24 hr for 5 days or as indicated by patient responses. 0.25 to 0.5 Gm once or twice weekly as maintenance dose.

Dilution: A single daily dose must be diluted in 300 ml of saline or dextrose for infusion.

Rate of administration: 20 drops/min for the first 15 minutes; then increase rate to complete infusion within 1 hour of starting time.

Actions: An estrogen hormone. In the diphosphate form there are fewer side effects, and large doses can be given. May be directly cytotoxic to malignant cells or may simply slow the growth. Does decrease the percentage of cells actively proliferating in a tumor mass.

Indications and uses: Palliative treatment of prostatic or breast carcinoma. Particularly useful in advanced stages.

Precautions: (1) IV route is used when oral route is ineffective or not practical. (2) Will cause salt and water retention. Monitor weight and encourage a low-salt diet. (3) Used with other antineoplastic drugs to achieve tumor remission. (4) Feminization in the male and uterine bleeding in postmenopausal women are expected. (5) Use caution in cardiac, liver, or renal disease and diabetes.

Contraindications: Markedly impaired liver function, a past history of or active thrombophlebitis, thromboembolic disorders or cerebral apoplexy, estrogen-dependent neoplasia.

Incompatible with: Sufficient information not available. Calcium gluconate.

Side effects: Burning and local pain in the perineal region and metastatic sites are expected and last only a few moments. Other side effects are abdominal cramps, anemia, decreased libido, dizziness, elevated prothrombin time, hypercalcemia, myocardial infarction, nausea, pulmonary embolism, thrombophlebi-

tis, and vomiting. All side effects associated with estrogens are possible.

Antidote: Notify the physician of all side effects. Most
will be treated symptomatically. Hypercalcemia is reversible when detected early (limit oral calcium, push
fluids, record output, and ambulate to keep calcium in
the bones). There is no specific antidote. Supportive
therapy as indicated will help sustain the patient in
toxicity.

DIGITOXIN

(Crystodigin)

Usual dose: 1.2 to 1.6 mg (6 to 8 ml) for digitalization. Initial dose of 0.6 mg (3 ml) followed by 0.4 mg (2 ml) in 4 to 6 hours and 0.2 mg (1 ml) every 4 to 6 hours until digitalized (approximately 12 hours). Maintenance dose is usually about 0.1 to 0.3 mg. Dosage must be adjusted to the specific patient.

Pediatric dose: Newborn, 0.022 mg/kg of body weight; under 1 year of age, 0.045 mg/kg; 1 to 2 years, 0.04 mg/kg; children 2 to 12 years, 0.03 mg/kg. Divide digitalizing dose into three or more doses and administer every 6 to 8 hours. Maintenance dose is usually one tenth the initial dose. Continuous monitoring is recommended.

Dilution: May be given undiluted but may be further diluted with 10 ml normal saline for injection. May not be mixed with infusion fluids. Give through Y tube or three-way stopcock of IV infusion set.

Rate of administration: 0.2 mg (1 ml) or fraction thereof over 1 minute.

Actions: A slow-acting crystalline cardiac glycoside obtained from *Digitalis purpurea*. Onset of action is within 30 minutes to 2 hours and lasts 2 to 4 days. It has positive inotropic action, increasing the strength of myocardial contraction. It also alters the electrical behavior of heart muscle through actions on myocardial automaticity, conduction velocity, and refraction. Results are a slower, stronger beat with increased cardiac output. Venous pressure falls, coronary circulation is increased, and heart size may become more normal. Considerably bound to plasma protein and metabolized in the liver, it is widely distributed throughout the body and slowly excreted in the urine.

Indications and uses: (1) Congestive heart failure, (2) atrial fibrillation, (3) atrial flutter, (4) paroxysmal tachycardia.

Precautions: (1) Do not give digitalized patients calcium; death has occurred. (2) Not the drug of choice for rapid digitalization in emergencies. (3) IV administration is the preferred route. (4) Potassium depletion makes the heart sensitive to digitalis intoxication; check electrolytes during therapy. (5) Use with caution in patients with hypercalcemia or liver or kidney disease. (6) Reduce dose in partially digitalized patients. (7) Potentiated by phenytoin (Dilantin), thyroid preparations, reserpine, quinidine, propranolol, verapamil, diuretics, pressor agents (epinephrine), and others. (8) Inhibited by potassium salts, spironolactone (Aldactone), triamterene (Dyrenium), and others. (9) ECG monitoring is suggested.

Contraindications: Digitalis intoxication. Not absolute: Adams-Stokes syndrome, carotid sinus hypersensitivity, heart block, myocardial infarction, ventricular tachycardia.

Incompatible with: Acids, alkalies, calcium chloride, calcium disodium edetate, calcium gluceptate, calcium gluconate, chloramphenicol (Chloromycetin), chlorothiazide (Diuril), methylprednisolone (Solu-Medrol).

Side effects: May persist for 4 to 6 days after drug is discontinued. Any form of digitalis may cause partial or AV block and almost any arrhythmia, including paroxysmal tachycardia, atrial tachycardia, fibrillation, or standstill. *First electrocardiographic signs of toxicity* are ST segment sagging, PR prolongation, and possible bigeminal rhythm. *Clinical signs of toxicity* are mostly gastrointestinal and visual: abdominal discomfort or pain, anorexia, blurred vision, confusion, diarrhea, disturbed color (yellow) vision, headache, nausea, salivation, vomiting, and weakness.

Antidote: Discontinue the drug at the first sign of toxicity and notify the physician. Dosage may be decreased or discontinued. For severe toxicity use one or more of the following, depending on symptoms: atropine, phenytoin (Dilantin), potassium salts (potassium chloride), procainamide (Pronestyl), or disodium edetate (EDTA disodium). Treatment with Fab fragments is new and still investigational. Resuscitate as necessary.

DIGOXIN INJECTION
pH 6.6 to 7.4

(Lanoxin)

Usual dose: 0.5 to 1 mg (2 to 4 ml) for digitalization. 0.25 to 0.5 mg (1 to 2 ml) as the initial dose, followed by 0.25 to 0.5 mg (1 to 2 ml) at 4- to 6-hour intervals until digitalized (approximately 4 to 6 hours). Maintenance dose is usually 0.125 to 0.5 mg daily.

Pediatric dose: Infants to 2 years: 0.04 to 0.06 mg/kg of body weight. Over 2 years, 0.02 to 0.04 mg/kg, give one half of total daily dose initially then two doses of one-fourth total daily dose at 8 hour intervals. Maintenance dose: one fifth of total daily dose divided and given every 12 hours. Individualized doses.

Dilution: May be given undiluted or each 1 ml may be diluted in 4 ml sterile water, normal saline, or 5% dextrose for injection. Less diluent will cause precipitation. Use diluted solution immediately. Give through Y tube or three-way stopcock of IV infusion set.

Rate of administration: Each single dose over a minimum of 5 minutes.

Actions: A crystalline cardiac glycoside obtained from *Digitalis lanata*, this is a fast-acting hydrolytic product of lanatoside C. Onset of action is within 5 to 10 minutes and lasts 2 to 3 days. It has positive inotropic action, increasing the strength of myocardial contraction. It also alters the electric behavior of heart muscle through actions on myocardial automaticity, conduction velocity, and refraction. Results are a slower, stronger beat with increased cardiac output. Venous pressure falls, coronary circulation is increased, and heart size may become more normal. Widely distributed throughout the body and rapidly excreted in the urine. Excretion reduces toxicity period in overdigitalization.

Indications and uses: (1) Congestive heart failure; (2) atrial fibrillation; (3) atrial flutter; (4) paroxysmal tachycardia; (5) cardiogenic shock; (6) ventricular arrhythmias with congestive heart failure; (7) preoperative, intraoperative, and postoperative need for digitalis because of stress on the heart.

Precautions: (1) IV administration is the preferred route. (2) Do not give digitalized patients calcium. Death has occurred. (3) Potassium depletion makes the heart sensitive to digitalis intoxication. Check electrolytes during therapy. (4) Use with caution in patients with hypercalcemia or liver or kidney disease. (5) Reduce dose in partially digitalized patients and impaired kidney function. (6) Potentiated by phenytoin (Dilantin), thyroid preparations, reserpine, quinidine, propranolol, verapamil, diuretics, pressor agents (epinephrine), and others. (7) Inhibited by potassium salts, spironolactone (Aldactone), triamterene (Dyrenium), and others. (8) EKG monitoring is suggested.

Contraindications: Digitalis intoxication. Not absolute. Used in ventricular paroxysmal tachycardia or ventricular fibrillation only if heart failure is present and the etiology is not digitalis intoxication.

Incompatible with: Acids, alkalies, calcium chloride, calcium disodium edetate, calcium gluceptate, calcium gluconate.

Side effects: Seldom last more than 3 days after drug is discontinued. Any form of digitalis may cause partial or AV block and almost any arrhythmia, including paroxysmal tachycardia, atrial tachycardia, fibrillation, or standstill. *First electrocardiographic signs of toxicity* are ST segment sagging, PR prolongation, and possible bigeminal rhythm. *Clinical signs of toxicity* are mostly abdominal discomfort or pain, blurred vision, confusion, diarrhea, disturbed color (yellow) vision, headache, nausea, vomiting, weakness.

Antidote: Discontinue the drug at the first sign of toxicity and notify the physician. Dosage may be decreased or discontinued. For severe toxicity use one or more of the following depending on symptoms: atropine, phenytoin (Dilantin), potassium salts (potassium chloride), procainamide (Pronestyl), or disodium edetate (EDTA disodium). Treatment with Fab fragments is new and still investigational. Resuscitate as necessary.

DIHYDROERGOTAMINE MESYLATE
(D.H.E. 45)

Usual dose: 1 mg (1 ml). May be repeated in 1 hour. No more than two doses (2 mg total) may be given IV in 24 hours. Do not exceed 6 mg in 1 week.

Dilution: May be given undiluted.

Rate of administration: 1 mg or fraction thereof over 1 minute.

Actions: A vasoconstrictor, it probably acts on distended cerebral arteries. It also paralyzes the effector cells connected with adrenergic nerves. Probably detoxified in the liver and excreted in the urine.

Indications and uses: Vascular headaches (migraine, histamine cephalalgia). Being used experimentally to enhance heparin effects in preventing postoperative deep vein thrombosis after total hip replacement.

Precautions: (1) IM use is preferred but may be given IV to obtain a more rapid effect. (2) Protect the ampoules from light and heat.

Contraindications: Advanced arteriosclerosis, hepatic disease, hypersensitivity, obliterative vascular disease, pregnancy, sepsis.

Incompatible with: Any other drug in syringe or solution.

Side effects: Rare in therapeutic doses but may include angina pectoris, blindness, gangrene, muscle pains, muscle weakness, nausea, numbness and tingling of the fingers and toes, thirst, uterine bleeding, and vomiting.

Antidote: Discontinue the drug and notify the physician of any side effects. Another drug will probably be chosen if further treatment is indicated. Vasodilators (nitroprusside) and CNS stimulants (caffeine, sodium benzoate, etc.) are indicated as an antidote.

DIMENHYDRINATE   pH 6.8 to 7.2

(Dramamine, Dimate, Dommanate, Dramilin, Dramocen, Dramoject, Dymenate, Hydrate, Marmine, Reidamine, Wehamine)

Usual dose: 50 to 100 mg every 4 hours.

Pediatric dose: 5 mg/kg of body weight divided into four equal doses over 24 hours. Do not exceed 300 mg.

Dilution: Each 50 mg (1 ml) must be diluted in 10 ml of sodium chloride injection.

Rate of administration: Each 50 mg or fraction thereof, properly diluted, is injected over 2 minutes.

Actions: An antihistamine and CNS depressant. Specific mode of aciton is not exactly known, but depression of hyperstimulated labrynthine functions and associated neural pathways does occur. Threshold of susceptibility, especially to motion sickness, is raised. Excreted in changed form in the urine.

Indications and uses: Treatment of motion sickness, nausea and vomiting, vertigo, and diseases affecting the vestibular system (labyrinthitis and Meniere's disease).

Precautions: (1) Will induce drowsiness; this is often a desirable reaction. (2) Will cause irreversible ototoxicity because of masking of infection or toxicity symptoms when given in conjunction with some antibiotics such as dihydrostreptomycin, gentamicin (Garamycin), kanamycin (Kantrex), neomycin, streptomycin, and vancomycin (Vancocin). (3) Reduce dosage for the elderly and debilitated. (4) Alcohol and CNS depressants will produce an additive effect. (5) Use caution in prostatic hypertrophy, peptic ulcer, pyloroduodenal obstruction, bladder neck obstruction, narrow angle glaucoma, cardiac arrhythmias, and asthma. (6) Antimuscarinic effect may inhibit lactation.

Contraindications: None absolute.

Incompatible with: Alkaline solutions, aminophylline, ammonium chloride, amobarbital (Amytal), clordiazepoxide (Librium), chlorpromazine (Thorazine), diphenhydramine (Benadryl), glycopyrrolate (Robinul), heparin, hydrocortisone (Solu-Cortef), hydroxyzine (Vistaril), pentobarbital (Nembutal), phenobarbital

172

(Luminal), phenytoin (Dilantin), prednisolone (Hy-deltrasol), prochlorperazine (Compazine), promazine (Sparine), promethazine (Phenergan), tetracyclines, thiopental (Pentothal), trifluoperazine (Stelazine).

Side effects: Rare when used as indicated. The primary side effect is drowsiness. Toxic doses produce CNS excitation in children, convulsions, hyperpyrexia, marked irritability, death.

Antidote: For exaggerated drowsiness or other major side effects, discontinue the drug and notify the physician. Side effects will usually subside within a few hours or may be treated symptomatically. Anticonvulsant barbiturates will increase toxicity. Resuscitate as necessary.

DIPHENHYDRAMINE HYDROCHLORIDE

pH 5.0 to 6.0

(Benadryl, Benahist, Bendylate, Benoject, Dihydrex, Hyrexin, Nordryl, Wehdryl 50)

Usual dose: 10 to 50 mg. Up to 100 mg may be given. Total dosage should not exceed 400 mg/24 hr.

Pediatric dose: Children after neonatal period: 5 mg/kg of body weight/24 hr. Divide this into four equal doses. Never exceed a total dosage of 300 mg/24 hr.

Dilution: May be given undiluted.

Rate of administration: 25 mg or fraction thereof over 1 minute. Extend injection time in nonemergency situations.

Actions: A potent antihistamine, it is capable of blocking the effects of histamines at various receptor sites, either eliminating allergic reaction or greatly modifying it. It is also an anticholinergic (antispasmodic), an antiemetic, and has sedative effects. Readily absorbed, widely distributed, and easily metabolized, it is excreted in changed form in the urine.

Indications and uses: (1) Supplemental therapy to epinephrine in anaphylaxis and angioneurotic edema, (2) preoperative sedation, (3) antidote for parkinsonism-like syndrome caused by some phenothiazines (prochlorperazine [Compazine], etc.), (4) severe nausea and vomiting, (5) motion sickness.

Precautions: (1) IV administration is used only in emergency situations. (2) Avoid subcutaneous or perivascular injection. (3) Will induce drowsiness. (4) Use with extreme caution in infants, children, elderly, and debilitated individuals. (5) Increases effectiveness of epinephrine and is often used in conjunction with it. (6) Potentiates anticholinergics (Atropine), alcohol, hypnotics, sedatives, tranquilizers, and other CNS depressants (reserpine, antipyretics), thioridazine (Mellaril), and others. (7) Inhibits anticoagulants, corticosteroids, and others. (8) Effectiveness of many drugs is reduced in combination with dephenhydramine because of increased metabolism.

Contraindications: Asthmatic attack, bladder neck obstruction, hypersensitivity to diphenhydramine, narrow angle glaucoma, patients receiving MAO inhibitors (pargyline [Eutonyl], etc.), pregnancy and lactation, premature or newborn infants, prostatic hypertrophy, pyloroduodenal obstruction, stenosing peptic ulcer.

Incompatible with: Amobarbital (Amytal), amphotericin B (Fungizone), cephalothin (Keflin), dexamethasone (Decadron), furosemide (Lasix), methylprednisolone (Solu-Medrol), pentobarbital (Nembutal), phenobarbital (Luminal), phenytoin (Dilantin), secobarbital (Seconal), thiopental (Pentothal).

Side effects: Rare when used as indicated: anaphylactic shock, blurring of vision; confusion; constipation; diarrhea; difficulty in urination; diplopia; drowsiness; drug rash; dryness of mouth, nose and throat; epigastric distress; headache; hemolytic anemia; hypotension; insomnia; nasal stuffiness; nausea; nervousness; palpitations; photosensitivity; restlessness; thickening of bronchial secretions; tightness of the chest and wheezing; tingling; weakness, heaviness of hands; urticaria; vertigo; vomiting.

Antidote: For exaggerated drowsiness or other disturbing side effects, discontinue the drug and notify the physician. Side effects will usually subside within a few hours or may be treated symptomatically. Anticonvulsant barbiturates will increase toxicity. Resuscitate as necessary.

DIPHTHERIA ANTITOXIN

Usual dose: Testing for sensitivity to horse serum is required before use (see precautions). Suggested ranges for adults and children are to be given as a single dose.
Pharyngeal or laryngeal disease of 48 hours' duration: 20,000 to 40,000 units.
Nasopharyngeal lesions: 40,000 to 60,000 units.
Extensive disease (3 or more days' duration or anyone with brawny swelling of the neck): 80,000 to 120,000 units.

Dilution: May be given undiluted as an IV infusion. May be warmed to 32° to 35° C (90° to 95° F).

Rate of administration: To be given as a slow intravenous infusion. Titrate carefully to patient reaction.

Actions: A sterile solution of purified antitoxic substances prepared from the blood serum of horses immunized against diphtheria toxin. Neutralizes the toxins produced by *Corynebacterium diphtheriae.*

Indications and uses: Treatment of patients with clinical symptoms of diphtheria.

Precautions: (1) Read drug literature supplied with antitoxin completely before use. Essential to evaluate symptoms and individual status of each patient. (2) Determine patient response to any previous injections of serum of any type and history of any allergic type reactions. (3) Hospitalize patient if possible. (4) Test every patient for sensitivity to horse serum without exception (1 ml vial of 1:10 dilution horse serum supplied). Skin test and conjuctival test are recommended for maximum safety.
Skin test: Inject 0.02 ml of 1:10 horse serum into (not under) skin (intracutaneous). A like injection of normal saline can be used as a control. An urticarial wheal surrounded by a zone of erythema is a positive reaction. Compare in 20 minutes.
Conjunctival test: Instill 1 drop of 1:10 horse serum into conjunctival sac for adults (1 drop of 1:100 dilution for children). Itching, redness, burning, and/or lacrimation within 30 minutes is a positive reaction. A drop of normal saline in the opposite eye is used as

a control and should be asymptomatic. Reverse adverse effects of positive reaction with 1 drop of epinephrine ophthalmic solution. Other testing methods may be used. Use at least two. (5) Bacteriological confirmation of the disease is not necessary to initiate treatment. Begin treatment as soon as possible. Each hour delay increases dosage requirements and decreases effectiveness. (6) Continue treatment until all symptoms are controlled or bacteriological confirmation of another disease entity is confirmed. (7) Use of full therapeutic doses of antimicrobial agents is recommended in conjunction with diphtheria antitoxin. (8) All contacts must be evaluated and immunized if necessary.

Contraindications: Hypersensitivity to horse serum unless only treatment available for life-threatening situation. Several techniques including preload of antihistamines and/or desensitization may be considered (see literature).

Incompatible with: Specific information not available. Do not mix with any other drug in syringe or solution due to specific use.

Side effects: Acute anaphylaxis with urticaria, respiratory distress, and vascular collapse. Serum sickness may occur. Usually appears in 7 to 12 days. Local pain, local erythema, and urticaria without systemic reaction can occur.

Antidote: Discontinue the drug and notify the physician of all side effects. Treat anaphylaxis immediately. Epinephrine (Adrenalin) and diphenhydramine (Benadryl), oxygen, vasopressors (dopamine), corticosteroids, and ventilation equipment must always be available. Resuscitate as necessary.

(EDTA disodium, Endrate chealamide, Sodium Versenate)

Usual dose: 50 mg/kg of body weight/24 hr as indicated. Total dose should not exceed 3 Gm/24 hr.

Pediatric dose: 40 mg/kg of body weight/24 hr as indicated. Do not exceed 70 mg/kg/24 hr or adult dose, whichever is less.

Dilution: Recommended dose must be diluted in 500 ml of dextrose or isotonic saline solution and given as IV infusion. A 0.5% solution will reduce the risk of thrombophlebitis.

Rate of administration: Must not exceed more than 15 mg of actual medication over 1 minute. Total dose is usually given over 3 to 4 hours. Reduce rate and further dilute solution for pain at injection site.

Actions: A calcium-chelating agent. Attracts calcium ions immediately on injection and becomes calcium disodium edetate. Capable of severely depleting the body of calcium stores. It is well distributed in extracellular fluids and rapidly excreted in the urine.

Indications and uses: (1) Cardiac arrhythmias (atrial and ventricular, especially when caused by digitalis toxicity); (2) hypercalcemia.

Precautions: (1) Used only when the severity of disease indicates necessity. (2) May produce hypocalcemia quickly, especially if used for purposes other than chelating calcium. (3) Use repeatedly only with caution because of potential for nephrotoxicity and mobilization of extracirculatory calcium stores. (4) Monitor vital signs and EKG before and during therapy. (5) Routine electrolyte panel (potassium deficiency) and urine specimens for casts and cells are necessary during therapy. (6) Inhibits coagulation of blood (transient). (7) Use caution in diabetes, severe renal disease, liver disease, and congestive heart failure (1 Gm of sodium in each 5 Gm). (8) Inhibits mannitol. (9) Potentiates neuromuscular blocking antibiotics (gentamicin [Garamycin], etc.). (10) Obtain blood for serum calcium levels just before beginning a new infusion. Specific laboratory methods must be used for accurate evaluation. (11) Keep patient in supine position during and after administration (15 to 30 minutes) to avoid postural hypotension.

Contraindications: Active or healed tuberculosis, anuria, known sensitivity to disodium edetate.

Incompatible with: Will chelate any metal. Not recommended to mix in syringe or solution with any other drug.

Side effects: *Minor:* anorexia, arthralgia, circumoral paresthesias, fatigue, fever, glycosuria, headache, hypotension, malaise, nasal congestion, nausea, sneezing, tearing, thirst, thrombophlebitis, urinary urgency, vomiting. *Major:* anaphylaxis, anemia, dermatitis, hemorrhage, hypocalcemic tetany, prolonged QT interval, renal tubular destruction (reversible), death.

Antidote: Notify the physician of any side effect. For progression of minor side effects or any major side effect, discontinue drug immediately and notify the physician. Calcium gluconate is the antidote of choice and should be available for infusion at all times. Treat anaphylaxis and resuscitate as necessary.

DOBUTAMINE HYDROCHLORIDE
(Dobutrex)

pH 2.5 to 5.5

Usual dose: 2.5 to 10 μg/kg of body weight/min initially. Adjust rate to effect desired response. Up to 40 μg/kg/min has been used in some instances.

Dilution: Each 250 mg ampoule should be initially diluted with 10 ml of sterile water or 5% dextrose for injection. An additional 10 ml may be used if necessary to completely dissolve. Must be further diluted to at least 50 ml. Any amount of infusion solution desired above 50 ml may be used. Adjust to fluid requirements of the patient. Use of 5% dextrose, 0.9% sodium chloride, or sodium lactate is recommended.

Rate of administration: Begin with recommended dose for body weight and seriousness of condition. Gradually increase to effect desired response. May take up to 10 minutes to achieve peak effect of a specific dose. Maintain at correct therapeutic level with microdrop (60 gtt/ml) or infusion pump. Half-life of dobutamine is only about 2 minutes.

Actions: A synthetic catecholamine, chemically related to dopamine, it is a direct-acting inotropic agent possessing beta stimulator activity. Induces short-term increases in cardiac output by improving stroke volume with minimal increases in rate and blood pressure, minimal rhythm disturbances, and decreased peripheral vascular resistance. Usually most effective for only a few hours. May improve atrioventricular conduction. Peak effect is obtained in 2 to 10 minutes. Has a very short duration of action and is excreted in the urine.

Indications and uses: Short-term inotropic support in cardiac decompensation due to depressed contractility (organic heart disease or cardiac surgical procedures). *Investigational use:* To increase cardiac output in children with congenital heart disease undergoing cardiac catheterization.

Precautions: (1) Observe patient's response continuously; monitor heart rate, ectopic activity, blood pressure, urine flow, and central venous pressure. Measure pulmonary wedge pressure and cardiac output if possible. (2) Use digitalis preparation before starting dobutamine in patients with atrial fibrillation with rapid ventricular response. (3) Compatible through common tubing with dopamine, lidocaine, tobramycin, nitroprusside, potassium chloride, and protamine sulfate. (4) Correct hypovolemia and acidosis as indicated before initiating treatment. (5) May be ineffective if beta blocking drugs (propranolol [Inderal], etc.) have been given. (6) Use extreme caution in myocardial infarction; may increase size of infarction. (7) Produces higher cardiac output and lower pulmonary wedge pressure when given concomitantly with nitroprusside. (8) May cause serious arrhythmias in presence of cyclopropane or halogen anesthetics, severe hypertension with oxytocic drugs. Use extreme caution and reduced dose, one tenth of calculated amount, in patients taking MAO inhibitors (isocarboxazid [Marplan], etc.). (8) Will produce severe hypotension and seizures with phenytoin (Dilantin). (9) May increase insulin requirements in diabetics. (10) Refrigerate reconstituted solution up to 48 hours or keep at room temperature 6 hours. When mixed in infusion solution, use within 24 hours. (9) Pink coloring of solution does not affect potency; will crystallize if frozen.

Contraindications: Idiopathic hypertrophic subaortic stenosis. Safety in pregnancy and children not established.

Incompatible with: Alkaline solutions (sodium bicarbonate, etc.), calcium gluconate, cefamandole (Mandol), cefazolin (Kefzol), cephalothin (Keflin), heparin, hydrocortisone, penicillin, potassium phosphate, sodium ethacrynate (Edecrin).

Side effects: Anginal pain, chest pain, headache, hypertension, increased ventricular ectopic activity, nausea, palpitations, shortness of breath, and tachycardia.

Antidote: Notify physician of all side effects. Decrease infusion rate and notify physician immediately if number of PVCs increases or there is a marked increase in pulse rate (30 or more beats) or blood pressure (50 or more mm Hg systolic). For accidental overdosage reduce rate or temporarily discontinue until condition stabilizes.

(Intropin)

Usual dose: 2 to 5 μg/kg of body weight/min initially in patients likely to respond to minimal treatment. 5 to 10 μg/kg/min may be required initially to correct hypotension in the seriously ill patient. Gradually increase by 5 to 10 μg/kg/min at 10- to 30-minute increments until optimum response occurs. Average dose is 20 μg/kg/min, over 50 μg/kg/min has been required in some instances.

Dilution: Each 5 ml (200 mg) ampoule must be diluted in 250 to 500 ml of the following IV solutions and given as an infusion: normal saline, 5% dextrose in water, 5% dextrose in 0.9% or 0.45% sodium chloride, 5% dextrose in lactated Ringer's injection, 1/6 molar sodium lactate, or lactated Ringer's injection. Diluted in 250 ml of solution, each milliliter contains 800 μg of dopamine. Diluted in 500 ml of solution, each milliliter contains 400 μg of dopamine. More concentrated solutions may be used if absolutely necessary to reduce fluid volume.

Rate of administration: Begin with recommended dose for body weight and seriousness of condition. Gradually increase by 5 to 10 μg/kg of body weight/min to effect desired response. Use slowest possible rate to maintain adequate or preset systolic blood pressure. Use a microdrop (60 gtt/ml) or an infusion pump and optimum urine flow for correct evaluation of dosage.

Actions: Dopamine is a chemical precursor of epinephrine, possessing alpha and beta receptor–stimulating actions. Increases cardiac output with minimum increase in myocardial oxygen consumption. Dilates renal and mesenteric blood vessels at doses lower than those required to elevate systolic blood pressure. Therapeutic doses effect little change on diastolic blood pressure. Has short duration of action and is promptly excreted in changed form in the urine.

Indications and uses: To correct hemodynamic imbalances including hypotension resulting from shock syndrome of myocardial infarction, trauma, endotoxic septicemia, open heart surgery, renal failure, and chronic cardiac decompensation.

Precautions: (1) Recognition of signs and symptoms and prompt treatment with dopamine will improve prognosis. (2) Alkaline solutions including sodium bicarbonate inactivate dopamine. (3) Check blood pressure every 2 minutes until stabilized at the desired level. Check every 5 minutes thereafter during therapy. Avoid hypertension. Check central venous pressure or pulmonary wedge pressure before administration and as ordered thereafter. (4) Use larger veins (antecubital fossa) and avoid extravasation; may cause necrosis and sloughing of tissue. (5) If possible, correct hypovolemia with whole blood or plasma as indicated; correct acidosis if present. (6) Discard diluted solution after 24 hours. (7) Use caution in pregnancy, children, and presence of cyclopropane or other similar anesthetics. (8) Monitor urine flow continuously. (9) Reduce dose to one tenth of the calculated amount for individuals being treated with MAO inhibitors (isocarboxazid [Marplan], etc.) and other sympathomimetics. (10) May cause severe hypertension with ergonovine or oxytocin. (11) Antagonizes effects of morphine, reducing analgesic effect. (12) Potentiated by tricyclic antidepressants and diuretics. (13) Therapy may be continued until the patient can maintain his own hemodynamic and renal functions. (14) Beta receptor effects are blocked by propranolol (Inderal), and dopamine antagonizes beta blocking effects of propranolol. (15) Will cause severe bradycardia and hypotension with phenytoin (Dilantin).

Contraindications: Pheochromocytoma, uncorrected tachyarrhythmias, ventricular fibrillation.

Incompatible with: Alkaline solutions, amphotericin B, sodium bicarbonate.

Side effects: Aberrant conduction, anginal pain, azotemia, bradycardia, dyspnea, ectopic beats, headache, hypertension, hypotension, nausea, palpitation, piloerection, tachycardia, vasoconstriction, vomiting, widened QRS complex.

Antidote: Notify the physician of all side effects. Decrease infusion rate and notify the physician immediately for

decrease in established urine flow rate, disproportion-
ate rise in diastolic blood pressure, increasing tachycardia, or new dysrhythmias. For accidental overdosage with hypertension, reduce rate or temporarily discontinue until condition stabilizes. Phentolamine may
be required. To prevent sloughing and necrosis in
areas where extravasation has occurred, inject 5 to 10
mg of phentolamine (Regitine) diluted in 10 to 15 ml
normal saline liberally throughout the tissue in the
extravasated area with a fine hypodermic needle. Begin as soon as extravasation is recognized.

DOXAPRAM HYDROCHLORIDE

(Dopram)

Usual dose: 0.5 to 1.0 mg/kg of body weight. May be given as a single injection or divided and given as several injections at 5-minute intervals. Maximum dosage equals 2 mg/kg. Repeat every 1 to 2 hours as necessary to maintain respiration. *Do not exceed 3 Gm/24 hr. Minimum effective dosage is recommended.*
Chronic obstructive pulmonary disease: 400 mg in specific amount of diluent over no more than 2 hours.

Dilution: May be given undiluted, diluted with equal parts of sterile water for injection, or dilute 250 mg (12.5 ml) in 250 ml 5% or 10% dextrose in water or normal saline solution and give as an infusion.
Chronic obstructive pulmonary disease: dilute 400 mg in 180 ml of infusion fluid (2 mg/ml).

Rate of administration: Total desired dose of undiluted medication over 1 minute. Infusion rate may start at 5 mg/min, decrease to 1 to 3 mg/min with observance of respiratory response. Use an infusion pump or microdrip (60 gtt/ml) for accuracy.
Chronic obstructive pulmonary disease: specific dose over a 2-hour period. Begin at 1 mg/min. *Do not exceed 3 mg/min.*

Actions: An analeptic CNS stimulant. Affects medullary respiratory center to increase the depth of respiration and slightly increase the rate. Achieves maximum effect in 2 minutes and lasts about 10 to 12 minutes with a single dose. Elevates blood pressure and heart rate. Rapidly metabolized.

Indications and uses: Respiratory stimulation and return of protective reflexes (laryngopharyngeal) postanesthesia, CNS depressant drug overdosage (except muscle relaxant and narcotic overdose), and chronic obstructive pulmonary disease with acute hypercapnia (to prevent CO_2 retention).

Precautions: (1) Maintain an adequate airway at all times. Oxygen and facilities for controlled ventilation must be available. (2) Observe patient continuously and monitor blood pressure, pulse, and deep tendon reflexes during therapy until 1 hour after doxapram is discontinued. (3) Arterial blood gas measurements are desirable to determine effective ventilation. (4) Failure to respond to treatment may indicate CNS source for sustained coma; requires neurological evaluation. (5) Not effective for muscle relaxant–or narcotic-induced respiratory depression. (6) Adjunctive therapy only. Does not inhibit depressant drug metabolism. (7) Stimulates systemic epinephrine increase. (8) Use care in agitation, asthma, cardiac arrhythmias or disease, cerebral edema, gastric surgery, hyperthyroidism, increased intracranial pressure, pheochromocytoma, tachycardia, and ulcers. (9) Potentiated by MAO inhibitors (pargyline [Eutonyl], etc.) and inhalant anesthetics (halothane, cyclopropane, etc.). (10) Confirm patency of vein; vascular extravasation and thrombophlebitis can result from extended usage. (11) In chronic obstructive pulmonary disease, arterial blood gases before administration and every 30 minutes are mandatory; do not use in conjunction with mechanical ventilation. Adjust rate of infusion and oxygen concentration as indicated by arterial blood gases and patient response. Consider increased work of breathing.

Contraindications: Cerebrovascular accidents, children under 12 years, convulsive states of any etiology, coronary artery disease, head injury, hypertension, inadequate ventilation capacity, known hypersensitivity to doxapram, pregnancy, severe pulmonary dysfunction.

Incompatible with: Alkaline drugs, aminophylline, pentobarbital (Nembutal), phenobarbital (Luminal), secobarbital (Seconal), sodium bicarbonate, thiopental (Pentothal).

Side effects: *Minor:* confusion, cough, diaphoresis, dizziness, dyspnea, fever, hiccups, hyperactivity, nausea, salivation, urinary retention or urgency, vomiting, warmth. *Major:* aggravated deep tendon reflexes, bilateral Babinski sign, bronchospasm, convulsions, hypertension, hypotension, laryngospasm, premature ventricular contractions, respiratory alkalosis, skeletal muscle spasm, tachycardia.

Antidote: Notify the physician of any side effect. Depending on severity, physician may elect to continue the drug at a reduced rate of administration or discontinue it. Discontinue doxapram with onset of sudden hypotension or dyspnea. IV diazepam (Valium) or pentobarbital sodium (Nembutal) may be useful in overdose. Resuscitate as necessary.

DOXORUBICIN
HYDROCHLORIDE   pH 3.8 to 6.5

(Adriamycin)

Usual dose: 60 to 75 mg/M^2 of body surface as a single injection every 21 days.
   Alternate dose schedule: 30 mg/M^2 of body surface as a single injection each day for 3 days. Repeat every 4 weeks. Normal liver and kidney function are required.

Pediatric dose: 30 mg/M^2 of body surface as a single injection each day for 3 days. Repeat every 4 weeks.

Dilution: *Specific techniques required, see precautions.* Each 10 mg must be diluted with 5 ml of sodium chloride for injection. An additional 5 ml of diluent for each 10 mg is recommended. Shake to dissolve completely. Do not use bacteriostatic diluent.

Rate of administration: A single dose of properly diluted medication over 3 to 5 minutes. Do not add to IV solutions. Should be given through Y tube or three-way stopcock of a free-flowing infusion of normal saline or 5% dextrose.

Actions: A highly toxic antibiotic antineoplastic agent that is cell cycle specific for the S phase. Rapidly cleared from plasma, it interferes with cell division by binding with DNA to slow production of RNA. Tissue levels remain constant for 7 to 10 days. Slowly excreted in bile and urine.

Indications and uses: To suppress or retard neoplastic growth. Regression has been produced in soft tissue, osteogenic, and other sarcomas; Hodgkin's disease; non Hodgkin's lymphomas; acute leukemias; breast, genitourinary, thyroid, lung, and stomach carcinoma; neuroblastoma; and many other carcinomas.

Precautions: (1) Follow guidelines for handling cytotoxic agents recommended by the National Study Commission on Cytotoxic Exposure (see Appendix, p. 528). (2) Usually administered in hospital by or under the direction of the physician specialist. (3) Determine absolute patency of vein; a stinging or burning sensation indicates extravasation; severe cellulitis and tissue necrosis will result. Discontinue injection, use another vein. (4) Diluted solution is stable 24 hours at room temperature, 48 hours if refrigerated; then discard. (5) Protect from sunlight. (6) Urine will be reddish in color for several days (from dye, not hematuria). (7) Monitoring of white blood cells, red blood cells, platelet count, uric acid levels, liver function, kidney function, EKG, chest x-ray, and echocardiogram is necessary before and during therapy. (8) Wash thoroughly if powder or solution contacts skin or mucosa. (9) Used with other antineoplastic drugs to achieve tumor remission. (10) Will produce teratogenic effects on the fetus. Toxic to embryo with mutagenic potential. Give with caution in men and women capable of conception. (11) Many drug interactions are possible; observe patient closely. (12) Do not administer any vaccines or chloroquine to patients receiving antineoplastic drugs. (13) Increased toxicity including skin redness and exfoliative changes is possible when given concurrent with or after radiation. (14) Maintain adequate hydration. (15) Allopurinol may prevent formation of uric acid crystals. (16) Be alert for signs of bone marrow depression, bleeding, or infection.

Contraindications: Myelosuppression resulting from treatment with other antineoplastic agents, impaired cardiac function, or previous treatment with complete cumulative doses of doxorubicin and/or daunorubicin.

Incompatible with: Aminophylline, cephalothin (Keflin), dexamethasone, diazepam (Valium), fluorouracil, heparin, hydrocortisone sodium succinate, and methotrexate. Should be considered incompatible with any other drug due to toxicity and specific use.

Side effects: Acute cardiac failure, alopecia (complete), bone marrow depression, diarrhea, esophagitis, gonadal suppression, hyperpigmentation of nail beds and dermal creases, hyperuricemia, nausea, stomatitis, vomiting.

Antidote: Most side effects will either be tolerated or treated symptomatically. Keep the physician informed. Hematopoietic toxicity may require cessation of therapy. Acute cardiac failure occurs suddenly (most common when total cumulative dosage approaches 500 mg/M^2) and frequently does not respond to currently available treatment. There is no specific antidote. Supportive therapy as indicated will help sustain the patient in toxicity. For extravasation inject long-acting dexamethasone (Decadron-LA) or hyaluronidase (Wydase) throughout extravasated tissue. Use a 27- or 25-gauge needle. Apply heat.

DOXYCYCLINE HYCLATE   pH 2.8 to 4.0

(Vibramycin)

Usual dose: Adults and children over 45 kg: 200 mg the first day in one or two infusions followed by 100 to 200 mg/24 hr on subsequent days, depending on severity of the infection.

Pediatric dose: Children under 45 kg (but over 8 years): 4.4 mg/kg of body weight/24 hr in two equally divided doses. Follow with 2.2 mg/kg of body weight/24 hr given once daily or in two equally divided doses on subsequent days.

Dilution: Each 100 mg or fraction thereof is diluted with 10 ml of sterile water or normal saline for injection. Further dilute with 100 to 1,000 ml of a compatible infusion solution such as sodium chloride, 5% dextrose injection, Ringer's injection, 10% invert sugar in water, or lactated Ringer's injection with or without 5% dextrose.

Rate of administration: Each 100 mg or fraction thereof, properly diluted, over a minimum of 1 to 4 hours. 100 mg diluted in 100 ml equals 1 mg/ml and must be given over a minimum of 2 hours. 100 mg diluted in 200 ml equals 500 µg/ml and can be given in 1 hour if absolutely necessary. Infusion must be completed in 6 hours when diluted in Ringer's lactate injection with or without dextrose 5% and in 12 hours when diluted in other compatible solutions.

Actions: A broad-sprectrum antibiotic that is bacteriostatic against many gram-positive and gram-negative organisms. Thought to interfere with the protein synthesis of microorganisms. Well distributed in most body tissues and often bound to plasma protein, tetracyclines are concentrated in the liver and excreted through the bile to urine and feces in a biologically active state. Crosses the placental barrier. Excreted in breast milk.

Indications and uses: (1) Infections caused by susceptible strains or organisms, such as rickettsiae, spirochetal agents, viruses, and many other gram-negative and gram-positve bacteria; (2) to substitute for contraindicated penicillin or sulfonamide therapy; (3) drug of choice when a tetracycline is indicated for treatment of an extrarenal infection in patients with renal impairment.

Precautions: (1) Initiate oral therapy as soon as possible. (2) Check expiration date. Outdated ampoules may cause nephrotoxicity. (3) Must be stored away from heat and light; protect from direct sunlight during infusion. (4) Buffered with ascorbic acid. (5) After reconstitution, must be stored at 2° to 8° C (36° to 46° F) and used within 72 hours. (6) Sensitivity studies are indicated to determine the susceptibility of the causative organism to doxycycline. (7) Avoid prolonged use of drug; superinfection caused by overgrowth of nonsusceptible organisms may result. (8) Use caution in impaired liver function, pregnancy, postpartum women, and lactation. Doxycycline serum concentrations and liver function tests are indicated. (9) May cause skeletal retardation in the fetus and infants and permanent tooth discoloration in children under 8 years, including in utero or through mother's milk. (10) Inhibits bactericidal action of penicillin, ampicillin, oxacillin, methicillin, etc. May be toxic with sulfonamides. (11) May potentiate digoxin and anticoagulants; reduced dosage of these drugs may be necessary. (12) Potentiated by alcohol and hepatotoxic drugs; severe liver damage may result. (13) Inhibited by alkalinizing agents, barbiturates, calcium, iron, and magnesium salts, cimetidine (Tagamet), hydantoins (phenytoin, etc.), riboflavin, sodium bicarbonate, and others. (14) Alert patient to photosensitive skin reaction. (15) Determine patency of vein; avoid extravasation. (16) Organisms resistant to one tetracycline are usually resistant to others.

Contraindications: Known hypersensitivity to tetracyclines. Not recommended in children under 8 years.

Incompatible with: Adequate research not completed. Cephalothin. 5% dextrose in lactated Ringer's and lactated Ringer's injection may present compatibility problems with some drugs. Administer separately.

Side effects: Relatively nontoxic in average doses. More toxic in large doses or if given too rapidly. *Minor:* anogenital lesions, anorexia, blood dyscrasias, diarrhea, dysphagia, enterocolitis, nausea, skin rashes, vomiting. *Major:* hypersensitivity reactions including anaphylaxis; liver damage; photosensitivity; systemic moniliasis; thrombophlebitis.

Antidote: Notify the physician of all side effects. If minor side effects are progressive or any major side effect occurs, discontinue the drug, treat allergic reaction, or resuscitate, as necessary.

DROPERIDOL

(Inapsine)

Usual dose: *Antiemetic:* 0.5 mg every 4 hours. May increase dose if required.

    Premedication: 2.5 to 10 mg 30 to 60 minutes preoperatively.

    Induction of anesthesia: 2.5 mg/10 to 12 kg of body weight.

    Maintenance of anesthesia: 1.25 to 2.5 mg as indicated.

Pediatric dose: Children 2 to 12 years: 1 to 1.5 mg/10 to 12 kg of body weight. Decrease dose to avoid excessive CNS depression when the patient is under the effects of another CNS depressant.

Dilution: Given undiluted. Do not mix with infusion fluids. Give through Y tube or three-way stopcock of infusion set.

Rate of administration: 10 mg or fraction thereof over 1 minute. Titrate by desired patient response.

Actions: An antianxiety agent that produces marked tranquilization and sedation. Has an antiemetic action also. It is an alpha adrenergic blocker and produces peripheral vascular dilation. May decrease an abnormally high pulmonary arterial pressure. Effective in 3 to 10 minutes with maximum results in 30 minutes. Lasts 2 to 4 hours. Some effects persist for 12 hours.

Indications and uses: (1) Preoperative sedation, (2) induction and maintenance of anesthesia, regional or general. Frequently given concurrently with narcotic analgesics such as fentanyl (Sublimaze). (3) Antiemetic, frequently recommended for cisplatin chemotherapy.

Precautions: (1) Primarily used by or under direct observation of the anesthesiologist. (2) A potent drug. Monitor the patient closely. Resuscitation equipment, a narcotic antagonist (if a narcotic has been used concurrently), IV infusion line, and drugs to manage hypotension must be readily available. (3) Reduce dose of narcotics and all CNS depressants to one fourth or one third of usual dose before, during, and for 24 hours after injection of droperidol. (4) If other CNS depressants (narcotics, etc.) have been given, reduce dose of droperidol. (5) Reduce dose for elderly, debilitated, poor-risk patients, impaired kidney or liver function. (6) Use caution with known Parkinson's disease. (7) Orthostatic hypotension is common; move and position patients with care. (8) EEG patterns may be slow in returning to normal postoperatively.

Contraindications: Known hypersensitivity to droperidol, children under 2 years, pregnancy.

Incompatible with: Barbiturates, epinephrine.

Side effects: *Minor:* abnormal EEG, chills, dizziness, hallucinations, hypotension, restlessness, shivering, tachycardia. *Major:* apnea, extrapyramidal symptoms, hypotension (severe), respiratory depression.

Antidote: Notify the physician of any side effect. Minor side effects will probably be transient; for major side effects discontinue the drug, treat symptomatically, and notify the physician. Treat hypotension with fluid therapy (rule out hypovolemia) and vasopressors such as dopamine hydrochloride (Intropin) or levarterenol (Levophed). Epinephrine is contraindicated for hypotension. Further hypotension will occur. Treat extrapyramidal symptoms with benztropine mesylate (Cogentin) or diphenhydramine hydrochloride (Benadryl). Resuscitate as necessary.

EDROPHONIUM CHLORIDE   pH 5.4

(Tensilon)

Usual dose: 1 to 10 mg (0.1 to 1 ml) at specified intervals depending on usage. Maximum dose should never exceed 40 mg (four doses of 10 mg each).

Myasthenia gravis diagnosis: 10 mg (1 ml) in tuberculin syringe. Give 2 mg (0.2 ml). If no reaction occurs in 45 seconds, give remaining 8 mg (0.8 ml). Test may be repeated after 30 minutes.

Myasthenia treatment evaluation: 1 to 2 mg (0.1 to 0.2 ml) 1 hour after oral intake of drug being used for treatment.

Myasthenia crisis evaluation: 2 mg (0.2 ml) in tuberculin syringe. Give 1 mg (0.1 ml). If the patient's condition does not deteriorate, give 1 mg (0.1 ml) after 60 seconds. Improvement in cardiac status and respiration should occur.

Curare antagonist: 10 mg (1 ml). May be repeated as necessary up to four doses.

Antiarrhythmic: 5 to 10 mg. Repeat once in 10 minutes if necessary.

Pediatric dose: *Myasthenis gravis diagnosis:* 1 mg for children under 34 kg; if no response in 30 to 45 seconds give 1 mg every 30 to 45 seconds up to 5 mg. Over 34 kg, give 2 mg; if no response in 30 to 45 seconds give 1 mg every 30 to 45 seconds up to 10 mg.

Antiarrhythmic: 2 mg administered slowly.

Dilution: May be given undiluted. In the treatment of myasthenia crisis, this drug may be given as a continuous IV drip. Use an infusion pump or microdrop (60 gtt/ml).

Rate of administration: 2 mg (0.2 ml) or fraction thereof over 15 to 30 seconds. As a curare antagonist give a single dose over 30 to 45 seconds.

Actions: An anticholinesterase and antagonist of skeletal muscle relaxants. Inhibits the enzyme cholinesterase, allowing acetylcholine to accumulate at the myoneural junction. Restores normal transmission of nerve impulses. Acts within 30 to 60 seconds and has an extremely short duration of action, seldom exceeding 10 minutes. Produces vagal stimulation, shortens re-

197

fractory period of atrial muscle, and slows conduction through the AV node.

Indications and uses: (1) Diagnosis of myasthenia gravis; (2) evaluation of adequate treatment of myasthenia gravis; (3) treatment of myasthenia crisis; (4) an antagonist to curare, tubocurarine, gallamine triethiodide (Flaxedil), and dimethyl tubocurarine; (5) termination of supraventricular tachycardia.

Precautions: (1) Atropine 1 mg must be available and ready for injection at all times. (2) A physician should be present when this drug is used. (3) Anticholinesterase insensitivity may develop; withhold drugs and support respirations as necessary. (4) Use caution in patients with bronchial asthma, cardiac arrhythmias, or myasthenia gravis treated with anticholinesterase drugs. (5) Potentiated by colistimethate (Coly-Mycin M). (6) Antagonizes neuromuscular blocking effects of dihydrostreptomycin, kanamycin (Kantrex), neomycin, and streptomycin. Prolongs muscle relaxant effect of succinylcholine chloride (Anectine). (7) May cause bradycardia with digitalis glycosides. (8) Continuously observe patient reactions.

Contraindications: Apnea, known hypersensitivity to anticholinesterase agents, mechanical intestinal and urinary obstructions, patients taking mecamylamine, pregnancy.

Incompatible with: An extremely specific drug. Should be considered incompatible in syringe or solution with any other drug.

Side effects: Abdominal cramps, anorexia, anxiety, bradycardia, bronchiolar spasm, cardiac arrhythmias and arrest, cold moist skin, contraction of the pupils, convulsions, diarrhea, dysphagia, fainting, increased lacrimation, increased pulmonary secretion, increased salivation, insomnia, irritability, laryngospasm, muscle weakness, nausea, perspiration, ptosis, respiratory arrest (either muscular or central), urinary frequency and incontinence, vomiting.

Antidote: If side effects occur, discontinue the drug and notify the physician. Atropine sulfate in doses of 0.4 to 0.5 mg IV will counteract most side effects and may be repeated every 3 to 10 minutes. Pralidoxime chloride 50 to 100 mg/min to 1 Gm may be used as a cholinesterase reactivator with extreme caution. Endotracheal intubation or tracheostomy is considered prophylactic in anesthesia or crises. Artificial ventilation, O_2 therapy, cardiac monitoring, adequate suctioning, and treatment of shock or convulsions must be instituted and maintained as necessary.

Usual dose: 25 to 50 mg, may be repeated every 3 to 4 hours. 150 mg/24 hr is the maximum total dose. Smaller doses, 5 to 25 mg, are encouraged for IV use.

Pediatric dose: Rarely used IV in children, but the dose is 3 mg/kg of body weight/24 hr divided into 4 to 6 hour doses.

Dilution: May be given undiluted. Not usually added to IV solutions. May be injected through Y tube or three-way stopcock of infusion set.

Rate of administration: Each 10 mg or fraction thereof over 1 minute.

Actions: An alkaloid sympathomimetic drug, a CNS stimulant; it is less potent but longer acting than epinephrine. It has positive inotropic action, increasing the strength of myocardial contraction. It increases the heart rate and elevates the blood pressure. Some arteriolar vasoconstriction occurs. Relaxes the smooth muscle of the bronchi and dilates the pupils. Metabolic rate and respiratory rate are increased. Widely distributed in body fluids, ephedrine crosses the blood-brain barrier. It is excreted in urine.

Indications and uses: (1) Pressor agent during spinal anesthesia, (2) Stokes-Adams syndrome, (3) allergic disorders (epinephrine is preferred), (4) narcotic, barbiturate, and alcoholic poisoning.

Precautions: (1) Check blood pressure every 5 minutes. (2) Note label; only specific solutions can be given IV. (3) Use caution in heart disease, angina, diabetes, hyperthyroidism, and prostatic hypertrophy. (4) Has a cumulative effect. (5) Hypertensive crisis may occur in conjunction with MAO inhibitors (e.g., pargyline [Eutonyl], etc.). (6) May cause cardiac arrhythmias with digitalis. (7) May cause severe hypertension with ergonovine or oxytocin, hypotension and bradycardia with hydantoins (phenytoin [Dilantin], etc.). (8) Interacts with many other drugs. (9) Tolerance may develop, but effectiveness is usually restored if the drug is discontinued temporarily. (10) Potentiated by tricyclic antidepressants and urinary alkalinizers.

Contraindications: Known hypersensitivity to ephedrine, labor and delivery if maternal blood pressure exceeds 130/80 mmHg. Do not use to treat overdosage of phenothiazines (chlorpromazine [Thorazine], etc.). A further drop in blood pressure and irreversible shock may result.

Incompatible with: Alkaline solutions, hydrocortisone (Solu-Cortef), pentobarbital (Nembutal), phenobarbital (Luminal), secobarbital (Seconal), thiopental (Pentothal).

Side effects: Rare in therapeutic doses: anorexia, cardiac arrhythmias, headache, insomnia, nausea, nervousness, painful urination, palpitations, precordial pain, sweating, tachycardia, urinary retention, vertigo, vomiting. Confusion, delirium, euphoria, and hallucinations may occur with higher doses.

Antidote: If side effects occur, discontinue the drug and notify the physician. Side effects may be treated symptomatically. Resuscitate as necessary.

EPINEPHRINE HYDROCHLORIDE

(Adrenalin chloride)

Usual dose: 0.2 to 0.5 mg of 1:10,000 solution. May be repeated as necessary.

Cardiac arrest: 0.5 to 1.0 mg of 1:10,000 solution IV; may repeat every 5 minutes. 0.5 mg of 1:10,000 solution intracardiac.

Maintenance dose: 1 to 8 µg/min.

Pediatric dose: *Cardiac arrest:* 5 to 10 µg/kg of body weight of 1:10,000 solution by IV or intracardiac administration.

Dilution: Each 1 mg (1 ml) of 1:1,000 solution must be diluted in at least 10 ml of normal saline for injection to prepare a 1:10,000 solution. For maintenance may be further diluted in 500 ml of 5% dextrose plus water. Give through Y tube or three-way stopcock of infusion set.

Rate of administration: Each 1 mg or fraction thereof over 1 minute or longer. May be given more rapidly in cardiac resuscitation.

Actions: A naturally occurring hormone secreted by the adrenal glands. A sympathomimetic drug, it imitates almost all actions of the sympathetic nervous system. It is a vasoconstrictor and delays the absorption of many drugs; a potent cardiac stimulant, it strengthens myocardial contraction (positive inotropic effect) and increases cardiac rate (positive chronotropic effect). A potent dilator or relaxant of smooth muscle, especially bronchial muscle. Decreases blood supply to the abdomen and increases blood supply to skeletal muscles. Elevates systolic blood pressure, lowers diastolic pressure, and increases pulse pressure. It is seldom used as a vasopressor because of its short duration of action. It is rapidly inactivated in the body by various enzymes and excreted in changed form in the urine.

Indications and uses: (1) Drug of choice for anaphylactic shock; (2) antidote of choice for histamine overdose and allergic reactions including bronchial asthma, urticaria, and angioneurotic edema; (3) cardiac resuscitation; (4) Stokes-Adams syndrome.

Precautions: (1) Usual route of choice is subcutaneous or IM. (2) Effects are instantaneous IV. Start with a small dose, giving only as much of the drug as required to alleviate undesirable symptoms, and repeat as necessary, gradually increasing the dose depending on the need. Check blood pressure every 5 minutes. (3) Deteriorates rapidly. Protect from light. Do not use if brown in color or if a sediment is present. (4) Check the label. Not all epinephrine solutions can be given IV. (5) Intracardiac injection or IV injection in cardiac arrest must be accompanied by cardiac massage to perfuse drug into the myocardium and permit effective defibrillation. (6) Use caution in elderly people, diabetic patients, hypotension (except in anaphylactic shock), patients receiving thyroid preparations, and those with long-term emphysema or bronchial asthma. (7) May be used alternately with isoproterenol (Isuprel), *but they may not be used together.* Both are direct cardiac stimulants and death will result. An adequate interval between doses must be maintained. (8) Simultaneous use with oxytocics or MAO inhibitors (pargyline [Eutonyl], etc.) may cause hypertensive crisis, with propranolol (Inderal) will cause hypertension. (9) Interacts with many other drugs, such as insulin, ergonovine, methylphenidate (Ritalin), tricyclic antidepressants, antihistamines, etc. (10) Often used with corticosteroids in treatment of anaphylactic shock.

Contraindications: Anesthesia with inhalant anesthetics (chloroform, trichloroethylene, cyclopropane, etc.), cerebral arteriosclerosis, during labor, hypertension, hyperthyroidism, narrow angle glaucoma, nervous instability, organic brain damage, patients receiving digitalis, shock. Do not use to treat overdosage of adrenergic blocking agents (phenoxybenzamine [Dibenzyline], etc.), phenothiazines (chlorpromazine [Thorazine], etc.), methotrimeprazine (Levoprome); a further drop in blood pressure will occur and irreversible shock may result.

Incompatible with: Any other drug in a syringe. Readily

destroyed by alkalies, alkaline solutions, and oxidizing agents. Unstable in any solution with a pH over 5.5, mephentermine (Wyamine), warfarin (Coumadin).

Side effects: Often transitory and sometimes occur with average doses. *Average dose:* anxiety, dizziness, dyspnea, glycosuria, pallor, palpitations. *Overdose* (frequently caused by too-rapid injection): cerebrovascular hemorrhage, collapse (rapid), fibrillation, headache (severe), hypertension, hypotension (irreversible), pulmonary edema, pupillary dilation, restlessness, tachycardia, weakness, death.

Antidote: If side effects from the average dose become progressively worse, discontinue the drug and notify the physician. IM or subcutaneous route may be preferable. For a severe reaction caused by toxicity, treat the patient for shock and administer neostigmine (Prostigmin) or an antihypertensive agent such as phentolamine (Regitine) or nitroprusside (Nipride). Treat cardiac arrhythmias with a beta adrenergic blocker (propranolol [Inderal]).

(Ergotrate maleate)

Usual dose: 1 ml (0.2 mg or gr ⅟₃₀₀). Repeat in 2 to 4 hours if necessary.

Dilution: May be given undiluted. Do not add to IV solutions. Give through Y tube or three-way stopcock of infusion set.

Rate of administration: 0.2 mg or fraction thereof over 1 minute.

Actions: An oxytocic, it exerts a direct stimulation on the smooth muscle of the uterus, causing contraction of the uterus itself and vasoconstriction of uterine vessels. In therapeutic doses the prolonged initial contraction is followed by periods of relaxation and contraction. Effective within 1 minute for up to 3 hours. The least toxic of the ergot derivatives, it is probably detoxified in the liver and excreted in bile and urine.

Indications and uses: Prevents or controls postpartum or postabortal hemorrhage.

Precautions: (1) Not recommended for use prior to the delivery of the placenta. (2) IV administration is for emergency use only. IM or oral route is preferred and should be used after the initial IV dose. (3) Monitor blood pressure. (4) Uterine response may be poor in calcium-deficient patients, will require calcium replacement for effective response. (5) Should be refrigerated; may not be stored at room temperature more than 60 days. (6) Check expiration date on vial. Ergonovine deteriorates with age. (7) Severe hypertension and cerebrovascular accidents can result in the presence of regional anesthesia (caudal or spinal) and with ephedrine, epinephrine, methoxamine (Vasoxyl), and other vasopressors. Chlorpromazine (Thorazine) IV will reduce this hypertension. (8) Use caution in patients with cardiac, renal, or liver disease and in febrile or septic states, (9) Potentiated by nitrates.

Contraindications: Known hypersensitivity to ergot alkaloids and pregnancy prior to the third stage of labor.

Incompatible with: Amobarbital (Amytal), ampicillin (Polycillin), cephalothin (Keflin), chloramphenicol (Chloromycetin), chlortetracycline (Aureomycin), epi-

205

nephrine (Adrenalin), heparin, methicillin (Staph-cillin), nitrofurantoin (Ivadantin), pentobarbital (Nem-butal), sulfadiazine, sulfisoxazole, thiopental (Pento-thal), warfarin (Coumadin).

Side effects: Rare in therapeutic doses, but may include the following: *Average dose:* allergic phenomena, blindness, confusion, diarrhea, dilated pupils, dizzi-ness, headache, hypertension, hypotension, nausea, numb and/or cold extremities, vomiting, weakness. *Overdose:* abortion, convulsions, excitement, gan-grene, hypercoagulability, shock, tachycardia, thirst, tremor, uterine bleeding.

Antidote: Discontinue the drug immediately at the onset of any side effect and notify the physician. Most side effects are transient unless there is severe toxicity and will be treated symptomatically. Severe poisoning is treated with vasodilator drugs, sedatives, calcium gluconate to relieve muscular pain, and other sup-portive treatment. Heparin is used to control hyper-coagulability.

ERYTHROMYCIN LACTOBIONATE: ERYTHROMYCIN GLUCEPTATE

pH 6.5 to 7.5

(Erythrocin; Ilotycin)

Usual dose: 15 to 20 mg/kg of body weight/24 hr in divided doses every 6 hours or preferably in a continuous infusion. Up to 4 Gm/24 hr has been given.

Pediatric dose: 10 to 20 mg/kg of body weight/24 hr in divided doses every 6 hours is recommended.

Dilution: Each 500 mg or fraction thereof must be diluted with 10 ml of sterile water for injection without preservatives to form a 5% solution and avoid precipitation. To administer direct IV, further dilute in at least 80 ml of a compatible IV fluid (normal saline, lactated Ringer's, or Normosol-R). Most often further diluted to 1 mg/ml in above infusion solutions or dextrose in water or saline and given as a continuous infusion.

Rate of administration: 1 Gm or fraction thereof in at least 100 ml over 20 to 60 minutes. Slow infusion rate for pain along injection site. IV infusion of a 0.1% to 0.2% solution by continuous drip over 6 hours is preferable.

Actions: Bacteriostatic antibiotic used as a substitute for penicillin. Effective against a number of gram-positive and some gram-negative organisms. Very effective against penicillin-resistant staphylococci. Well distributed in body fluids, except for spinal fluid. Excreted in urine and bile. Crosses placental barrier. Excreted in breast milk.

Indications and uses: (1) Staphylococci, pneumococci, and streptococci infections, (2) prophylaxis against endocarditis preoperatively in patients with a history of rheumatic fever or congenital heart disease, (3) gonorrhea, (4) syphilis in penicillin-sensitive patients, (5) active diphtheria in conjunction with antitoxin, (6) Legionnaire's disease.

Precautions: (1) Sensitivity studies are indicated to determine the susceptibility of the causative organism to erythromycin. (2) Begin oral therapy as soon as

207

practical. (3) Superinfection caused by overgrowth of nonsusceptible organisms is rare unless this drug is given in combination with other antibacterial agents. (4) Not stable if final pH is less than 5.5. Give within 4 hours or use 1 ml of sodium bicarbonate (Neut) to 100 ml of solution to stabilize. (5) Use caution in impaired liver function, pregnancy, and lactation. (6) Refrigerate after dilution. Maintains potency for up to 7 days. (7) Antagonized by clindamycin and lincomycin. (8) Inhibits penicillins. (9) Will increase serum levels of digoxin and theophyllines.

Contraindications: Known erythromycin sensitivity.

Incompatible with: Do not add any drug to solution unless effects on chemical and physical stability are determined. Amikacin (Amikin), aminophylline, ascorbic acid, carbenicillin (Geopen), cephalothin (Keflin), cephapirin (Cefadyl), chloramphenicol (Chloromycetin), colistimethate (Coly-Mycin M), heparin, lincomycin (Lincocin), metaraminol (Aramine), oxytetracycline (Terramycin), pentobarbital (Nembutal), phenobarbital (Luminal), phenytoin (Dilantin), prochlorperazine (Compazine), secobarbital (Seconal), sodium chloride solutions until after initial dilution, sodium salts, tetracycline (Achromycin), thiopental (Pentothal), vancomycin (Vancocin), vitamin B complex with C, warfarin (Coumadin).

Side effects: Relatively free from side effects when given as directed. Urticaria and mild local venous discomfort. Increased incidence of reversible ototoxicity with larger doses. Anaphylaxis may occur.

Antidote: Notify the physician of early or mild symptoms. For severe symptoms, discontinue the drug, treat allergic reactions, or resuscitate as necessary and notify physician.

(Sodium Edecrin)

Usual dose: 0.5 to 1 mg/kg of body weight. 50 mg for average adult. Do not exceed 100 mg in a single dose.

Dilution: Add 50 ml of sodium chloride injection to reconstitute; 5% dextrose may be used if pH adjusted upward. Do not add to IV solutions. May be injected through Y tube or three-way stopcock of infusion set.

Rate of administration: Each 10 mg or fraction thereof (approximately 10 ml) may be given over 1 minute. Infusion of total dose over 30 minutes is preferred.

Actions: A saluretic-diuretic agent. Extremely potent and has a rapid onset of action. Effectiveness is noted within 5 to 10 minutes; peak effect noted in 1 to 2 hours after administration and may last for 8 hours. Has a mild hypotensive effect. Apparently acts on the proximal and distal ends of the tubule and the ascending limb of the loop of Henle to excrete sodium, chlorides, and potassium. Will produce diuresis in alkalosis or acidosis. Rapidly absorbed and distributed, it is excreted in the urine.

Indications and uses: (1) Congestive heart failure, (2) acute pulmonary edema, (3) renal edema, (4) hepatic cirrhosis with ascites, (5) nephrotic syndrome in children, (6) edema unresponsive to other diuretic agents, (7) ascites due to malignancy, (8) short-term management of hospitalized pediatric patients with congenital heart disease.

Precautions: (1) For IV use only. (2) Use a new injection site for each dose to avoid thrombophlebitis. (3) May precipitate excessive diuresis with water and electrolyte depletion. (4) Routine checks on electrolyte panel, CO_2, and BUN are necessary during therapy. Potassium chloride replacement may be required. (5) Do not give simultaneously with whole blood or its derivatives. (6) Discard reconstituted solution after 24 hours. (7) Use caution in patients with advanced cirrhosis of the liver, electrolyte imbalance, or hepatic encephalopathy. (8) May precipitate an acute attack of gout. (9) Has caused permanent deafness when given in conjunction with other ototoxic drugs (dihydrostreptomycin, gentamicin, etc.). (10) Potentiates antihypertensive drugs, oral antidiabetics, oral anticoagulants, and some muscle relaxants (curare, tubocurarine, etc.). (11) May cause cardiac arrhythmias with digitalis or furosemide (Lasix). (12) Not recommended for use in children except for specialized indications.

Contraindications: Anuria; infants; pregnancy and lactation; severe, progressive renal disease with increasing azotemia and oliguria; severe watery diarrhea; women during childbearing years.

Incompatible with: Any other drug in a syringe, whole blood and its derivatives, drugs and solutions with pH below 5.0, Normosol-M.

Side effects: Usually occur with prolonged therapy or in seriously ill patients. *Minor:* anorexia, deafness (transient), dysphagia, hyperglycemia, hyperuricemia, hypochloremic alkalosis, hypokalemia, muscle cramps, nausea, thirst, vomiting, weakness. *Major:* blood volume reduction, circulatory collapse, deafness (permanent), dehydration, diarrhea (watery), embolism, hypokalemia (severe), vascular thrombosis, death.

Antidote: If minor side effects are noted, discontinue the drug and notify the physician, who may treat the side effects symptomatically and continue the drug. If side effects are progressive or any major side effect occurs, discontinue the drug immediately and notify the physician. Treatment of major side effects is symptomatic and aggressive. Resuscitate as necessary.

FACTOR IX COMPLEX (HUMAN)   pH 7.0 to 7.4

(Konyne, Profilnine, Proplex, Proplex SX)

Usual dose: Completely individualized, depending on specific factor deprivation (II, VII, IX, X), appropriate and ongoing coagulation assays, and patient's condition.

Dilution: Use a minimum of 1 ml of sterile water for injection to dilute each 50 units (50 units/ml). This is a maximum concentration for administration, and a more dilute solution is preferred (2 ml of sterile water for injection to dilute each 50 units [25 units/ml]). pH is 7.0 to 7.4 diluted with 20 ml of sterile water. Diluent is usually provided.

Rate of administration: Completely individualized according to patient's condition. Decrease rate of administration for side effects such as chills, fever, flushing, headache, or tingling. Never exceed 10 ml/minute.

Actions: A lyophilized concentrate of human coagulation factors: IX (plasma thromboplastin and antihemophilic factor B, 400 to 625 units), II (prothrombin, 300 to 600 units), VII (proconvertin, 250 units), and X (Stuart-Prower factor, 250 units). Obtained from fresh human plasma and prepared, irradiated, and dried by a specific process. Concentration of 25 units/1 ml is 25 times greater than normal plasma. Also contains 500 mg of total protein in each vial.

Indications and uses: Elevation of demonstrated deficiency of one or more specific coagulation factors (IX, II, VII, X), especially in hemophilia B (Christmas disease). May be required to correct or prevent a dangerous bleeding episode or to perform surgery. Proplex may be used for bleeding episodes in patients who have inhibitors to factor VIII.

Precautions: (1) Used only when plasma infusions would result in hypervolemia and/or proteinemia or when blood volume or red blood cell replacement is not indicated. (2) Store lyophilized powder at 2° to 8° C (36° to 46° F); do not freeze. (3) Note expiration date. (4) Stable for 12 hours after reconstitution, but administer promptly with aseptic technique to avoid bacterial contamination. (5) Monitor the patient's levels of all four coagulation factors before, between, and after administrations. *Do not overdose.* (6) Use extreme caution in newborns, infants, and patients with liver disease; hepatitis is possible. May be a necessary risk. (7) Observe for signs and symptoms of postoperative thrombosis or disseminated intravascular coagulation.

Contraindications: Known liver disease with suspicion of intravascular coagulation or fibrinolysis.

Incompatible with: All protein precipitants. Sufficient information not available.

Side effects: *Minor:* chills, fever, flushing, headache, tingling. *Major:* anaphylaxis, disseminated intravascular coagulation, hepatitis, postoperative thrombosis.

Antidote: Decrease rate of administration for minor side effects. If any major symptoms appear, discontinue drug and notify physician. Treat allergic reactions as indicated. For thrombosis or disseminated intravascular coagulation, anticoagulation with heparin may be indicated.

5-FLUOROURACIL

(Adrucil, 5 FU Fluorouracil)

Usual dose: 12 to 15 mg/kg of body weight/24 hr for 4 days. Total dose should not exceed 800 mg/24 hr. If no toxicity is observed, one-half dose (6 to 7.5 mg/kg) is given on the even days for four doses. No medication is given on the odd days following the initial four doses. Dosage regime is reduced by one half or more throughout a course of therapy for poor-risk patients or those in a poor nutritional state. The most common form of maintenance therapy is to repeat the entire course of therapy beginning 30 days after the previous course is completed or 10 to 15 mg/kg/week; not to exceed 1 Gm. Adjustments are made depending on side effects and tolerance.

Dilution: *Specific techniques required, see precautions.* May be given undiluted. Do not add to IV solutions. May inject through Y tube or three-way stopcock of a free-flowing infusion.

Rate of administration: A single dose over 1 to 3 minutes.

Actions: An antimetabolite. A fluorinated pyrimidine antagonist, cell cycle phase nonspecific, that interferes with the synthesis of DNA and RNA. Through various chemical processes this deprivation acts more quickly on rapidly growing cells and causes their death. Complete metabolism occurs within 3 hours. Excretion is through the urine and as respiratory CO_2.

Indications and uses: To suppress or retard neoplastic growth considered incurable by surgery or other means. Response has been experienced in carcinoma of the colon, rectum, breast, ovary, head and neck, urinary bladder, stomach, and pancreas, either alone or in combination with other drugs.

Precautions: (1) Follow guidelines for handling cytotoxic agents recommended by the National Study Commission on Cytotoxic Exposure (see Appendix, p. 528). (2) Usually administered in the hospital by or under the direction of the physician specialist. (3) Confirm patency of vein. Avoid extravasation. (4) Protect from light. May be slightly discolored without affecting safety and potency. (5) Use caution in patients who

213

have had high-dose pelvic irradiation, previous anti-metabolic drugs, metastatic tumor involvement of the bone marrow, and impaired hepatic or renal function. (6) Not to be considered adjunctive to surgical treatment. (7) May produce teratogenic effects on the fetus. Has a mutagenic potential. Give with caution in men and women capable of conception. (8) Often used with other antineoplastic drugs in reduced doses to achieve tumor remission. (9) Dosage based on average weight in presence of edema or ascites. (10) Potentiates anticoagulants. (11) Be alert for signs of bone marrow depression or infection. (12) Do not administer any vaccines or chloroquine to patients receiving antineoplastic drugs. (13) Prophylactic antiemetics may reduce nausea and vomiting and increase patient comfort. (14) Toxicity is increased by stress, poor nutrition, and bone marrow depression. Obtain a WBC and differential before each dose.

Contraindications: Potentially serious infections; depressed bone marrow function; poor nutritional state.

Incompatible with: Cytarabine (ARA-C), diazepam (Valium), methotrexate (Amethopterin). Give separately.

Side effects: Alopecia (reversible), cerebellar syndrome, dermatitis, diarrhea, dry lips, erythema, esophago-pharyngitis, euphoria, hemorrhage from any site, increased skin pigmentation, leukopenia, mouth soreness and ulceration, nausea, photophobia, stomatitis, thrombocytopenia, vomiting.

Antidote: Discontinue the drug and notify physician of side effects. Death may occur from the progression of most of these side effects. There is no specific antidote; supportive therapy as indicated will help to sustain patient in toxicity.

FOLIC ACID

(Folvite)

Usual dose: 1 mg daily. Up to 5 mg will be used infrequently.

Dilution: May be given direct IV undiluted or added to most IV solutions and given as an infusion.

Rate of administration: 5 mg or fraction thereof over 1 minute in undiluted form.

Actions: Folic acid (pteroylglutamic acid) is part of the vitamin B complex. It can be synthesized by intestinal bacteria. It is an important growth factor for many cells and is involved in the synthesis of amino acids and DNA. Stimulates the production of red blood cells, white blood cells, and platelets. Excreted in urine.

Indications and uses: Macrocytic anemias of malnutrition seen in alcoholism, sprue, steatorrhea, celiac disease, pregnancy, developmental or surgical anomalies of the gastrointestinal tract, and fish tapeworm infestation.

Precautions: (1) Folic acid is not commonly administered by the IV route in adults and *never* in children. Oral or IM administration provides adequate absorption in most cases. (2) Obscures the peripheral blood picture and prevents the diagnosis of pernicious anemia. May actually aggravate the neurological symptoms. (3) Toxic effects of antineoplastic folic acid antagonists are blocked by folinic acid (leucovorin) but not by folic acid IV. (4) Refrigerate and protect from light. (5) Therapeutic dose is higher than actually needed because small doses have not proved effective. (6) Increases hydantoin metabolism (phenytoin [Dilantin], etc.); seizures may result.

Contraindications: IV route contraindicated in children; pernicious anemia unless used in combination with diagnostic testing; liver extracts, etc.; aplastic anemia and iron-deficiency anemia.

Incompatible with: Calcium salts, chlorpromazine hydrochloride (Thorazine), heavy metal ions, iron sulfate, oxidizing agents, reducing agents, vitamin B complex with C.

Side effects: Almost nonexistent. Some slight flushing or feeling of warmth; anaphylaxis can occur.

Antidote: Discontinue drug and notify physician if anaphylaxis occurs. Treat anaphylaxis or resuscitate as necessary.

(Lasix)

Usual dose: 20 to 40 mg. May be repeated in 1 to 2 hours. If necessary, increase dosage by 20 mg increments (under close medical supervision and no sooner than 2 hours after previous dose) until desired diuresis is obtained. Maximum human dose is 600 mg/24 hr. After the initial diuresis the minimum effective dose may be given once or twice every 24 hours as required for maintenance.

Pediatric dose: 1 to 2 mg/kg of body weight; increase by 1 mg/kg increments to effect desired response. Do not exceed 6 mg/kg.

Dilution: May be given undiluted. May be given through Y tube or three-way stopcock of infusion set. Not usually added to IV solutions but large doses may be added to 5% dextrose in water or normal saline and given and an infusion. pH of solution must be over 5.5.

Rate of administration: Each 20 mg or fraction thereof should be given over 1 minute. High dose therapy in an infusion should not exceed a rate of 4 mg/minute.

Actions: A sulfonamide diuretic, antihypertensive, and antihypercalcemic agent related to the thiazides. Extremely potent and has a rapid onset of action. Effectiveness is noted within 5 minutes and may last for 2 hours. Apparently acts on the proximal and distal ends of the tubule and the ascending limb of the loop of Henle to excrete water, sodium, chlorides, and potassium. Will produce diuresis in alkalosis or acidosis. Rapidly absorbed and distributed, it is excreted unchanged in the urine.

Indications and uses: (1) Congestive heart failure, (2) acute pulmonary edema, (3) cirrhosis of the liver with ascites, (4) renal disease including the nephrotic syndrome, (5) edema unresponsive to other diuretic agents, (6) hypercalcemia.

Precautions: (1) May be used concurrently with aldosterone antagonists (spironolactone [Aldactone], etc.) for more effective diuresis and to prevent excessive potassium loss. (2) Discontinue at least 2 days prior to elective surgery. (3) May precipitate excessive diuresis with water and electrolyte depletion. Routine checks on electrolyte panel, CO_2, and BUN are necessary during therapy. Potassium chloride replacement may be required. (4) Use caution and improve basic condition first in hepatic coma, electrolyte depletion, and advanced cirrhosis of the liver. (5) Causes excessive potassium depletion with corticosteroids and spironolactone hydrochlorothiazide (Aldactazide). (6) Potentiates antihypertensive drugs, salicylates, muscle relaxants (curare, tubocurarine, etc.), and hypotensive effect of other diuretics and MAO inhibitors (pargyline [Eutonyl], etc.). (7) May cause transient deafness in doses exceeding the usual or in conjunction with ototoxic drugs (dihydrostreptomycin, gentamicin, etc.). (8) May increase blood glucose and has precipitated diabetes mellitus, lower serum calcium level, causing tetany, and rarely precipitates an acute attack of gout. (9) Inhibits oral anticoagulants and pressor amines. (10) May cause cardiac arrhythmias with digitalis or ethacrynic acid (Edecrin). (11) If diluted in compatible infusion solution (5% dextrose in water, isotonic saline, lactated Ringer's solution), discard after 24 hours. (12) Higher doses may be required in nephrosis or chronic renal failure. Hepatic necrosis may result.

Contraindications: Anuria, severe progressive renal disease with increasing azotemia and oliguria; not used in children, pregnancy and lactation, known sulfonamide sensitivity.

Incompatible with: Acidic solutions, ascorbic acid, corticosteroids, diphenhydramine (Benadryl), epinephrine (Adrenalin), levarterenol (Levophed), meperidine (Demerol), reserpine, spironolactone hydrochlorothiazide (Aldactazide), tetracyclines, any drug in a syringe.

Side effects: Usually occur in prolonged therapy, seriously ill patients, or following large doses. *Minor:* anemia, anorexia, blurring of vision, deafness (reversible), diarrhea, dizziness, hyperglycemia, hyperuricemia, hypokalemia, leg cramps, lethargy, leukopenia, mental confusion, paresthesia, postural hypotension, pruritus, tinnitus, urinary frequency, urticaria, vomiting, weakness. *Major:* anaphylactic shock, blood volume reduction, circulatory collapse, dehydration, excessive diuresis, hypokalemia, metabolic acidosis, vascular thrombosis and embolism.

Antidote: If minor side effects are noted, discontinue the drug and notify the physician, who may treat the side effects symptomatically and continue the drug. If side effects are progressive or any major side effect occurs, discontinue the drug immediately and notify the physician. Treatment of major side effects is symptomatic and aggressive. Resuscitate as necessary.

GALLAMINE TRIETHIODIDE

pH 6.5 to 7.5

(Flaxedil)

Usual dose: Must be individualized, depending on previous drugs administered and degree and length of muscle relaxation required. 0.5 to 1.0 mg/kg of body weight initially. Repeat every 30 to 40 minutes as required.

Dilution: May be given undiluted.

Rate of administration: A single dose over 30 to 60 seconds.

Actions: A skeletal muscle relaxant. Causes paralysis by interfering with neural transmission at the myoneural junction. Onset of action is immediate and lasts about 30 minutes. Duration of action is dose dependent. Has a cumulative action. Excreted in the urine.

Indications and uses: (1) Adjunctive to general anesthesia, (2) management of patients undergoing mechanical ventilation.

Precautions: (1) Administered only by or under the direct observation of the anesthesiologist. (2) This drug produces apnea. Controlled artificial respiration with oxygen must be continuous and under direct observation at all times. Maintain a patent airway. (3) Repeated doses may produce a cumulative effect. (4) Impaired pulmonary function or respiratory deficiencies can cause critical reactions. Use caution in impaired liver or kidney function. (5) Myasthenia gravis increases sensitivity to drug. Reaction may be fatal (see contraindications). (6) Potentiated by inhalant anesthetics (ether, etc.), neuromuscular blocking antibiotics (kanamycin [Kantrex], etc.), carbon dioxide, digitalis, diuretics, diazepam (Valium) and other muscle relaxants, lidocaine, magnesium sulfate, MAO inhibitors, propranolol (Inderal), quinidine, and others. Markedly reduced dose of gallamine must be used with caution. (7) Antagonized by anticholinesterases and potassium ions. Hyperkalemia may cause cardiac arrhythmias. (8) Patient may be conscious and completely unable to communicate by any means. Gallamine has no analgesic properties. Respiratory depression with narcotics may be preferred in some patients requiring mechanical ventilation. (9) Action is altered by dehydration, electrolyte imbalance, body temperature, and acid-base imbalance. (10) Use a peripheral nerve stimulator to monitor response to gallamine and avoid overdosage.

Contraindications: Myasthenia gravis, known hypersensitivity to gallamine or to iodides, impaired renal function or shock, infants under 5 kg; if tachycardia, would increase the severity of an existing condition.

Incompatible with: Considered incompatible in a syringe with any other drug. Evaluation of predictable results is imperative.

Side effects: Prolonged action resulting in respiratory insufficiency or apnea; airway closure caused by relaxation of epiglottis, pharynx, and tongue muscles; tachycardia; anaphylaxis.

Antidote: All side effects are medical emergencies. Treat symptomatically. Controlled artificial ventilation must be continuous. Edrophonium and neostigmine methylsulfate with atropine may help to reverse muscle relaxation. Not effective in all situations. Treat allergic reactions and resuscitate as necessary.

GENTAMICIN SULFATE

(Apogen, Bristagen, Garamycin, Jenamicin)

Usual dose: 3 mg/kg of body weight/24 hr equally divided into three or four doses. Up to 5 mg/kg may be given if indicated. Reduce to usual dose as soon as feasible. Normal renal function is necessary for all recommended doses.

Pediatric dose: 6 to 7.5 mg/kg of body weight/24 hr (2 to 2.5 mg/kg every 8 hours).

Newborn dose: 7.5 mg/kg of body weight/24 hr (2.5 mg/kg every 8 hours).

Dilution: Prepared solutions equal 10 or 40 mg/ml. Further dilute each single dose in 50 to 200 ml of IV normal saline or 5% dextrose in water. Must be diluted to a 0.1% solution (1 mg/ml) or less. Decrease volume of diluent for children, but maintain 0.1% solution. Commercially diluted solutions are available.

Rate of administration: Each single dose, properly diluted, over 30 to 60 minutes; up to 2 hours in children.

Actions: An aminoglycoside antibiotic with neuromuscular blocking action. Bactericidal against specific gram-positive and gram-negative bacilli, including *Escherichia coli*, *Klebsiella*, *Proteus*, and *Pseudomonas*. Not effective for fungal or viral infections. Well distributed throughout all body fluids; serum and urine levels remain adequate for 6 to 12 hours. Crosses the placental barrier. Excreted through the kidneys.

Indications and uses: (1) Treatment of serious infections of the CNS; gastrointestinal, respiratory, and urinary tracts; and skin and soft tissue and septicemia; (2) primarily used when penicillin and other less toxic antibiotics are ineffective or contraindicated; (3) to treat suspected infection in the immunosuppressed patient.

Precautions: (1) Use extreme caution if therapy is required over 7 to 10 days. (2) Sensitivity studies are indicated to determine the susceptibility of the causative organism to gentamicin. (3) Reduce daily dose commensurate with the amount of renal impairment. Intervals between injections should also be increased. (4) Watch for decrease in urine output and rising BUN and serum creatinine. Dosage may require decreasing. Routine serum levels and evaluation of hearing are recommended. (5) Use caution in infants, children, and the elderly. (6) Potentiated by anesthetics, other neuromuscular blocking antibiotics (kanamycin, streptomycin, etc.), anticholinesterases (edrophonium [Tensilon], etc.), antineoplastics (nitrogen mustard, cisplatin, etc.), barbiturates, muscle relaxants (tubocurarine, etc.), phenothiazines (promethazine [Phenergan], etc.), procainamide, quinidine, and sodium citrate. *Apnea can occur.* (7) Also potentiated by other ototoxic drugs (ethacrynic acid [Edecrin], etc.) and all potent diuretics. An elevated serum level of gentamicin may occur, increasing nephrotoxicity and neurotoxicity. (8) Superinfection may occur from overgrowth of nonsusceptible organisms. (9) Maintain good hydration.

Contraindications: Known gentamicin sensitivity, pregnancy, renal failure.

Incompatible with: Inactivated in solution with carbenicillin, other penicillins, and most cephalosporins. Amphotericin B, cefamandole (Mandol), cephalothin (Keflin), dopamine (Intropin), heparin. Administer all drugs separately.

Side effects: Occur more frequently with impaired renal function, higher doses, or prolonged administration. *Minor:* anorexia, burning, dizziness, fever, headache, hypertension, hypotension, itching, lethargy, muscle twitching, nausea, numbness, rash, roaring in ears, tingling sensation, tinnitus, urticaria, vomiting, and weight loss. *Major:* blood dyscrasias; convulsions; elevated bilirubin, BUN, serum creatinine, SGOT, and SGPT; hearing loss; laryngeal edema; and oliguria.

Antidote: Notify the physician of all side effects. If minor side effects persist or any major symptom appears, discontinue the drug and notify the physician. Treatment is symptomatic. Hemodialysis or peritoneal dialysis may be indicated.

GLUCAGON HYDROCHLORIDE   pH 2.5 to 3.0

Usual dose: *Hypoglycemia:* 0.5 to 1 mg. May be repeated in 20 minutes for two doses if indicated. Up to 2 mg has been given as initial dose.
Diagnostic aid: 0.5 mg.

Dilution: Dilute 1 unit (1 mg) of glucagon powder with 1 ml of its own diluting solution. Do not add to IV solutions. May be given through Y tube or three-way stopcock of infusion set if a dextrose solution is infusing.

Rate of administration: 1 unit or fraction thereof over 1 minute.

Actions: A pancreatic extract from the alpha cells of the islets of Langerhans. Blood glucose is raised by activating phosphorylase, which converts glycogen to glucose in the liver. Glucagon acts only on liver glycogen. Produces relaxation of the smooth muscle of the stomach, duodenum, small bowel, and colon.

Indications and uses: (1) Treatment of hypoglycemic reactions during insulin therapy in the management of diabetes mellitus and in induced insulin shock during psychiatric therapy. (2) Induction of a hypotonic state and smooth muscle relaxation in the radiological examination of the stomach, duodenum, small bowel, and colon. (3) Experimental uses: may be helpful in reversing adverse effects of propranolol (Inderal), or may be used to enhance digitalis effects in heart failure.

Precautions: (1) Should awaken the patient in 5 to 20 minutes. Prolonged hypoglycemic reactions may result in severe cortical damage. (2) Emesis on awakening is common. Prevent aspiration by turning the patient face down. (3) Dose may be repeated if necessary. Supplement with IV glucose (50%) to precipitate awakening. Utilize oral sugars after awakening to prevent secondary hypoglycemia. (4) Easily absorbed IM or subcutaneously. (5) Potentiates oral anticoagulants. (6) If glucagon and glucose do not awaken the patient, coma is probably caused by a condition other than hypoglycemia. (7) Not as effective in the juvenile diabetic patient; supplement with carbohydrate as soon as possible. (8) Use caution in patients with insulinoma and/or pheochromocytoma. (9) As a smooth muscle relaxant, it is as effective as anticholinergic drugs with fewer side effects.

Contraindications: Known hypersensitivity to protein compounds.

Incompatible with: Any other drug in the syringe. Solutions containing sodium chloride, potassium chloride, or calcium chloride. Not soluble in any solution with a pH range of 3.0 to 9.5.

Side effects: Rare in recommended doses: anaphylaxis, hyperglycemia (excessive dosage), hypersensitivity reactions, hypertension (rare), hypotension (rare), nausea, and vomiting.

Antidote: Nausea and vomiting are tolerable and do occur in hypoglycemia. For any other side effects, discontinue the drug and notify the physician. Treat allergic reactions and resuscitate as necessary. Insulin administration *may* be indicated in *acute* overdose.

GLYCOPYRROLATE

(Robinul)

Usual dose: *Gastrointestinal disorders:* 0.1 to 0.2 mg at 4-hour intervals three to four times a day.

Reversal of neuromuscular blockade: 0.2 mg for each 1 mg of neostigmine or equivalent dose of pyridostigmine. Administer IV simultaneously. May be mixed in the same syringe.

Intraoperative medication: 0.1 mg as needed, may repeat every 2 to 3 minutes.

Dilution: May be given undiluted. Administer through Y tube or three-way stopcock of infusion tubing.

Rate of administration: 0.2 mg or fraction thereof over 1 to 2 minutes.

Actions: A synthetic anticholinergic agent. It inhibits the action of acetylcholine. It reduces the volume and free acidity of gastric secretions and controls excessive pharyngeal, tracheal, and bronchial secretions. Antagonizes cholinergic drugs. Onset of action is within 1 minute. Some effects last 2 to 3 hours.

Indications and uses: Adjunctive therapy in peptic ulcer, reversal of neuromuscular blockade (usually intraoperatively), and other intraoperative uses controlled by the anesthesiologist (counteract drug-induced or vagal traction reflexes and associated arrhythmias).

Precautions: (1) Use IV only when immediate drug effect is essential. (2) Not recommended for peptic ulcer therapy in children. (3) Urinary retention can be avoided if the patient voids just prior to each dose. (4) Use extreme caution in autonomic neuropathy, asthma, pregnancy, lactation, cardiac arrhythmias, congestive heart failure, coronary artery disease, hepatic or renal disease, hiatal hernia, hypertension, hyperthyroidism. (5) Potentiated by alkalinizing agents, synthetic narcotic analgesics, tricyclic antidepressants (amitryptyline [Elavil], etc), antihistamines, MAO inhibitors (pargyline [Eutonyl], etc.), nitrates, phenothiazines (chlorpromazine [Thorazine], etc.), and many others. (6) Antagonized by histamine, reserpine, and others. (7) Potentiates digoxin.

Contraindications: Known hypersensitivity to glycopyrrolate, glaucoma, obstructive uropathy, obstructive disease of the gastrointestinal tract, paralytic ileus, unstable cardiovascular status in acute hemorrhage, severe ulcerative colitis, megacolon, myasthenia gravis.

Incompatible with: Alkaline solutions, chloramphenicol, diazepam (Valium), dimenhydrinate (Dramamine), methohexital (Brevital), methylprednisolone (Solu-Medrol), pentazocine (Talwin), pentobarbital (Nembutal), phenothiazines (Compazine, etc), secobarbital (Seconal), sodium bicarbonate, thiopental (Pentothal.

Side effects: Anaphylaxis, blurred vision, constipation, decreased sweating, drowsiness, dry mouth, heat prostration, impotence, increased ocular tension, loss of taste, muscular weakness, nervousness, paralysis, tachycardia, urinary hesitancy and retention.

Antidote: Notify the physician of all side effects. May be treated symptomatically or drug may be discontinued. 1 mg of neostigmine for each 1 mg of glycopyrrolate administered may be used for overdose. Resuscitate as necessary.

HEMIN

(Panhematin)

Usual dose: A single dose of 1 to 4 mg/kg of body weight/ 24 hr for 3 to 14 days. This dose could be repeated in 12 hours for severe cases. Never exceed a total dose of 6 mg/kg/24 hr. Length of treatment dependent on severity of symptoms and clinical response.

Dilution: Each vial containing 313 mg of hemin must be diluted with 43 ml of sterile water for injection. Shake well for 2 to 3 minutes to ensure dilution. Each 1 ml contains 7 mg of hematin. Each 0.14 ml contains 1 mg of hematin. May be given directly from vial as an infusion or through Y tube or three-way stopcock of infusion set. Use of a 0.45 or smaller filter is recommended.

Rate of administration: A single dose evenly distributed over 10 to 15 minutes.

Actions: An iron-containing metalloporphyrin enzyme inhibitor extracted from red blood cells. Inhibits rate of prophyria/heme biosynthesis in the liver and bone marrow by an unknown mechanism. Induces remission of symptoms only; not curative. Some excretion occurs in urine and feces.

Indications and uses: To control symptoms of recurrent attacks of acute intermittent porphyria in selected patients (often related to the menstrual cycle in susceptible women).

Precautions: (1) Confirm diagnosis of acute porphyria before use (positive Watson-Schwartz or Hoesch test). (2) Alternate therapy of 400 Gm glucose/24 hr for several days should be tried before use of hemin is initiated. (3) Keep frozen until reconstituted immediately before use. Contains no preservatives, decomposes rapidly; discard unused solution. (4) Must be given before irreversible neuronal damage of porphyria has begun. (5) Use of a large arm vein or central venous catheter is recommended to avoid phlebitis. (6) Effectiveness is monitored by decrease in urine concentration of ALA, UPG, or PBG. (7) Action is inhibited by estrogens, barbiturates, and steroid metabolites. Avoid concurrent use. (8) Potentiates anticoagulants. (9) Use extreme caution in pregnancy, lactation, and children.

Contraindications: Hypersensitivity to hemin; prophyria cutanea tarda.

Incompatible with: Specific information not available. Do not mix with other drugs.

Side effects: Almost nonexistent with usual dosage and appropriate technique. Fever, phlebitis, reversible renal shutdown.

Antidote: Discontinue temporarily if known or questionable side effect appears and notify physician. Treat anaphylaxis (antihistamines, epinephrine, and corticosteroids) and resuscitate as necessary.

(Heparin Lock-Flush, Hep-Lock, Heprinar, Lipo-Hepin, Liquaemin sodium, Panheprin, Panheprin Lok)

Usual dose: *Intermittent injection:* 10,000 units initially. Dosage is adjusted according to clotting time and repeated every 4 to 6 hours.

Intravenous infusion: 20,000 to 40,000 units/24 hr in 1,000 ml of isotonic saline or other compatible infusion solution.

Open heart surgery: 150 to 400 units/kg of body weight during surgical procedure.

Maintain patency of infusion needle: 1,000 to 1,500 units to each 1,000 ml of IV fluid.

Maintain patency of heparin plug needle: 10 to 100 units diluted in 0.5 to 1 ml normal saline after each medication injection or every 8 to 12 hours.

Dilution: May be given undiluted or diluted in any given amount of isotonic sodium chloride, dextrose, or Ringer's solution for infusion and given direct IV or as an intermittent IV injection or continuous IV infusion.

Rate of administration: First 1,000 units or fraction thereof over 1 minute. After this test dose, any single injection (5,000 units or fraction thereof) may be given over 1 minute. A continuous IV infusion may be given over 4 to 24 hours, depending on specific dosage of heparin required, amount of heparin added, and amount of infusion fluid used as a diluent. Continuous IV infusion is the preferred method of administration. Use an infusion pump for accuracy.

Actions: An anticoagulant with immediate and predictable effects on the blood. Heparin combines with other factors in the blood to inhibit the conversion of prothrombin to thrombin and fibrinogen to fibrin. Adhesiveness of platelets is reduced. Well-established clots are not dissolved, but their growth is prevented and newer clots may be dissolved. Duration of action is short, about 4 to 6 hours. Does not cross the placental barrier. Metabolized in the liver and excreted in the kidneys. Has a wide margin of safety.

Indications and uses: (1) Prevention and/or treatment of all types of thromboses and emboli; (2) treatment of disseminated intravascular coagulation; (3) prevention of clotting in surgery of the heart or blood vessels, blood transfusion, and hemodialysis; (4) maintain patency of needle during prolonged IV infusion; (5) maintain patency of heparin lock needle for intermittent medication injection or vein access.

Precautions: (1) Read label carefully. Comes in many strengths. (2) Unit to milligram conversions are not consistent. (3) Whole blood clotting time or activated partial thromboplastin time must be done before initial injection. Often done before each injection on the first day of treatment. Usually repeated daily thereafter during IV therapy and more often if indicated. Depending on the test chosen, the desired therapeutic level is approximately two to three times greater than the control level. Confirm desired control level with physician. Obtain test just prior to next dose due in intermittent injection. Notify the physician if APTT or clotting time is above therapeutic level. (4) Use with caution during pregnancy. Hemorrhage is most likely to occur during the last trimester or postpartum. (5) Decrease dosage gradually. Abrupt withdrawal may precipitate increased coagulability. (6) Potentiated by chloramphenicol (Chloromycetin), salicylates, and others. (7) Inhibited by antihistamines, barbiturates, digitalis, calcium disodium edetate, hyaluronidase, hydroxyzine (Vistaril), penicillin, phenothiazines, and others, some of which may cause increased heparin absorption or result in withdrawal bleeding when discontinued. (8) Potentiates oral anticoagulants, phenytoin (Dilantin), thyroxine, and others. (9) To avoid precipitation, irrigate heparin plug catheters with normal saline before injecting acidic solutions. (10) Use caution if administering ACD converted blood (variable). (11) Use extensive precautionary methods to prevent bleeding if patient requires IM injection, arterial puncture, or venipuncture.

Contraindications: Active bleeding, blood dyscrasias, history of bleeding, hypersensitivity to heparin (derived from animal protein), inadequate laboratory facili-

231

ties, liver disease with hypoprothrombinemia, recent neurosurgical procedures, subacute bacterial endocarditis.

Incompatible with: Amikacin (Amikin), ampicillin (Amcil), atropine, cephalothin (Keflin), chlordiazepoxide (Librium), chlorpromazine (Thorazine), chlortetracycline (Aureomycin), codeine, daunorubicin (Cerubidine), erythromycin (Ilotycin, Erythrocin), ergonovine, gentamicin (Garamycin), hyaluronidase, hydrocortisone (Solu-Cortef), hydroxyzine (Vistaril), insulin (aqueous), kanamycin (Kantrex), levorphanol (Levo-Dromoran), meperidine (Demerol), metaraminol (Aramine), methadone, methicillin (Staphcillin), morphine sulfate, oxytetracycline (Terramycin), penicillin G, polymyxin B (Aerosporin), procainamide (Pronestyl), prochlorperazine (Compazine), promazine (Sparine), promethazine (Phenergan), streptomycin, sulfisoxazole (Gantrisin), tetracycline (Achromycin), vancomycin (Vancocin).

Side effects: Allergic reactions (rare), alopecia (rare), bruising, epistaxis, hematuria, prolonged coagulation time (in excess of two to three times the control level), tarry stools, or any other signs of bleeding. Allergic reactions including anaphylaxis do occur.

Antidote: Discontinue the drug and notify the physician of any side effects. Protamine sulfate is a heparin antagonist and specifically indicated in overdose or desired heparin reversal.

232

HETASTARCH

(Hespan)

Usual dose: *Shock:* Variable, depending on amount of fluid loss and resultant hemoconcentration. Initially 500 ml (30 Gm). Total dose should not exceed 1,500 ml/24 hr or 20 ml/kg of body weight.

Leukapheresis: 250 to 700 ml in continuous flow centrifugation procedures.

Dilution: Available as a 6% solution in 500 ml bottles properly diluted in normal saline and ready for use. Calculated osmolarity is approximately 310 mOsm/L.

Rate of administration: Variable, depending on indication, present blood volume, and patient response. Initial 500 ml may be given at rates approaching 20 ml/kg of body weight/hr. Reduce rate in burns or septic shock. If additional hydroxyethyl starch is required, reduce flow to lowest rate possible to maintain hemodynamic status.

Leukapheresis: usually infused at a constant ratio to venous whole blood, i.e., 1 to 8.

Actions: A synthetic polymer with properties similar to dextran. Approximates colloidal properties of human albumin. Provides hemodynamically significant plasma volume expansion in excess of the amount infused for about 24 hours. Dilutes total serum protein and hematocrit values. Increases erythrocyte sedimentation rate. Granulocyte collection by centrifuging becomes more efficient. Enzymatically degraded to molecules small enough to be excreted through the kidneys attached to glucose units.

Indications and uses: (1) As an adjunct in treatment of shock due to burns, hemorrhage, surgery, or trauma; (2) adjunct in leukapheresis to improve harvesting and increase yield of granulocytes.

Precautions: (1) For IV use only. (2) Not a substitute for whole blood or plasma proteins. (3) Monitor pulse, blood pressure, central venous pressure, and urine output every 5 to 15 minutes for the first hour and hourly thereafter while indicated. (4) Maintain adequate hydration of patient with additional IV fluids. (5) Change IV tubing or flush with normal saline before

233

imposing blood. (6) Use caution in heart disease, renal shutdown, congestive heart failure, pulmonary edema, and liver disease. (7) May reduce coagulability of the circulating blood, Observe patient for increased bleeding. (8) Does not interfere with blood typing or cross-matching. (9) Hemoglobin, hematocrit, electrolyte, and serum protein evaluation are necessary during therapy. During leukapheresis also monitor leukocyte and platelet count, leukocyte differential, prothrombin time, and partial thromboplastin time.

Contraindications: Severe bleeding disorders, severe congestive heart failure, renal failure with oliguria or anuria. No data are available pertaining to use in pregnancy or children.

Incompatible with: Specific information not available. See precautions.

Side effects: Chills, fever, headache, itching, muscle pains, peripheral edema, submaxillary and parotid glandular enlargement, urticaria, and vomiting. Anaphylaxis can occur.

Antidote: Notify the physician of any side effect. Discontinue the drug immediately at the first sign of an allergic reaction, provided other means of sustaining the circulation are available Antihistamines such as diphenhydramine (Benadryl) are helpful. Ephedrine or epinephrine (Adrenalin) may also be indicated. Resuscitate as necessary.

Usual dose: Must be given in specific sequence to determine validity of test results. 0.01 mg (10 μg) as initial dose. If no response after 5 minutes 0.05 mg (50 μg) may be given.

Dilution: May be given undiluted through tubing of an IV infusion of 5% dextrose in water or normal saline.

Rate of administration: Each single dose may be rapidly injected.

Actions: Histamine is a naturally occurring substance in the body. It acts to dilate even the smallest blood vessels, causing flushing, lowering peripheral resistance, and decreasing blood pressure. It has numerous other effects on the body.

Indications and uses: Presumptive diagnosis of pheochromocytoma. Indicated only for specific patients who have paroxysmal signs of excessive catecholamine secretion but have normal urinary values for assays of catecholamines and metabolites when asymptomatic.

Precautions: (1) Resting blood pressure must be 150/110 mm Hg or lower. (2) Have epinephrine available for hypotensive reaction and phentolamine (Regitine) available for hypertensive reaction. (3) Withhold antihypertensives, sympathomimetic agents, sedatives, and narcotics for 24 to 72 hours before the test. (4) Place patient on best rest. Start a slow IV infusion of 5% dextrose in water or normal saline. Record blood pressure until stable. Collect a 2-hour urine specimen for catecholamine assay. When completed give histamine through IV tubing rapidly. Collect another 2-hour urine specimen. Record blood pressure and pulse every 30 seconds for 15 minutes after histamine injection. Expected response includes headache, flushing, and a decrease in BP followed by an increase in BP within 2 minutes. (5) Very small doses can precipitate asthma in patients with bronchial disease. Use extreme caution. (6) Safety during pregnancy and lactation are not established.

Contraindications: Hypersensitivity to histamine products, hypotension, severe hypertension, vasomotor instability, history of bronchial asthma, history of urticaria, severe cardiac, pulmonary, or renal disease, the elderly.

Incompatible with: Specific information not available. Consider incompatible in syringe or solution due to specific use.

Side effects: Abdominal cramps, allergic reactions (including anaphylaxis), asthma, bronchial constriction, collapse with convulsions, diarrhea, dizziness, dyspnea, faintness, flushing, headache, hypertension, hypotension, metallic taste, nervousness, palpitations, syncope, tachycardia, urticaria, visual disturbances, vomiting.

Antidote: For accidental overdose, obstruct vein flow with tourniquet, use epinephrine and antihistamines (diphenhydramine [Benadryl], etc.). Treat anaphylaxis and resuscitate as necessary.

HYDRALAZINE HYDROCHLORIDE

pH 3.4 to 4.0

(Apresoline)

Usual dose: 10 to 40 mg. Begin with a low dose. Increase gradually as indicated. Repeat as necessary. Maximum dose is 300 to 400 mg/24 hr.

Pediatric dose: 1.7 to 3.5 mg/kg of body weight/24 hr in divided doses every 4 to 6 hours.

Dilution: May be given undiluted. Do not add to IV solutions. May be given through Y tube or three-way stopcock of infusion set.

Rate of administration: Each 10 mg or fraction thereof over 1 minute.

Actions: A potent antihypertensive drug. It lowers blood pressure by direct relaxation of smooth muscle of arteries and arterioles. Peripheral vasodilation results. Stimulation of the carotid sinus reflex increases cardiac output and rate. Action begins 2 to 10 minutes after the drug is given. Renal blood flow is increased in some cases, while cerebral blood flow is maintained. Well absorbed; 90% bound to plasma protein. Some excretion in urine.

Indications and uses: (1) Hypertensive crises of azotemia, (2) toxemia of pregnancy, (3) acute glomerulonephritis, (4) vasodilation in cardiogenic shock.

Precautions: (1) Check blood pressure every 5 minutes until stabilized at the desired level. Check every 15 minutes thereafter throughout crises. Average maximal decrease occurs in 10 to 80 minutes. (2) IV use is recommended only when the oral route is not feasible. (3) Rarely the drug of choice for hypertension unless used in combination (effectiveness increased and side effects decreased) with spironolactone (Aldactone), reserpine (Serpasil), guanethidine (Ismelin), and thiazide diuretics. Sometimes used with a beta adrenergic blocking drug (propranolol [Inderal], etc.); use caution, may potentiate effects. (4) Tolerance is easily developed but subsides about 7 days after the drug is discontinued. (5) Color changes occur in most 10% dextrose solutions. (6) Tricyclic antidepressants (amitriptyline [Elavil], etc.) may be contraindicated; will require dosage adjustment. (7) Potentiated by anesthetics, ethacrynic acid (Edecrin), MAO inhibitors (pargyline [Eutonyl], etc.), and triamterene (Dyrenium). (8) Inhibits epinephrine, levarterenol (Levophed). (9) Use caution in advanced renal damage, cerebrovascular accidents, congestive heart failure, coronary insufficiency, headache, increased intracranial pressure, pregnancy, and tachycardia.

Contraindications: Hypersensitivity to hydralazine, coronary artery disease, mitral valvular rheumatic heart disease.

Incompatible with: Aminophylline, ampicillin, calcium disodium edetate, chlorothiazide (Diuril), ethacrynic acid (Edecrin), hydrocortisone (Solu-Cortef), mephentermine (Wyamine), methohexital (Brevital), phenobarbital (Luminal), 10% fructose, 10% dextrose in lactated Ringer's injection.

Side effects: *Minor:* anxiety, depression, dry mouth, flushing, headache, nausea, numbness, palpitations, paresthesia, postural hypotension, tachycardia, tingling, unpleasant taste, vomiting. *Major:* angina, blood dyscrasias, chills, coronary insufficiency, delirium, dependent edema, fever, ileus, lupus erythematosus (simulated), myocardial ischemia and infarction, rheumatoid syndrome (simulated), toxic psychosis.

Antidote: If minor side effects occur, notify the physician, who will probably treat them symptomatically. Ganglionic blocking agents (trimethaphan camsylate [Arfonad], etc.) will control tachycardia. Pyridoxine will relieve numbness, tingling, and paresthesia. Antihistamines, barbiturates, and salicylates may be required. Treat hypotension with a vasopressor that is least likely to precipitate cardiac arrhythmias (methoxamine [Vasoxyl]). If side effects are progressive or any major side effects occur, discontinue the drug immediately and notify the physician. Treatment is symptomatic. Resuscitate as necessary. Occasionally methyldopa (Aldomet) will be used as a substitute, since it is effective for the same indications but has fewer side effects.

HYDROCORTISONE PHOSPHATE

pH 7.5 to 8.5

(Hydrocortone phosphate)

Usual dose: 25 to 250 mg initially. May repeat as necessary every 4 to 6 hours. Total dose usually does not exceed 1 Gm (20 ml)/24 hr. Dosage individualized according to the severity of the disease and the response of the patient.

Acute adrenal insufficiency: 100 mg initially. Repeat every 8 hours in IV fluids.

Pediatric dose: 2 to 8 mg/kg of body weight/24 hr. Dose varies with disease.

Acute adrenal insufficiency: 1 to 2 mg/kg direct IV, then 150 to 250 mg/kg/24 hr in divided doses. Maximum of 150 mg/kg/24 hr in divided doses for infants.

Dilution: May be given without mixing or dilution. Always use a separate syringe for hydrocortisone. May be added to sodium chloride or dextrose injection and given by IV infusion. Solution must be used within 24 hours of dilution.

Rate of administration: 25 mg or fraction thereof over 1 minute. Decrease rate of injection if any complaints of burning or tingling along injection site.

Actions: The principal hormone secreted by the adrenal cortex. Very rapidly absorbed adrenocortical steroid with potent metabolic, antiinflammatory, and innumerable other effects. May be used in conjunction with other forms of therapy, such as epinephrine for acute allergic reactions or antibiotics in acute infections. It is absorbed primarily into the lymph stream at extremely high levels and probably excreted in the urine and feces. 75% excretion occurs within 24 hours, allowing use of very large doses with reasonable safety. Will appear in breast milk.

Indications and uses: (1) Adrenocortical insufficiency; total, relative, and operative; (2) supplementary therapy for severe allergic reactions; (3) shock unresponsive to conventional therapy; (4) acute exacerbation of disease for patients receiving steroid therapy; (5) acute life-threatening infections with massive antibiotic therapy; (6) to induce remissions of some malignancies; (7) viral hepatitis; (8) thyroid crisis.

Precautions: (1) Sensitive to heat. (2) May cause elevated blood pressure and salt and water retention. (3) Salt restriction and potassium and calcium replacement are necessary. (4) May mask signs of infection. (5) To avoid relative adrenocortical insufficiency, do not stop therapy abruptly. Taper off. Patient is observed carefully, especially under stress, for up to 2 years. The exception is very short-term therapy. (6) Maintain on ulcer regime and antacid prophylactically. (7) May increase insulin needs in diabetes. (8) Inhibited by anticonvulsants, some antihistamines, barbiturates, propranolol (Inderal), phenylbutazone (Butazolidin). (9) Do not vaccinate for smallpox during therapy.

Contraindications: *Absolute contraindications* except in life-threatening situations: tuberculosis (active or healed), ocular herpes simplex, acute psychoses. *Relative contraindications:* active or latent peptic ulcer, chickenpox, congestive heart failure, diabetes mellitus, diverticulitis, fresh intestinal anastomoses, hypertension, myasthenia gravis, osteoporosis, pregnancy, psychotic tendencies, renal insufficiency, thromboembolic tendencies, and vaccinia.

Incompatible with: Amobarbital (Amytal), calcium gluconate, cephalothin (Keflin), chloramphenicol (Chloromycetin), erythromycin, heparin, kanamycin (Kantrex), metaraminol (Aramine), methicillin (Staphcillin), nitrofurantoin (Ivadantin), oxytetracycline (Terramycin), pentobarbital (Nembutal), phenobarbital (Luminal), phytonadione (Aquamephyton), prochlorperazine (Compazine), promazine (Sparine), tetracycline, vancomycin (Vancocin), vitamin B complex with C, warfarin (Coumadin).

Side effects: Do occur but are usually reversible: alteration of glucose metabolism including hyperglycemia and glycosuria; Cushing's syndrome (moon face, fat pads, etc.); electrolyte and calcium imbalance; euphoria or other psychic disturbances; hypersensitivity reactions including anaphylaxis; increased blood pressure; increased intracranial pressure; masking of infection; menstrual irregularities; perforation and hemorrhage from aggravation of peptic ulcer; protein catabolism with negative nitrogen balance; spontaneous fractures; transitory burning or tingling, sweating, headache, or weakness; thromboembolism.

Antidote: Notify the physician of any side effect. Will probably treat the side effect if necessary. Resuscitate as necessary for anaphylaxis and notify physician. Keep epinephrine immediately available.

HYDROCORTISONE SODIUM SUCCINATE

pH 7.0 to 8.0

(A-Hydrocort, Solu-Cortef)

Usual dose: 100 to 500 mg initially. May be repeated every 1 to 6 hours as necessary. For severe shock, doses up to 2 Gm or more every 2 to 4 hours have been given. These massive doses should not be used longer than 48 to 72 hours. Dosage is individualized according to the severity of the disease and the response of the patient and is not necessarily reduced for children. Never give less than 25 mg/24 hr.

Dilution: Available in a Mix-O-Vial, which is reconstituted by removing the protective cap, turning the rubber stopper a quarter turn, and pressing down, allowing the diluent into the lower chamber. Agitate gently. Using sterile techniques, a needle can be easily inserted through the center of the rubber stopper to withdraw the solution. If a Mix-O-Vial is not available, reconstitute each 250 mg or fraction thereof with 2 ml of bacteriostatic water for injection. Agitate gently to mix solution. May be given direct IV, or each 100 mg (250 mg, 500 mg, etc.) may be further diluted in at least 100 ml (250 ml, 500 ml, etc.) but not more than 1,000 ml of suitable IV solution for infusion. Suitable solutions are 5% dextrose in water, isotonic saline, or 5% dextrose in isotonic saline.

Rate of administration: Direct IV each 500 mg or fraction thereof over 1 minute. Direct IV is usually the route of choice and eliminates the possibility of overloading the patient with IV fluids. At the discretion of the physician, a continuous infusion may be given, properly diluted, over the specified time desired.

Actions: The principal hormone secreted by the adrenal cortex. A rapidly absorbed adrenocortical steroid with potent metabolic, antiinflammatory, and innumerable other effects. May be used in conjunction with other forms of therapy, such as epinephrine for acute allergic reactions or antibiotics in acute infections. It is absorbed primarily into the lymph stream at extremely high levels and probably excreted in the urine and feces. 75% excretion occurs within 24 hours, allowing use of very large doses with reasonable safety. Will appear in breast milk.

Indications and uses: Situations requiring high doses of hydrocortisone in a small amount of diluent and a need for high blood levels in a short period of time, such as (1) acute adrenocortical insufficiency, (2) acute hypersensitivity reactions, (3) aspiration pneumonitis, (4) bilateral adrenalectomy, (5) overwhelming infections with severe toxicity, (6) severe shock, (7) systemic lupus erythematosus relapse, (8) chemotherapy.

Precautions: (1) Sensitive to heat and light. (2) Discard unused solutions after 3 days. (3) May cause elevated blood pressure and salt and water retention. (4) Salt restriction and potassium and calcium replacement are necessary. (5) May mask signs of infection. (6) To avoid relative adrenocortical insufficiency, do not stop therapy abruptly. Taper off. Patient is observed carefully, especially under stress, for up to 2 years. The exception is very short-term therapy. (7) Maintain on ulcer regime and antacid prophylactically. (8) May increase insulin needs in diabetes. (9) Inhibited by anticonvulsants, some antihistamines, barbiturates, propranolol (Inderal), phenylbutazone (Butazolidin). (10) Do not vaccinate for smallpox during therapy.

Contraindications: None in short-term therapy. *Absolute contraindications* in long-term therapy, except in life-threatening situations: tuberculosis (active or healed), ocular herpes simplex, acute psychoses. *Relative contraindications:* active or latent peptic ulcer, chickenpox, congestive heart failure, diabetes mellitus, diverticulitis, fresh intestinal anastomoses, hypertension, myasthenia gravis, osteoporosis, pregnancy, psychotic tendencies, renal insufficiency, thromboembolic tendencies, and vaccinia.

Incompatible with: Aminophylline, amobarbital (Amytal), ampicillin, chlorpromazine (Thorazine, colistimethate (Coly-Mycin M), dimenhydrinate (Dramamine), diphenhydramine (Bendryl), doxorubicin (Adriamycin), ephedrine, heparin, hyaluronidase, hydralazine (Apresoline), hydroxyzine (Vistaril), kanamycin (Kantrex), lobeline, meperidine (Demerol), metaraminol (Aramine), methicillin (Staphcillin, nafcillin, oxytetracycline (Terramycin), pentobarbital (Nembutal), phenobarbital (Luminal), prochlorperazine (Compazine), promazine (Sparine), promethazine (Phenergan), secobarbital (Seconal), tetracycline, thiamylal (Surital), tolazoline (Priscoline), vancomycin (Vancocin).

Side effects: Do occur but are usually reversible: alteration of glucose metabolism including hyperglycemia and glycosuria; Cushing's syndrome (moon face, fat pads, etc.); electrolyte and calcium imbalance; euphoria or other psychic disturbances; hypersensitivity reactions including anaphylaxis; increased blood pressure; increased intracranial pressure; masking of infection; menstrual irregularities; perforation and hemorrhage from aggravation of peptic ulcer; protein catabolism with negative nitrogen balance; spontaneous fractures; transitory burning or tingling, sweating, headache, or weakness; thromboembolism; and many others.

Antidote: Notify the physician of any side effect. Will probably treat the side effect if necessary. Resuscitate as necessary for anaphylaxis and notify the physician. Keep epinephrine immediately available.

HYDROMORPHONE HYDROCHLORIDE

pH 4.0 to 5.5

(Dilaudid)

Usual dose: 2 to 4 mg every 3 to 4 hours.

Dilution: Each dose should be diluted with 5 ml of sterile water or normal saline for injection. May give through Y tube or three-way stopcock of infusion set.

Rate of administration: 2 mg or fraction thereof properly diluted solution over 3 to 5 minutes. Frequently titrated according to symptom relief and respiratory rate.

Actions: An opium derivative and CNS depressant closely related to morphine. Provides potent analgesia without hypnotic effects. Five times more potent than morphine milligram for milligram. Onset of action is prompt and lasts 3 to 4 hours. Hydromorphone is detoxified in the liver and excreted in the urine. Crosses placental barrier. Excreted in breast milk.

Indications and uses: Moderate to severe, acute or chronic pain, especially in situations in which a hypnotic effect is not desirable, such as postoperatively or in some malignancies.

Precautions: (1) Oxygen and controlled respiratory equipment must be available. (2) Observe patient frequently and monitor vital signs. (3) Use caution in the elderly and in patients with impaired hepatic or renal function and emphysema. (4) Potentiated by phenothiazines and other CNS depressants, such as narcotic analgesics, alcohol, anticholinergics, antihistamines, barbiturates, hypnotics, sedatives, MAO inhibitors (isocarboxazid [Marplan], etc.), neuromuscular blocking agents (tubocurarine, etc.) and psychotropic agents. Reduced dosages of both drugs may be indicated. (5) Tolerance to hydromorphone gradually increases. Physical dependence can develop but is not a factor in the presence of chronic pain of malignancy.

Contraindications: Bronchial asthma, increased intracranial pressure, known hypersensitivity to opiates.

Incompatible with: Alkalies, bromides, iodides, pentobarbital (Nembutal), prochlorperazine (Compazine), sodium bicarbonate, thiopental (Pentothal).

Side effects: Nausea, vomiting, and drowsiness are less frequent than with morphine. *Minor:* anorexia, constipation, dizziness, skin rash, urinary retention, and urticaria. *Major:* anaphylaxis, hypotension, respiratory depression, somnolence.

Antidote: Notify the physician of any side effect. If minor side effects progress or any major side effect occurs, discontinue the drug and notify the physician. Treat anaphylaxis as indicated or resuscitate as necessary. Naloxone hydrochloride (Narcan) or levallorphan tartrate (Lorfan) will reverse serious respiratory depression.

HYDROXYSTILBAMIDINE ISETHIONATE

Usual dose: 225 mg every 24 hours until successful results are obtained. Total dose will vary from 5 to 25 Gm. Lower doses or two treatment periods with a rest in between may be used if usual dose causes side effects.

Dilution: Each 225 mg or fraction thereof must be diluted in 200 ml of 5% dextrose in water or sodium chloride for injection.

Rate of administration: A single dose should be evenly distributed over 2 to 3 hours.

Actions: An antiinfective agent. Active against specific organisms *(Leishmania donovani* and *Blastomyces dermatitidis)*. Combines with RNA after penetrating the cell nucleus. Concentrates in the liver and kidney. Deposited in most body tissues and slowly excreted in urine and bile. Therapeutic effects continue after drug is discontinued.

Indications and uses: Visceral leishmaniasis (kala-azar), American mucocutaneous leishmaniasis, and North American blastomycosis.

Precautions: (1) Specific use only; establish correct diagnosis. (2) Not effective if host-defense mechanism is not adequate. Amphotericin B (Fungizone) may be used as an alternate. (3) Open a new ampoule for each dose. Use only clear, freshly prepared solutions for each injection. (4) Protect from heat, sunlight, and ultraviolet light. Cover infusion bottle with foil, dark paper, or a heavy towel to prevent decomposition. (5) Determine liver and renal function previous to and during course of therapy.

Contraindications: Hypersensitivity to hydroxystilbamidine, pregnancy unless life threatening.

Incompatible with: Specific information not available. Consider incompatible in syringe or solution due to specific use.

Side effects: Anaphylaxis, anorexia, arthralgia, chills, diarrhea, dizziness, drowsiness, fever, headache, hypotension, leukopenia, nausea, paresthesias, pruritus, skin rash, thrombophlebitis, vomiting.

Antidote: Notify the physician of all side effects. Most will subside with reduced rate of infusion, reduced dosage, a rest between treatment periods, or an alternate drug. Resuscitate as necessary.

HYOSCINE HYDROBROMIDE

pH 4.0 to 6.0

(Scopolamine hydrobromide)

Usual dose: 0.3 to 0.6 mg (gr ¹⁄₂₀₀ to ¹⁄₁₀₀).

Pediatric dose: 6 μg (0.006 mg)/kg of body weight or 200 μg/M² as a single dose.

Dilution: Dilute desired dose in at least 10 ml of sterile water for injection.

Rate of administration: 0.6 mg or fraction thereof over 1 minute.

Actions: Parasympathic depressant. Anticholinergic. It dilates the pupils, decreases glandular secretions, relaxes smooth muscle tissue, temporarily increases rate of heartbeat, has a calming, sedative action that produces a partial amnesia, and produces less tenacious sputum postoperatively. It is widely distributed throughout the body. It undergoes changes in the body, but much is excreted unchanged in urine. Crosses the placental barrier. Excreted in breast milk.

Indications and uses: (1) Alone or with sedatives for preanesthetic medication, (2) asthma and rhinitis, (3) biliary or renal colic, (4) gastric hypermotility, (5) motion sickness, (6) combined with analgesic or hypnotics in obstetrics.

Precautions: (1) Most frequently used subcutaneously or IM. Rarely given IV. (2) Potentiated by alkalinizing agents, synthetic narcotic analgesics, tricyclic antidepressants (amitriptyline [Elavil], etc.) antihistamines, MAO inhibitors (pargyline [Eutonyl], etc.), nitrates, phenothiazines (chlorpromazine [Thorazine], etc.), and many others. (3) Antagonized by histamine, reserpine, and others. (4) Use with caution in the elderly, in infants and small children, and in debilitated patients with chronic lung disease. (5) Hyoscine does interact with many drugs and potentiates the effects of both. Sometimes this is a desired interaction, as with morphine. (6) Use with methotrimeprazine (Levoprome) may cause a drop in blood pressure and tachycardia. (7) Inhibits lactation.

Contraindications: Known sensitivity to hyoscine, acute glaucoma, pyloric stenosis, prostatic hypertrophy.

249

Incompatible with: Limited information available. Alkalies. Incompatibilities listed under atropine should be considered.

Side effects: Mild in therapeutic doses, aggravated with overdosage: delirium, dry mouth, excitement, fever (heat loss by evaporation is inhibited), flushing, hallucination, hypertension, restlessness, slow reaction of pupils to light, tachycardia, thirst, urinary retention. *Overdose:* coma, respiratory failure, and unconsciousness do occur.

Antidote: Wide margin of safety between therapeutic and lethal dosage. Notify physician of aggravated side effects. Neostigmine methysulfate, 0.5 to 1 mg IV, may be used for symptomatic treatment as may sedatives and barbiturates.

L-HYOSCYAMINE SULFATE

(Levsin)

Usual dose: *Gastrointestinal disorders:* 0.25 to 0.5 mg (0.5 to 1.0 ml) at 4-hour intervals 3 to 4 times/day.
Hypotonic duodenography: 0.25 to 0.5 mg 5 to 10 minutes prior to the diagnostic procedure.
Preanesthetic medication: 5 mg/kg of body weight 30 to 60 minutes before induction of anesthesia.
Intraoperative medication: 0.125 mg (0.25 ml) to counteract drug-induced bradycardia. Repeat as needed.
Reversal or neuromuscular blockade: 0.2 mg for each 1 mg of neostigmine or equivalent dose of physostigmine and pyridostigmine.

Dilution: May be given undiluted. Administer through Y tube or three-way stopcock of infusion tubing.

Rate of administration: A single dose over at least 1 minute.

Actions: A chemically pure anticholinergic/antispasmodic component of belladonna alkaloids. Affects peripheral cholinergic receptors in autonomic effector cells of smooth muscle, cardiac muscle, sinoatrial node, atrioventricular node, and exocrine glands. Does not affect autonomic ganglia. Inhibits gastrointestinal motility, reduces gastric secretions, and controls excessive pharyngeal, tracheal and bronchial secretions. Onset of action is prompt and lasts 4 to 6 hours. Metabolized in the liver and excreted in urine. Traces occur in breast milk.

Indications and uses: (1) Adjunctive therapy in peptic ulcer, spastic colitis, cystitis, pylorospasm, dysentery, diverticulitis, irritable bowel syndrome, and neurogenic bowel disturbances; (2) biliary and renal colic; (3) hypotonic duodenography; (4) antiarrhythmic to counteract drug-induced bradycardia in surgery; (5) antidote for anticholinesterase agents (reversal of neuromuscular blockade).

Precautions: (1) Urinary retention can be avoided if the patient voids just prior to each dose. (2) Use caution in autonomic neuropathy, cardiac arrhythmias (especially tachycardia), congestive heart failure, coronary artery disease, dehydration, hypertension, and hyperthyroidism. (3) Potentiated by alkalinizing agents, synthetic narcotic analgesics, tricyclic antidepressants (amitryptyline [Elavil], etc.), antihistamines, MAO inhibitors (pargyline [Eutonyl], etc.), nitrates, phenothiazines (chlorpromazine [Thorazine], etc.), and many others. (4) Antagonized by histamine, reserpine, and others. (5) Use caution with digoxin, cholinergics, diphenhydramine (Benadryl), levodopa, and neostigmine. (6) Will cause cardiac arrhythmias with cyclopropane anesthesia.

Contraindications: Glaucoma, hypersensitivity, intestinal atony of the elderly or debilitated, megacolon, myasthenia gravis, obstructive disease of the gastrointestinal tract, obstructive uropathy, paralytic ileus, ulcerative colitis, unstable cardiovascular status in acute hemorrhage.

Incompatible with: Specific information not available.

Side effects: Anaphylaxis, blurred vision, cycloplegia, decreased sweating, drowsiness, dry mouth, headache, heat prostration, increased ocular tension, mydriasis, nervousness, palpitations, suppression of lactation, tachycardia, urinary hesitancy and retention, urticaria, weakness.

Antidote: Notify the physician of all side effects. May be treated symptomatically, or the drug may be discontinued. For overdose, physostigmine 0.5 to 2 mg IV up to 5 mg may be used. Thiopental sodium (Pentothal sodium) 2% may be required to decrease excitement. Mechanical ventilation equipment must be available. Treat fever with cooling measures. Treat anaphylaxis and resuscitate as necessary.

IMMUNE GLOBULIN INTRAVENOUS

(Gamimune)

Usual dose: 100 mg/kg of body wieght (2 ml/kg) as a single dose intravenous infusion. May be repeated monthly if indicated. If adequate IgG levels in the circulation or clinical response are not achieved, may be increased to 200 mg/kg (4 ml/kg) or lesser dose given at 2-week intervals.

Dilution: May be given undiluted but is usually diluted with a given amount of 5% dextrose for injection to facilitate slow and accurate rate of infusion. An infusion pump or microdrip (60 gtt/ml) would be appropriate.

Rate of administration: 0.01 to 0.02 ml/kg of body weight/minute of actual immune globulin for the first 30 minutes (0.7 to 1.4 ml/min of undiluted drug for a 70 kg individual). If no discomfort or adverse effects, may be increased to 0.02 to 0.04 ml/kg/min.

Actions: An immune serum containing 5% immune globulin. Obtained, purified, and standardized from human serum or plasma. Provides immediate antibody levels that last for about 3 weeks.

Indications and uses: Maintenance and treatment of individuals unable to produce adequate amounts of IgG antibodies, especially in the following situations: need for immediate increase in intravascular immunoglobulin levels, small muscle mass or bleeding tendencies that contraindicate IM injection, and selected disease states (congenital agammaglobulinemia, common variable hypogammaglobulinemia, or combined immunodeficiency).

Precautions: (1) Check label; must state for intravenous use. (2) Skin testing is not required. (3) Monitor vital signs and observe patient continuously during infusion. Anaphylaxis can occur at any time. Emergency equipment and supplies must be at bedside. (4) Keep refrigerated and discard partially used vials. Do not use if turbid or has been frozen. (5) Use extreme caution in individuals with isolated immunoglobulin A deficiency or a history of prior systemic allergic reactions. Incidence of anaphylaxis may be increased especially with repeated injections. (6) Use with caution in pregnancy; no adverse effects are documented, but adequate studies are not available. (7) Do not administer live virus vaccines for at least 3 months.

Contraindications: Individuals known to have an allergic response to gamma globulin or preexisting antiimmunoglobulin A (IgA) antibodies.

Incompatible with: Should be considered incompatible in syringe or solution with any other drug or solution (except 5% dextrose in water) due to specific use and potential for anaphylaxis.

Side effects: Full range of allergic symptoms including anaphylaxis is possible. Angioedema, erythema, fever, and urticaria are most frequently observed. A precipitous hypotensive reaction can occur and is most frequently associated with too-rapid rate of injection.

Antidote: Discontinue the drug and notify the physician of all side effects. May be treated symptomatically, and infusion resumed at slower rate if symptoms subside. Treat anaphylaxis immediately. Epinephrine (Adrenalin), diphenhydramine (Benadryl), oxygen, vasopressors (dopamine [Intropin], etc.), corticosteroids, and ventilation equipment must always be available. Resuscitate as necessary.

INSULIN INJECTION (REGULAR)   pH 7.4

(Actrapid, Beef Regular Iletin II, Humulin R, Pork Regular Iletin II, Purified Pork Insulin, Regular Iletin I, Velosulin)

Usual dose: Varies greatly. 50 to 100 units/hr as indicated by patient's condition and response. *Low-dose treatment:* 20 to 30 units initially then 3 to 8 units/hr.

Dilution: May be given undiluted either directly into the vein or through a Y tube or three-way stopcock. Insulin is compatible with commonly used IV solutions and may be given as an infusion; however, insulin potency may be reduced by at least 20% to 80% via the glass or plastic infusion container and plastic IV tubing before it actually reaches the venous system in an infusion. The percentage absorbed is inversely proportional to the concentration of insulin.

Rate of administration: Each 50 units or fraction thereof over 1 minute. When given in an IV infusion, the rate should be ordered by the physician, depending on insulin and fluid needs.

Actions: An aqueous solution that acts as a catalyst in carbohydrate metabolism in combination with adrenal, anterior pituitary, and thyroid hormones. This action is thought to occur at the cell membrane, facilitating glucose entry into peripheral tissues and lowering the blood glucose level. Also affected is the transport and incorporation of amino acids into protein. Release of free fatty acids from adipose tissue is inhibited. Insulin promotes storage of carbohydrate in liver and muscle cells and reduces the liver's capacity to put glucose into the blood. Potassium is also deposited in the liver with lower blood levels. Rapidly absorbed and readily distributed throughout the body; excretion, if any, is in changed form in the urine.

Indications and uses: (1) Diabetic coma, (2) ketoacidosis, (3) in combination with glucose to treat hyperkalemia, (4) induction of insulin shock for psychotherapy.

Precautions: (1) Regular insulin *only* may be given IV. Humulin R is the newest product (recombinant DNA origin). (2) Store in refrigerator. Discard any open vial not used for several weeks. (3) Use only if water clear. (4) Response to insulin measured by blood glucose, blood pH, acetone, BUN, sodium, potassium, chloride, and carbon dioxide levels. (5) Each voiding should be tested for sugar and acetone. (6) Hypovolemia is a common complication of diabetic acidosis. (7) Insulin is inactivated at pH above 7.5. (8) Combination of insulin and MAO inhibitors (pargyline [Eutonyl], etc.) or alcohol is hazardous and may be lethal. (9) Potentiated by beta adrenergic blockers (propranolol [Inderal], etc.), anabolic steroids (nandrolone [Durabolin], etc.), anticoagulants (warfarin [Coumadin], etc.), antineoplastics (methotrexate, etc.), isoniazid, pyrazalone compounds (phenylbutazone [Butazolidin], etc.), salicylates, sulfonamides, and many others. (10) Inhibited by corticosteroids, thiazide diuretics, epinephrine (Adrenalin), furosemide (Lasix), thyroid preparations, and others.

Contraindications: There are no contraindications when insulin is indicated as a lifesaving measure.

Incompatible with: Aminophylline, amobarbital (Amytal), chlorothiazide (Diuril), heparin, nitrofurantoin (Ivadantin), penicillin G potassium, pentobarbital (Nembutal), phenobarbital (Luminal), phenytoin (Dilantin), secobarbital (Seconal), sodium bicarbonate, sulfisoxazole (Gantrisin), thiopental (Pentothal).

Side effects: Hypoglycemia with overdose. *Early:* ashen color, clammy skin, drowsiness, faintness, fatigue, headache, hunger, nausea, nervousness, sweating, tremors, weakness. *Advanced:* coma, convulsions, disorientation, hypokalemia (with EKG changes), psychic disturbances, unconsciousness, hypersensitivity reactions including anaphylaxis; death is rare.

Antidote: Discontinue the drug immediately and notify the physician. *Glucagon* is the specific antidote for insulin overdose. It may be supplemented by glucose 50% IV and oral carbohydrates, such as orange juice, etc. Oral carbohydrates may be sufficient to combat the early symptoms of hypoglycemia. Allergic reactions will usually respond to symptomatic treatment.

INTRAVENOUS FAT EMULSION

(Intralipid 10%, Intralipid 20%, Liposyn 10% Liposyn 20%, Travamulsion 10%)

Usual dose: 500 ml on the first day. Increase dose gradually each day. Do not exceed 60% of the patient's total caloric intake or 2.5 Gm/kg of body weight.

Pediatric dose: 1 Gm/kg of body weight. Increase dose gradually each day. Do not exceed 60% of total caloric intake or 4 Gm/kg.

Dilution: Must be given as prepared by manufacturer.

Rate of administration: *Adult:* 1 ml/min for the first 15 to 30 minutes. If no untoward effects, increase rate to administer 500 ml equally distributed over 4 hours. *Pediatric:* 0.1 ml/min for the first 10 to 15 minutes. If no untoward effects, increase rate to administer 1 Gm/ kg of body weight (total usual dose) equally distributed over 4 hours. An infusion pump is recommended.

Actions: A parenteral nutrient. Has an osmolarity of 280 mOsm/L and contains emulsified fat particles about 0.5 μm in size. Total caloric value (fat, phospholipid, and glycerol) is 1.1 cal/ml. Metabolized and used as a source of energy. Increases heat production and oxygen consumption. Decreases respiratory quotient. Cleared from the bloodstream by a not fully understood process.

Indications and uses: (1) To provide calories and essential fatty acids for patients requiring parenteral nutrition over extended periods (over 5 days usually). (2) To prevent essential fatty acid deficiency.

Precautions: (1) May be administered by a peripheral vein or central venous infusion. (2) Infuse separately from any other intravenous solution or medication. Do not disturb emulsion. (3) May be administered via a Y tube or three-way stopcock near the infusion site. Rates of both solutions (fat emulsion and amino acid products) should be controlled by infusion pumps. (4) Do not use filters; will disturb emulsion. (5) Use only freshly opened solutions; discard remainder of partial dose. (6) Store under refrigeration. (7) Do not use if there appears to be an oiling out of the emulsion. (8)

Normal liver function is required. (9) Monitor lipids before each infusion; lipemia should clear daily. (10) Monitor platelet count in neonates. Use extreme caution in neonates; death from intravascular fat accumulation in the lungs has occurred. (11) Use caution in pulmonary disease, anemia, or blood coagulation disorders, or when there is any danger of fat embolism.

Contraindications: Any condition that disturbs normal fat metabolism, such as pathological hyperlipemia, lipoid nephrosis, and acute pancreatitis with hyperlipemia.

Incompatible with: Do not mix with any electrolyte or other nutrient solution. No additives or medications are to be placed in bottle or tubing (see precautions).

Side effects: Anaphylaxis, back pain, chest pain, cyanosis, dizziness, dyspnea, elevated temperature, flushing, headache, hypercoagulability, hyperlipemia, nausea and vomiting, pressure over eyes, sepsis (from contamination of IV catheter), sleepiness, sweating, thrombophlebitis (from concurrent hyperalimentation fluids), a delayed overloading syndrome (focal seizures, fever, leukocytosis, splenomegaly, shock), and many others.

Antidote: Notify physician of all side effects. Many will be treated symptomatically. Treat allergic reaction promptly and resuscitate as necessary.

(Imferon IM/IV, Proferdex)

Usual dose: *Direct IV:* 0.5 ml (25 mg) on the first day as a test dose. Wait 1 hour. If no adverse reactions, may be increased gradually to 2 ml (100 mg)/24 hr and repeated daily until results are achieved or maximum calculated dosage is reached (see literature).

Infusion: Up to the maximum calculated dose may be given in one or more infusions (not FDA approved).

Infant dose: 0.5 ml (25 mg)/24 hr maximum dose for infants under 5 kg.

Pediatric dose: 1 ml (50 mg)/24 hr maximum dose for children under 10 kg.

Dilution: Given undiluted or up to the total desired dose may be further diluted in 50 to 250 ml normal saline for infusion.

Rate of administration: 1 ml (50 mg) or fraction thereof over 1 minute or more.

Infusion: Test dose of 25 mg over 5 minutes. If no adverse reactions, infuse remaining dose over 1 to 2 hours. Discontinue IV infusion solutions during administration of iron dextran injections.

Actions: The iron-dextran complex is separated into smaller molecules by cellular systems in the bone marrow, liver, spleen, etc. By chemical processes usable iron can then be absorbed into the hemoglobin. After the hemoglobin needs of the blood are met, iron is stored in the body for reserve use. Small amounts of unabsorbed iron are excreted in the urine, feces, and bile.

Indications and uses: (1) Iron-deficiency anemia *only*, (2) insufficient muscle to allow repeated deep IM injection, (3) impaired muscle absorption, (4) hemophilia, (5) intermittent or repetitive substantial blood loss (familial telangiectasia, renal hemodialysis).

Precautions: (1) Check vial carefully, must state "for IV use." (2) Discontinue oral iron before starting iron dextran. (3) Use only when truly indicated to avoid excess storage of iron. (4) Increases joint pain and swelling in patients with rheumatoid arthritis. (5) Keep patient lying down after injection to prevent postural hypotension. (6) Use caution with history of asthma or allergies. (7) Use only if absolutely necessary in liver disease, early pregnancy, or childbearing years. Known hazard to fetus. (8) Monitor serum ferritin assays in prolonged therapy. Consider possibility of false results for months after injection due to delayed utilization. (9) Inhibits doxycycline (Vibramycin). (10) Inhibited by chloramphenicol.

Contraindications: Manifestation of allergic reaction, any anemia other than iron deficiency.

Incompatible with: Any other drug in syringe or solution.

Side effects: *Minor:* headache, itching, nausea, rash, shivering, transitory paresthesias. *Major:* anaphylaxis, arthritic reactivation, hypotension, leukocytosis, local phlebitis, lymphadenopathy, peripheral vascular flushing especially with too-rapid injection.

Antidote: Discontinue the drug and notify the physician of early symptoms. For severe symptoms, discontinue drug, treat allergic reactions, or resuscitate as necessary and notify physician. Epinephrine (Adrenalin) and diphenhydramine (Benadryl) should always be available. In acute poisoning an iron-chelating drug (deferoxamine), 1 to 2 Gm in 5% dextrose solution, may be given by slow IV drip over 24 hours. Deferoxamine can remove the iron from transferrin but not from the hemoglobin itself.

ISOPROTERENOL HYDROCHLORIDE

(Isuprel hydrochloride, Iprenol)

Usual dose: *Infusion:* 1 to 5 µg/min of a 1:250,000 solution.

Direct IV: 0.02 to 0.06 mg (1 to 3 ml of a 1:50,000 solution) as initial dose. Repeat as necessary.

Intracardiac: 0.02 mg (0.1 ml) of a 1:5,000 solution (rarely used).

Bronchospasm: 0.01 to 0.02 mg (0.5 to 1 ml of a 1:50,000 solution as initial dose. Repeat as necessary.

Pediatric dose: One tenth to one half the adult dose. Adjust to patient response.

Dilution: *Infusion:* 2 mg (10 ml) of a 1:5,000 solution in 500 ml of 5% dextrose in water. 4 µg equals 1 ml in this 1:250,000 solution. Use an infusion pump or microdrip (60 gtt/ml) to administer. Less diluent may be used to reduce fluid intake.

Direct IV or bronchospasm: dilute 0.2 mg (1 ml) of a 1:5,000 solution with 10 ml of normal saline for injection to make a 1:50,000 solution.

Intracardiac: 1:5,000 solution undiluted.

Rate of administration: *Infusion:* each 1 ml of a 1:250,000 (4 µg) solution over 1 minute. May be increased if necessary. Adjust to patient response.

Direct IV: each 1 ml of a 1:50,000 (0.02 mg) solution or fraction thereof over 1 minute.

Intracardiac: each 0.1 ml of a 1:5,000 solution over 1 second.

Actions: A synthetic cardiac beta receptor stimulant (sympathomimetic amine) similar to epinephrine and levarterenol. Has positive inotropic and chronotropic actions more potent than those of epinephrine. It increases stroke volume, cardiac output, cardiac work, coronary flow, and venous return. Improves atrioventricular conduction. Stimulates only the higher ventricular foci, allowing a more normal cardiac pacemaker to take over, thus suppressing ectopic pacemaker activity. Decreases peripheral vascular resistance by relaxing arterial smooth muscle and is a most effective bronchial smooth muscle relaxant. Onset of action is immediate and lasts 1 to 2 hours. Excreted in urine.

Indications and uses: (1) Atrioventricular heart block (Stokes-Adams syndrome) and cardiac standstill; (2) some ventricular arrhythmias, including ventricular tachycardia if increased inotropic activity is required for treatment; (3) bronchospasm during anesthesia; (4) management of shock (effective only with normal or elevated central venous pressure); (5) cardiac catheterization to simulate exercise; (6) on occasion as an antidote to reverse severe hypotension caused by tricyclic antidepressants (amitriptyline [Elavil], etc.).

Precautions: (1) Decrease rate of infusion as necessary. Ventricular rate generally should not exceed 110 beats/min. Maintain adequate blood volume and correct acidosis. (2) Intracardiac or IV injection in cardiac standstill must be accompanied by cardiac massage to perfuse drug into the myocardium. (3) Continuous cardic monitoring, central venous pressure readings, and blood pressure and urine flow measurements are advisable during therapy with isoproterenol. (4) May be used alternately with epinephrine (Adrenalin), *but they may not be used together.* Both are direct cardiac stimulants, and death will result. An adequate interval between doses must be maintained. (5) Use extreme caution when inhalant anesthetics (cyclopropane, etc.) are being administered and supplementary to digitalis administration. (6) Use caution in coronary insufficiency, diabetes, hyperthyroidism, known sensitivity to sympathomimetic amines, and preexisting cardiac arrhythmias with tachycardia. (7) Simultaneous use with oxytocics or MAO inhibitors (pargyline [Eutonyl], etc.) may cause hypertensive crisis. (8) Antagonized by propranolol (Inderal). Tachycardia and hypotension secondary to peripheral vasodilation may occur. (9) Potentiated by tricyclic antidepressants. (10) Severe hypotension and bradycardia may occur with hydantoins (Dilantin, etc.). (11) Do not use if pink or brown in color or contains a precipitate.

Contraindications: Patients with tachycardia caused by digitalis intoxication.

Incompatible with: Barbiturates, carbenicillin (Geopen), diazepam (Valium), epinephrine (Adrenalin).

Side effects: Anginal pain, cardiac arrhythmias, flushing, headache, nausea, nervousness, palpitations, sweating, tachycardia, vomiting. Cardiac dilation, marked hypotension, pulmonary edema, and death occur with prolonged use or overdose.

Antidote: Notify the physician of any side effect. Treatment will probably be symptomatic. For ventricular rate over 110 beats/min, decrease rate of infusion or discontinue drug. For accidental overdose, discontinue drug immediately, resuscitate and sustain patient, and notify physician.

KANAMYCIN SULFATE   pH 4.5

(Kantrex, Klebcil)

Usual dose: Up to 15 mg/kg of body weight/24 hr equally divided into two to four doses. Do not exceed a total adult dose of 1.5 Gm by all routes in 24 hours.

Dilution: Each 500 mg or fraction thereof must be diluted with at least 100 ml of 5% dextrose in water, 5% dextrose in normal saline, or normal saline for infusion.

Rate of administration: Do not exceed a rate of 3 to 4 ml/min diluted solution. Give total dose over 30 to 60 minutes.

Actions: An aminoglycoside antibiotic with neuromuscular blocking action. Bactericidal against many gram-negative organisms resistant to other antibiotics. Well distributed through all body fluids; crosses the placental barrier. Excreted in high concentrations through the kidneys. Cross-allergenicity does occur between aminoglycosides.

Indications and uses: Short-term treatment of serious infections caused by susceptible organisms. Concurrent therapy with a penicillin or cephalosporin is sometimes indicated.

Precautions: (1) Most frequently given by the IM route. (2) Discard partially used vials after 48 hours. (3) Use extreme caution if therapy is required over 7 to 10 days. (4) Sensitivity studies are necessary to determine the susceptibility of the causative organism to kanamycin. (5) Reduce daily dose for renal impairment; intervals between injections should also be increased. (6) Watch for decrease in urine output, rising BUN, and serum creatinine, and declining creatinine clearance levels. Dosage may need to be decreased. Routine serum levels and evaluation of hearing are necessary. (7) Use caution in infants, children, and the elderly and during pregnancy. (8) Potentiated by anesthetics, other neuromuscular blocking antibiotics (gentamicin, streptomycin, etc.), anticholinesterases (edrophonium [Tensilon], etc.), antineoplastics (cisplatin, nitrogen mustard, etc.), barbiturates, muscle relaxants (tubocurarine, etc.), phenothiazines (promethazine [Phenergan], etc.), procainamide, quini-

dine, and sodium citrate. *Apnea can occur.* (9) Ototoxicity may be potentiated by loop diuretics (furosemide [Lasix], etc.). Concurrent use is not
recommended. (10) Inhibited by penicillins. (11) Digoxin dose may need adjustment. (12) Superinfection
may occur from overgrowth of nonsusceptible organisms. (13) Maintain good hydration.

Contraindications: Known kanamycin sensitivity, prior
hearing damage by kanamycin or other ototoxic
agents unless infection is life threatening.

Incompatible with: Administer separately. Amphotericin
B, ampicillin, carbenicillin (Geopen), cefoxitin (Mef-
oxin), cephalothin (Keflin), cephapirin (Cefadyl), chlorpheniramine (Chlor-Trimeton), colistimethate (Coly-
Mycin M), heparin, hydrocortisone (Solu-Cortef),
methohexital (Brevital), penicillins.

Side effects: *Minor:* fever, headache, paresthesias, skin
rash, thrombophlebitis. *Major:* apnea, azotemia, elevated BUN, NPN, creatinine, hearing loss, oliguria,
proteinuria, tinnitus, vertigo.

Antidote: Notify the physician of all side effects. If minor
symptoms persist or any major symptom appears, discontinue the drug and notify the physician. Treatment
is symptomatic, or a reduction in dose may be required. Hemodialysis or peritoneal dialysis may be
indicated. Resuscitate as necessary.

(Citrovorum factor, folinic acid)

Usual dose: *Folinic acid rescue:* For high-dose methotrexate, an IV infusion of leucovorin is initiated anywhere from 0 to 36 hours after methotrexate and continued for 36 to 96 hours, depending on the dose of methotrexate, serum levels, and creatinine clearance of patient. Many schedules have been used. Examples are: (a) 10 to 40 mg/M^2 IV 24 hours after methotrexate followed by 10 to 25 mg/M^2 IM or IV every 6 hours for 72 hours. (b) 6 to 15 mg/M^2 every 6 hours for 72 hours beginning 2 hours after methotrexate. Dose regime depends on methotrexate dose.

Overdose of methotrexate: Milligram for milligram or greater than dose of methotrexate. Administer within first hour or up to 75 mg as an IV infusion within 12 hours of methotrexate dose. Follow with 12 mg IV every 6 hours for four doses.

Dilution: A single dose should be diluted in 100 to 500 ml of any common IV infusion solution. 1 ml (3 mg) ampoules may be given undiluted.

Rate of administration: A single dose equally distributed over 15 minutes to 1 hour. May be given more rapidly if patient's condition warrants. For massive-dose folinic acid rescue total dose may be infused equally distributed over a 6-hour period.

Actions: Potent agent for neutralizing immediate toxic effects of methotrexate (and folic acid antagonists) on the hematopoietic system. Preferentially rescues normal cells without reversing the oncolytic effect of methotrexate.

Indications and uses: (1) Investigational (not FDA approved but in common use): folinic acid rescue to prevent or decrease the toxicity of massive doses of methotrexate used to treat resistant neoplasms. (2) Treatment of accidental methotrexate overdose.

Precautions: (1) Usually administered in the hospital by or under the direction of the physician specialist. (2) Permits use of massive doses of methotrexate. (3) Do not discontinue leucovorin until methotrexate serum levels fall below toxic levels. (4) Monitor serum blood levels of methotrexate and serum creatinine levels. Death can occur in 5 to 10 days if methotrexate remains at toxic levels longer than 48 hours. (5) Minimum fluid intake of 3 L/24 hr and alkalinization of urine with oral sodium bicarbonate is recommended. Begin 12 hours before methotrexate dose is administered and continue for 48 hours after final dose in each sequence. (6) Much less effective in accidental overdose after a 1-hour delay. (7) May inhibit phenytoins (Dilantin, etc.).

Contraindications: None when used as indicated.

Incompatible with: Specific information not available. Consider incompatible in solution with any other drug due to specific use.

Side effects: Almost nonexistent. Some slight flushing or feeling of warmth may occur.

Antidote: Keep physician informed of patient's condition. Symptomatic treatment indicated.

LEVALLORPHAN TARTRATE   pH 4.0 to 4.5
(Lorfan)

Usual dose: 1 mg followed by 0.5 mg every 10 to 15 minutes for one or two doses. Do not exceed a total dose of 3 mg.

Pediatric dose: 0.02 mg/kg of body weight; may repeat 0.01 to 0.02 mg/kg of body weight in 10 to 15 minutes.

Neonatal dose: 0.05 to 0.1 mg or one tenth of the adult dose into umbilical vein.

Dilution: May be given undiluted. For infants, dilute a single dose in 2 to 3 ml of normal saline for injection. May be administered in the same syringe with the narcotic when used as a preventive measure.

Rate of administration: 1 mg or fraction thereof over 1 minute.

Actions: A potent narcotic antagonist, 10 times as potent as naloxone (Narcan). Prevents or overcomes narcotic-induced respiratory depression without abolishing analgesia. Onset of action occurs within 1 minute and lasts 4 to 5 hours. Readily absorbed into the body, it is inactivated by the liver.

Indications and uses: (1) Reversal of narcotic depression; (2) antidote for natural and synthetic narcotics, butorphanol (Stadol), methadone, nalbuphine (Nubain), and propoxyphene (Darvon). Not indicated for pentazocine (Talwin).

Precautions: (1) If used without a narcotic, levallorphan may actually cause respiratory depression. (2) Not effective against respiratory depression caused by barbiturates, anesthetics, other nonnarcotic agents or pathological conditions. (3) May be injected into the infant's umbilical vein immediately after delivery. (4) Symptomatic treatment with oxygen and artificial respiration as necessary should be continued until levallorphan is effective. (5) Will precipitate acute withdrawal symptoms in narcotic addicts. (6) Repeated doses result in decreasing effectiveness. (7) Will increase respiratory depression of pentazocine (Talwin). (8) Use caution in neonates of narcotic-dependent mothers.

Contraindications: Mild respiratory depression. Do not use for patients who have been bitten by a scorpion; potentiates toxicity of scorpion venom.

Incompatible with: Methicillin (Staphcillin), phenytoin (Dilantin), prochlorperazine (Compazine), sulfisoxazole (Gantrisin), trifluoperazine (Stelazine).

Side effects: Occur only with large doses: drowsiness, dysphoria, lethargy, nausea, pallor, sense of heaviness in the limbs, sweating, tachyarrhythmias, visual hallucinations. Irritability and a tendency toward increased crying may occur in the neonate.

Antidote: Any and all side effects are treated symptomatically. Notify the physician. Facilities for artificial respiration, oxygen therapy, and other supportive measures should be available.

LEVARTERENOL BITARTRATE   pH 3.0 to 4.5

(Levophed, norepinephrine)

Usual dose: 0.25 to 0.5 ml (0.5 to 1 mg of 0.2% solution)/
10 kg of body weight. Average dose is 4 ml (8 mg of
0.2% solution) to each 1,000 ml of diluent. More or
less may be added to each 1,000 ml of diluent, depending on clinical fluid volume requirements. Larger
doses may be given safely as long as the patient remains hypotensive and blood volume depletion is corrected.

Dilution: Must be diluted in 500 to 1,000 ml of 5% dextrose in water or saline and given as an IV infusion.
Administration in a dextrose solution reduces loss of
potency that is caused by oxidation. Normal saline
without dextrose is not recommended.

Rate of administration: Begin with 2 to 3 ml/min of infusion. Use the slowest possible flow rate to correct
hypotension gradually and maintain adequate or preset blood pressure. Some response should be noted
within 1 to 2 minutes of IV administration. Use of an
infusion pump or microdrip (60 gtt/ml), is an aid to
correct evaluation of dosage.

Actions: Levarterenol is the levo-isomer of norepinephrine, a sympathomimetic drug and powerful vasoconstrictor. Greatly increases blood flow to all vital organs
without increasing the workload or output of the
heart. Dilates the coronary arteries more than twice
as much as epinephrine can. It is rapidly inactivated
in the body by various enzymes and excreted in
changed form in the urine.

Indications and uses: All hypotensive states, including
anesthesia, blood reactions, drug reactions, hemorrhage, myocardial infarction, pheochromocytomectomy, septicemia, surgery, sympathectomy, and
trauma.

Precautions: (1) Check blood pressure every 2 minutes
until stabilized at the desired level. Check every 5
minutes thereafter during therapy. Avoid hypertension. (2) Observe for hypovolemia and replace fluids
immediately. In an emergency, levarterenol can be
effective in a hypovolemic state before fluid replace-

ment has been accomplished. (3) Check flow rate and injection site constantly. (4) Infusion should be through a large vein, preferably the antecubital vein, to prevent complications of prolonged peripheral vasoconstriction. Avoid veins in the hands, ankles, and legs. Use of the femoral vein may be considered. (5) Causes severe tissue necrosis, sloughing, and gangrene. Always use a plastic IV catheter at least 6 or more inches long for administration. Insert well into vein to prevent extravasation into any surrounding tissue. (6) Blanching along the vein pathway is a preliminary sign of extravasation. Change the injection site. (7) Whole blood or plasma should be given in a separate IV site. May be given through Y tube connection. (8) Use caution in the elderly and in those with peripheral vascular disease. (9) Phentolamine (Regitine) 5 to 10 mg and/or heparin sodium 10 mg have been recommended by some authorities to prevent any sloughing, necrosis, and/or thrombosis from slight leakage along the vein pathway. These are added with the levarterenol to 500 ml of the diluent. (10) Therapy may be continued until the patient can maintain his own blood pressure. Decrease dosage gradually. (11) Hazardous when potentiated by amphetamines, antihistamines, tricyclic antidepressants (desipramine [Norpramine], etc.), MAO inhibitors (isocarboxazid [Marplan], etc.), rauwolfia alkaloids (reserpine, etc.), thyroid preparations, and methylphenidate (Ritalin). (12) Interacts in numerous and sometimes contradictory ways with many drugs. (13) May cause severe hypertension with ergot alkaloids. (14) Will cause hypotension and bradycardia with hydantoins (phenytoin [Dilantin], etc.).

Contraindications: Do not use in mesenteric or peripheral vascular thrombosis or cyclopropane or halothane (inhalant) anesthesias.

Incompatible with: Amobarbital (Amytal), ampicillin (Polycillin), ascorbic acid, cephalothin (Keflin), cephapirin (Cefadyl), chlorphenirmine (Chlor-Trimeton), chlorothiazide (Diuril), diazepam (Valium), heparin, metaraminol (Aramine), methicillin (Staphcillin), nitrofurantoin (Ivadantin), oxytocin (Pitocin, Syntocinon), pentobarbital (Nembutal), phenobarbital (Luminal), phenytoin (Dilantin), secobarbital (Seconal), sodium bicarbonate, sodium iodide, streptomycin, sulfisoxazole (Gantrisin), tetracycline (Achromycin), thiopental (Pentothal), warfarin (Coumadin), whole blood.

Side effects: Rare when used as directed. Bradycardia, chest pain, headache, ischemia, necrosis caused by extravasation, pallor, photophobia, vomiting.

Antidote: To prevent sloughing and necrosis in areas in which extravasation has occurred, inject 5 to 10 mg of phentolamine (Regitine) diluted in 10 to 15 ml of normal saline liberally throughout the tissue in the extravasated area with a fine hypodermic needle. Treatment should be started as soon as extravasation is recognized. Atropine may be used to counteract the bradycardia. Notify physician of any side effect. Should a sudden or uncontrolled hypertensive state occur, discontinue levarterenol, notify the physician, and treat with antihypertensive agents, such as phentolamine (Regitine) or phenoxybenzamine (Dibenzyline).

(Levo-Dromoran)

Usual dose: 2 to 3 mg every 4 to 6 hours.

Dilution: Each dose should be diluted with 5 ml of sterile water or normal saline for injection. Do not add to IV solutions. May give through Y tube or three-way stopcock of infusion set.

Rate of administration: 3 mg or fraction thereof properly diluted solution over 3 to 5 minutes.

Actions: A synthetic narcotic analgesic and CNS depressant closely related to morphine. Five times more potent than morphine milligram for milligram. Onset of action is immediate and lasts 6 to 8 hours. Levorphanol is detoxified in the liver and excreted in the urine. Crosses the placental barrier. Excreted in breast milk.

Indications and uses: (1) Relief of moderate to severe, acute, or chronic pain, such as pain of biliary or renal colic, cancer, myocardial infarction, severe trauma, or postoperatively; (2) preanesthetic sedation.

Precautions: (1) Oxygen and controlled respiratory equipment must be available. (2) Observe patient frequently and monitor vital signs. (3) Tolerance to levorphanol gradually increases. (4) Use caution in the elderly, in patients with impaired hepatic or renal function, emphysema, and during pregnancy or delivery. (5) Potentiated by phenothiazines (chlorpromazine [Thorazine], etc.) and other CNS depressants, such as narcotic analgesics, alcohol, anticholinergics, antihistamines, barbiturates, hypnotics, sedatives, MAO inhibitors (isocarboxazid [Marplan], etc.), neuromuscular blocking agents (tubocurarine etc.), and psychotropic agents. Reduced dosage of both drugs may be indicated. (6) IV is not the route of choice. Usually given subcutaneously. (7) Physical dependence can develop with abuse.

Contraindications: Acute alcoholism, anoxia, bronchial asthma, increased intracranial pressure, known hypersensitivity to levorphanol, respiratory depression.

Incompatible with: Aminophylline, ammonium chloride, amobarbital (Amytal), chlorothiazide (Diuril), heparin, methicillin (Staphcillin), nitrofurantoin (Ivadantin), pentobarbital (Nembutal), phenobarbital (Luminal), phenytoin (Dilantin), secobarbital (Seconal), sodium bicarbonate, sodium iodide, sulfisoxazole (Gantrisin), thiopental (Pentothal).

Side effects: Nausea, vomiting, and constipation are less frequent than with morphine. Other side effects are the following. *Minor:* dizziness, skin rash, urinary retention, urticaria. *Major:* anaphylaxis, cardiac arrhythmias, hypotension, respiratory depression.

Antidote: Notify the physician of any side effect. If minor side effects progress or any major side effect occurs, discontinue the drug and notify the physician. Treat anaphylaxis as indicated or resuscitate as necessary. Levallorphan (Lorfan) will reverse serious respiratory depression. It may be given with levorphanol in a 1:10 ratio (levallorphan 0.1 mg to levorphanol 1 mg) to prevent respiratory depression.

LEVOTHYROXINE SODIUM

(Levothroid, Noroxine, Synthroid, T₄, L-Thyroxine)

Usual dose: 0.2 to 0.5 mg as initial dose. 0.1 to 0.2 mg/24 hr may be repeated as indicated by patient response or serum PBI levels. 0.1 mg equals approximately 65 mg (gr 1) of thyroid. Maintain with oral medication.

Pediatric dose: *under 1 year:* 18 to 37 μg as a single daily dose. *Over 1 year:* 2 to 3.5 μg/kg of body weight as a single daily dose. Do not exceed adult dose.

Dilution: Diluent usually provided. Each 0.5 mg of lyophilized powder is diluted with 5 ml of sodium chloride for injection (without preservatives). Shake well to dissolve completely. 1 ml equals 0.1 mg. Do not add to IV solutions. May be given through Y tube or three-way stopcock of infusion set.

Rate of administration: 0.1 mg or fraction thereof over 1 minute.

Actions: A synthetic thyroid hormone. Effective replacement for decreased or absent thyroid function. Onset of action is slow. Up to 5 or 6 hours is required before any noticeable improvements occur, and 24 hours may be required to note full benefits. Thyroid is essential to many body functions, including rate of metabolism.

Indications and uses: (1) Hypothyroid states due to any cause, (2) an emergency measure in myxedematous coma.

Precautions: (1) Must be used immediately after dilution; any remaining solution is discarded. (2) Correct adrenocortical insufficiency before administration, or acute adrenal crisis and death will result. Corticosteroid therapy is also required concomitantly to prevent acute adrenal insufficiency in myxedematous coma or any preexisting manifestation of adrenal insufficiency. (3) Observe patient continuously and monitor vital signs. (4) Use caution in diabetes and cardiovascular disease. (5) Increases rate of metabolism and requires dosage adjustment for anticoagulants, antidepressants, oral antidiabetics, barbiturates, digitalis,

275

catecholamines (epinephrine, etc.), beta adrenergic blockers (propranolol, etc.), insulin, and others. Cardiac arrhythmias, hypoglycemia, and bleeding can occur with unadjusted dosage of some of these drugs.

Contraindications: Myocardial infarction, thyrotoxicosis.

Incompatible with: No specific references are available. Should be considered incompatible in the syringe with any other drug.

Side effects: Chest pain, diarrhea, heart palpitations, muscle cramps, nervousness, perspiration, tachycardia, vomiting.

Antidote: Notify the physician of any side effect. A reduction in dosage will usually decrease symptoms.

(Xylocaine)

Usual dose: 1 to 1.5 mg/kg of body weight, (70 to 100 mg
for a 70 kg person). May repeat in 5 minutes if indicated. Do not give more than three bolus doses in 1
hour. Follow with 1 to 4 mg/min as an IV infusion.
Do not exceed 4 mg/min rate.
Prophylactic dose: Initiate a keep-open IV of 5% dextrose in water. Give 75 mg as a bolus dose independent
of weight, height, or age. Repeat 50 mg bolus every 5
minutes if ventricular ectopic activity is present to a
maximum dose of 325 mg or every 10 minutes if no
ectopic activity to a maximum of 275 mg while en
route to hospital.

Pediatric dose: 0.5 to 1 mg/kg of body weight as a bolus
dose. May repeat at 5-minute intervals if necessary.
Do not exceed a total of 3 mg/kg. Follow with an infusion of 15 to 30 μg/kg/min.

Dilution: Bolus dose may be given undiluted. *Infusion:*
add 1 Gm of lidocaine to 500 ml of 5% dextrose in
water. Solution gives 2 mg/ml of lidocaine.

Rate of administration: *Bolus dose:* a single dose over 1
minute or less if indicated. Too-rapid injection may
cause seizures. *Infusion:* Using a microdrip (60 gtt/
ml) or an infusion pump delivers lidocaine in recommended doses. Adjust as indicated by progress in
patient's condition.

Actions: A local anesthetic agent. Exerts an antiarrhythmic effect similar to procainamide, but it is more
potent. Decreases ventricular excitability without depressing the force of ventricular contractions by increasing the stimulation threshold of the ventricle
during diastole. Decreases cell membrane permeability and prevents loss of sodium and potassium ions.
Onset of action should occur within 2 minutes and
last approximately 10 to 20 minutes. Crosses placental
barrier. Metabolized in the liver and excreted in the
urine.

Indications and uses: Ventricular arrhythmias, such as
premature ventricular contractions or ventricular

tachycardia, occurring during acute myocardial infarction and during cardiac and other surgery.

Precautions: (1) Label must state "for IV use." (2) Monitor flow rate and the patient's EKG continuously. (3) Discontinue lidocaine when patient's cardiac condition is stable or any signs of toxicity become apparent. (4) Oral antiarrhythmic drugs are preferred for maintenance. (5) Keep a bolus dose, 100 mg (5 ml), available at all times for emergency use in myocardial infarction. (6) Cross-sensitivity and/or potentiation may occur with procainamide or quinidine. (7) Use caution in severe liver or renal disease, hypovolemia, shock, all forms of heart block, and untreated bradycardia. (8) Reduce dose in congestive heart failure, reduced cardiac output, and the elderly. (9) Discard diluted solution after 24 hours. (10) Do not add lidocaine to blood transfusion tubings. (11) Potentiates succinylcholine (Anectine). (12) Potentiated by beta adrenergic blockers (propranolol [Inderal], etc.), and cimetidine (Tagamet).

Contraindications: Known sensitivity to lidocaine or any other local anesthetic of the amide type; Adams-Stokes syndrome or any other severe degree of first-, second-, or third-degree heart block.

Incompatible with: Methohexital (Brevital). Physically compatible with many drugs. However, combination is not practical because of extensive individualized rate adjustments to achieve desired effects.

Side effects: Transient because of short duration of action of lidocaine. *Minor:* apprehension; blurred vision; dizziness; drowsiness; euphoria; light-headedness; sensations of heat, cold, and numbness; tinnitus; vomiting. *Major:* anaphylaxis, bradycardia, cardiac arrest, cardiovascular collapse, convulsions, hypotension, PR interval prolonged, QRS widening, respiratory depression, tremors, twitching, unconsciousness.

Antidote: Notify the physician of any side effects. For major side effects, discontinue the drug immediately and institute appropriate measures. For anaphylactic shock use epinephrine and corticosteroids, etc. To correct CNS stimulation use diazepam (Valium), rapid short-acting barbiturates (pentobarbital [Nembutal], etc.), or short-acting muscle relaxants (succinylcholine [Anectine], etc.). Use vasopressors (dopamine [Intropin], etc.) to correct hypotension. Maintain and support patient; resuscitate as necessary.

LINCOMYCIN HYDROCHLORIDE   pH 3.0 to 5.5

(Lincocin)

Usual dose: 600 mg to 1 Gm every 8 to 12 hours. Total doses from 4 to 8 Gm/24 hr have been given in life-threatening infections.

Pediatric dose: Children over 1 month of age: 10 to 20 mg/kg of body weight/24 hr divided in two or three doses.

Dilution: Add 1 Gm or fraction thereof to a minimum of 100 ml of 5% glucose in water, normal saline, or other compatible solutions. If 4 Gm or more is to be given, add to 500 ml of solution.

Rate of administration: Give properly diluted solution as an infusion. Infusion rate must not exceed 100 ml/hr (1 Gm/hr).

Actions: Interferes with protein synthesis of bacterial organism. It may be bactericidal or bacteriostatic. Well distributed in most body tissues. Actively excreted in bile and urine. Crosses the placental barrier. Excreted in breast milk.

Indications and uses: Rarely used. (1) Infections caused by susceptible strains of streptococci, pneumococci, and staphylococci; (2) patients allergic to penicillin; (3) penicillin-resistant gram-positive infections.

Precautions: (1) Sensitivity studies are necessary to determine the susceptibility of the causative organism to lincomycin. (2) Keep patient lying down after injection to prevent hypotension. (3) Avoid prolonged use of drug; superinfection caused by overgrowth of nonsusceptible organisms may result. (4) Periodic blood cell counts and liver function studies are indicated in prolonged therapy. (5) Capable of causing severe, even fatal, colitis; observe for symptoms of diarrhea. (6) May potentiate other neuromuscular blocking agents (kanamycin, streptomycin, etc., and tubocurarine, etc.); *apnea can result*. (7) Severe hypotension and cardiac arrest can occur with too-rapid injection. (8) Use caution in allergic tendencies and in the elderly. Reduce dose to 30% in severe renal impairment. (9) Discard diluted solution after 24 hours.

(10) Dilution with other antibiotics in infusion solution may be possible. Consult pharmacist. Adhere to minimum rate of administration.

Contraindications: Colitis; known lincomycin, clindamycin, or erythromycin sensitivity; known monilial infections unless they are being treated concurrently; minor bacterial or viral infections; preexisting liver disease; pregnancy; newborns.

Incompatible with: Carbenicillin (Geopen), kanamycin (Kantrex), novobiocin (Albamycin), penicillin, phenytoin (Dilantin).

Side effects: Agranulocytosis, anaphylaxis, cardiac arrest, diarrhea, enterocolitis, hypotension, jaundice and elevated SGOT, leukopenia, neutropenia, pruritus ani, skin rashes, thrombocytopenic purpura, urticaria, vaginitis.

Antidote: Notify the physician of early symptoms. For severe symptoms including significant diarrhea, discontinue the drug, treat allergic reaction or resuscitate as necessary, and notify the physician.

LORAZEPAM

(Ativan)

Usual dose: 2 mg or 0.044 mg/kg of body weight, whichever is smaller, 15 to 20 minutes before procedure.
Maximum dose 2 mg for patients over 50 years old.
For greater lack of recall in patients under 50 years
old, 0.05 mg/kg up to 4 mg may be given.

Dilution: Must be diluted immediately before use with
an equal volume of sterile water, 5% dextrose, or 0.9%
sodium chloride for injection. May be given direct IV
or through the Y tube or three-way stopcock of infusion tubing.

Rate of administration: Each 2 mg or fraction thereof
over 1 minute.

Actions: A benzodiazepine that relieves anxiety, produces
sedation, and inhibits ability to recall events. Effective in 15 to 20 minutes. Lasts up to 16 hours. Widely
distributed in body fluids, some is slowly excreted in
urine. Crosses the placental barrier. Excreted in
breast milk.

Indications and uses: Preanesthetic medication for adult
patients.

Precautions: (1) Bed rest required for a minimum of 3
hours after IV injection and assistance required for
up to 8 hours. (2) To reduce incidence of thrombophlebitis, avoid smaller veins. Extravasation or arterial administration is hazardous. (3) Maintain patent airway. Respiratory assistance must be available.
(4) Potentiates narcotics, phenothiazines (prochlorperazine [Compazine], etc.), barbiturates, and MAO
inhibitors (pargyline [Eutonyl], etc.) for up to 48
hours. Potentiated by alcohol and other CNS depressants. (5) Reduce dosages for the elderly and debilitated and in those with impaired liver or renal function. (6) Scopolamine increases sedation, hallucinations, and irrational behavior. (7) Rarely given IV.
Rapidly and completely absorbed IM. (8) Refrigerate,
use only freshly prepared solutions, discard if discolored or precipitate forms. (9) Patient is able to respond
to simple instructions.

Contraindications: Hypersensitivity to benzodiazepines (diazepam [Valium], chlordiazepoxide [Librium], etc.), glycols, or benzyl alcohol. Acute narrow angle glaucoma, psychoses, pregnancy and lactation, children.

Incompatible with: Limited information available. Specific incompatibilities not documented.

Side effects: Airway obstruction, apnea, blurred vision, confusion, crying, delirium, depression, excessive drowsiness, hallucinations, restlessness.

Antidote: Notify physician of all symptoms. Treatment if indicated will be supportive. In overdose, maintain an adequate airway and ventilation. Promote excretion through fluid and electrolyte administration and osmotic diuretics (mannitol, etc.). Consider hemodialysis. Physostigmine 0.5 to 4 mg at 1 mg/minute may reverse symptoms of anticholinergic overdose (confusion, etc.).

LYMPHOCYTE IMMUNE GLOBULIN

(Anti-Thymocyte Globulin [Equine], Atgam)

Usual dose: Range is 10 to 30 mg/kg of body weight/24 hr. Actual potency and activity may vary from lot to lot. Given concomitantly with other immunosuppressive therapy (antimetabolites (Azathioprine [Imuran], etc. and corticosteroids). Skin test required (see precautions).

Delay onset of renal allograft rejection: 15 mg/kg/24 hr for 14 days then every other day for seven more doses. Initial dose should be given 24 hours before or after the transplant.

Treat allograft rejection: 10 to 15 mg/kg/24 hr for 14 days then every other day for 7 more doses (optional). Initial dose should be given when first rejection episode is diagnosed.

Pediatric dose: Range is 5 to 25 mg/kg of body weight/ 24 hr.

Dilution: Total daily dose must be further diluted with 0.45% to 0.9% saline for infusion. Invert saline while injecting drug so contact is not made with air in infusion bottle. Preferred minimum concentration is 1 mg of drug/1 ml of saline infusion solution. May be infused into a vascular shunt, AV fistula, or high-flow central vein. Use of a 0.2 to 1.0 μm filter recommended.

Rate of administration: A total daily dose equally distributed over a minimum of 4 hours.

Actions: A lymphocyte selective immunosuppressant. Reduces the number of thymus-dependent lymphocytes and contains low concentrations of antibodies against other formed elements in blood. Effective without causing severe lymphopenia. Supports an increase in the frequency of resolution of an acute rejection episode.

Indications and uses: (1) Management of allograft rejection in renal transplant patients, (2) adjunctive to other immunosuppressive therapy to delay onset of initial rejection episode.

Precautions: (1) Administered only under the direction of a physician experienced in immunosuppressive therapy and management of renal transplant patients in a facility with adequate laboratory and supportive medical resources. (2) Intradermal skin test is required previous to administration. Use 0.1 ml of a 1:1,000 dilution in normal saline and a saline control. If a systemic reaction (rash, dyspnea) occurs do not administer. If a limited reaction (10 mm wheal or erythema) occurs, proceed with extreme caution. Anaphylaxis can occur even if skin test is negative. (3) Keep refrigerated before and after dilution. Discard diluted solution after 12 hours. (4) Monitor carefully for signs of leukopenia, thrombocytopenia, or infection. Notify physician immediately so prompt treatment can be instituted and/or drug discontinued. (5) Masked reactions may occur as dosage of corticosteroids and antimetabolites is decreased. Observe carefully. (6) Anaphylaxis can occur at any time. Emergency equipment and supplies must be at bedside. (7) Not recommended for use during pregnancy. (8) Use caution in repeat courses of therapy.

Contraindications: Systemic hypersensitivity reaction to previous injection of lymphocyte immune globulin or any other equine gamma globulin preparation.

Incompatible with: Should be considered incompatible in syringe or solution with any other drug or solution (except 0.45% or 0.9% saline) due to specific use. Will precipitate with 5% dextrose in water or other acid infusion solutions.

Side effects: Full range of allergic symptoms including anaphylaxis is possible. Arthralgia, back pain, chest pain, chills, clotted AV fistula, diarrhea, dyspnea, fever, headache, hypotension, infusion site pain, leukopenia, nausea, night sweats, pruritus, rash, stomatitis, thrombocytopenia, thrombophlebitis, urticaria, vomiting, wheal and flare.

Antidote: Notify physician of all side effects. Discontinue if anaphylaxis, severe and unremitting thrombocytopenia, and/or severe and unremitting leukopenia occur. May be discontinued if infection or hemolysis is present even if appropriately treated. Clinically significant hemolysis may require erythrocyte transfusion, IV mannitol, furosemide, sodium bicarbonate, and fluids. Prophylactic or therapeutic antihistamines (diphenhydramine [Benadryl], etc.) or corticosteroids should control chills caused by release of endogenous leukocyte pyrogens. Treat anaphylaxis immediately. Epinephrine (Adrenalin), diphenhydramine (Benadryl), oxygen, vasopressors (dopamine [Intropin] etc.), corticosteroids, and ventilation equipment must always be available. Resuscitate as necessary.

Usual dose: *Convulsive states:* 1 to 2 Gm (10 to 20 ml) of a 10% solution. Repeat as indicated, observing all necessary precautions.

Hypomagnesemia (severe): 4 Gm (32 mEq) to 250 ml 5% dextrose in water or saline as an infusion.

Hyperalimentation: Adults, 8 to 24 mEq/24 hr. Infants, 2 to 10 mEq/24 hr.

Dilution: May be given undiluted. May be added to IV solutions. May be given through Y tube or three-way stopcock of infusion set.

Rate of administration: *Direct IV:* 1.5 ml of a 10% solution or its equivalent over 1 minute.

IV infusion in hypomagnesemia: A single dose infused over 3 hours. Do not exceed 3 ml/minute

.Actions: A CNS depressant as well as a depressant of smooth, skeletal, and cardiac muscle. It also possesses a mild diuretic effect. Onset of action is immediate and effective for about 30 minutes. Excreted in the urine. Crosses the placental barrier.

Indications and uses: (1) Convulsive states (eclampsia, glomerulonephritis, hypoparathyroidism); (2) severe hypomagnesemia; (3) nutritional supplementation in hyperalimentation; (4) cerebral edema; (5) uterine tetany, especially after large doses of oxytocin.

Precautions: (1) Discontinue IV administration when the desired therapeutic effect is obtained. (2) Test knee jerks before each additional dose. If the knee jerk is absent, do not give additional magnesium sulfate. (3) Equipment to maintain artificial respiration must be available at all times. Patient must be continuously observed. Maintain minimum of 100 ml of urine output every 4 hours. (4) Use caution in impairment of renal function and in patients receiving digitalis. (5) Inhibits tetracycline absorption. (6) Reduce dosage of other CNS depressants (narcotics, barbiturates, etc.) when given in conjunction with magnesium sulfate. (7) Potentiates neuromuscular blocking agents (tubocurarine [Curare], etc.).

Contraindications: Presence of heart block or myocardial damage.

Incompatible with: Alcohol, alkalies, (bicarbonates, carbonates, and hydroxides), arsenates, calcium gluconate, calcium gluceptate, chlorpromazine (Thorazine), clindamycin (Cleocin), hydrocortisone (Solu-Cortef), phosphates, polymyxin B (Aerosporin), phytonadione (Aquamephyton), procaine (Novocain), salicylates, sodium bicarbonate, strontium, tartrates, tobramycin (Nebcin), vitamin B complex.

Side effects: Absence of knee jerk reflex, cardiac arrest, circulatory collapse, flushing, hypotension, respiratory depression and failure, sweating.

Antidote: Discontinue the drug and notify the physician with the occurrence of any side effect. Calcium gluconate and calcium gluceptate are specific antidotes. Employ artificial respiration as necessary and resuscitate as necessary.

MANNITOL

pH 4.5 to 7.0

(Osmitrol)

Usual dose: Very flexible. 1 to 2 Gm/kg of body weight/24 hr. Do not exceed 6 Gm in 24 hours. 1 Gm is equal to approximately 5.5 mOsm. Available as:

25% solution (12.5 Gm/50 ml) (1,375 mOsm/L)

20% solution (50 Gm/250 ml, 100 Gm/500 ml) (1,100 mOsm/L)

15% solution (22.5 Gm/150 ml, 75 Gm/500 ml) (825 mOsm/L)

10% solution (50 Gm/500 ml, 100 Gm/L) (550 mOsm/L)

5% solution (50 Gm/L) (275 mOsm/L)

Pediatric dose: 1 to 2 Gm/kg of body weight or 30 to 60 Gm/M^2 of body surface as a 15% to 20% solution.

Dilution: No further dilution is necessary; however, if there are any crystals in the solution, they must be completely dissolved before administration. Warm ampoule or bottle in hot water (to 50° C [122° F]) and shake vigorously at intervals. Cool to at least body temperature before administration. Use an in-line filter for 15%, 20%, and 25% solutions.

Rate of administration: Each 1 to 2 Gm/kg of body weight as an individual dose should be given over 30 to 90 minutes. Up to 3 Gm/kg of body weight have been given over this time span. A test dose (see precautions) or loading doses may be given over 3 to 5 minutes. *Glomerular filtration rate:* 100 ml of a 20% solution (20 Gm) diluted with 180 ml of normal saline should be infused at a rate of 20 ml/min. Collect urine samples as ordered.

Actions: A sugar alcohol and most effective osmotic diuretic. It is a stable, inert, and nontoxic solution. Distribution in the body is limited to extracellular compartments. Mannitol is not reabsorbed by the tubules of the kidneys. It is excreted almost completely in the urine along with water. Reduction in cerebrospinal and intraocular fluid occurs within 15 minutes and lasts 4 to 8 hours. Rebound may occur within 12 hours.

Indications and uses: (1) Reduction of intracranial pressure and brain mass, (2) reduction of extremely high intraocular pressure, (3) treatment of oliguria resulting from transfusion reactions, (4) promotion of excretion of toxic substances from sedative overdose, (5) kidney function test (glomerular filtration, (6) reduction of generalized edema and ascites, (7) oliguric phase of acute renal failure, (8) (2.5% solution) irrigation in transurethral prostatic resection, (9) to prevent hemolysis and hemoglobin buildup in cardiopulmonary bypass procedures.

Precautions: (1) Use only freshly prepared solutions. Discard unused portions. (2) Test dose should be used in patients with impaired renal functions. Give 200 mg/kg of body weight over 3 to 5 minutes. 40 ml of urine should be produced in 1 hour. (3) Observe urine output continuously; should exceed 30 to 50 ml/hr. Insert Foley catheter if necessary. (4) Electrolyte depletion may occur. Check with laboratory studies and replace as necessary. (5) Observe infusion site to prevent infiltration. (6) May cause deafness with kanamycin. (7) Calcium disodium edetate will increase the amount of mannitol absorbed, an undesirable effect. (8) Maintain hydration; may obscure signs of inadequate hydration or hypovolemia. (9) Reduce dose by one half for small or debilitated patients. (10) Evaluate cardiac status to avoid fulminating congestive heart failure.

Contraindications: Anuria; edema associated with capillary fragility of membrane permeability; fluid and electrolyte depletion, some cases of metabolic edema; pregnancy; severe congestive heart failure; severe dehydration; severe renal impairment.

Incompatible with: Whole blood. If mannitol must be given in conjunction with whole blood, add 20 mEq of sodium chloride to each 1,000 ml to avoid pseudoagglutination. Should be considered incompatible in syringe or solution with any other drug or infusion.

Side effects: Rare when used as directed but may include backache, blurred vision, chest pain, chills, convulsions, decreased chloride levels, decreased sodium levels, dehydration, diuresis, dizziness, dryness of mouth, edema, fever, headache, hypertension, hypotension, nausea, pulmonary edema, rhinitis, tachycardia, thirst, thrombophlebitis, urinary retention.

Antidote: If side effects persist or if urine output is under 30 to 50 ml/hr, discontinue the drug and notify the physician.

MECHLORETHAMINE HYDROCHLORIDE

pH 3.0 to 5.0

(Mustargen, nitrogen mustard)

Usual dose: 0.4 mg/kg of body weight as a single dose is preferred or may be divided into 2 to 4 equal doses and given daily for 2 to 4 days. Allow about 3 to 6 weeks between courses of therapy. Confirm bone marrow recovery. Results with subsequent courses are rarely as satisfactory as the initial course.

Dilution: *Specific techniques required, see precautions.* Wear disposable mask, gown, and gloves for mixing. Safety glasses are appropriate. Dilute each 10 mg vial with 10 ml of sterile water or sodium chloride for injection. Do not remove needle and syringe. Hold securely and shake vial to dissolve completely. Withdraw desired dose. Contains 1 mg/ml. May be given direct IV, but administration through a Y tube or three-way stopcock of a free-flowing infusion is preferred.

Rate of administration: Total daily dose equally distributed over 3 to 5 minutes.

Actions: An alkylating agent, cell cycle phase nonspecific, with antitumor activity. It has a selective cytotoxic effect on rapidly growing cells. Palliative, not curative, in its effects; regression in the size of malignant tumor may occur; pain and fever subside; appetite, strength, and a sense of well-being are increased. Immediately absorbed and metabolized, it is excreted in changed form in the urine.

Indications and uses: To suppress or retard neoplastic growth. Good response is inconsistent but has been experienced in Hodgkin's disease, lymphosarcoma, bronchogenic carcinoma, specific types of chronic leukemia, polcythemia vera, and mycosis fungoides. Used in generalized metastasis and in patients refractory to radiation therapy.

Precautions: (1) Follow guidelines for handling cytotoxic agents recommended by the National Study Commission on Cytotoxic Exposure (see Appendix, p. 528). (2) Usually administered in the hospital by or under the direction of the physician specialist. (3) Highly toxic; must not be inhaled or come into contact with skin or any mucous membrane, especially the eyes, at any stage of mixing, administration, or destruction. For accidental contact, copious irrigation with water for at least 15 minutes is indicated. Follow with rinse of 2% sodium thiosulfate. Use an isotonic ophthalmic irrigation solution to irrigate if eye contamination occurs. (4) Dosage based on average weight in presence of edema or ascites. (5) Mix solution immediately before use. Very unstable. Neutralize unused portion with equal volume sodium thiosulfate–sodium bicarbonate solution and let stand 45 minutes. Then discard. (6) Do not use if solution is discolored or if droplets of water remain isolated in the vial. (7) Extremely narrow margin of safety; dosage is individual, and frequent blood examinations are mandatory. (8) Use precaution with radiation therapy, other chemotherapy, severe leukopenia, thrombocytopenia, anemia, and bone marrow infiltrated with malignant cells. (9) May produce teratogenic effects on the fetus. Has mutagenic potential. Give with caution in men and women capable of conception. (10) Alkylating agents interact with numerous drugs such as amphotericin B (Fungizone), radiation therapy, other antineoplastics, and many others to produce serious reaction. (11) Extravasation into surrounding tissue can cause sloughing and possible necrosis. (12) Often given in the late evening with antiemetics and sedatives to promote patient comfort. (13) Used in reduced doses with other chemotherapeutic agents to produce tumor remission. (14) Maintain adequate hydration. (15) Allopurinol may prevent formation of uric acid crystals. (16) Do not administer any vaccine or chloroquine to patients receiving antineoplastic drugs. (17) Observe closely for all signs of infection. (18) Specific tissue can be protected from the effects of this agent by temporary interruption of its blood supply during and immediately after injection.

Contraindications: Not recommended in terminal stages of malignancy or in leukemia with coexistent infectious granuloma.

Incompatible with: Any other drug in syringe or solution.

Side effects: Alopecia, anorexia, bleeding, bone marrow depression, cerebrovascular accidents, delayed catamenia, depression of formed elements in circulating blood, diarrhea, hemolytic anemia, hyperuricemia, jaundice, leukopenia, nausea, petechiae, sloughing, susceptibility to infection, tinnitus, thrombophlebitis, vertigo, vomiting, weakness, death.

Antidote: (1) For external contact and cleaning purposes, use a 2% sodium thiosulfate solution. (2) To prevent sloughing and necrosis in areas where extravasation has occurred, inject isotonic sodium thiosulfate with a fine hypodermic needle into the indurated area. Apply ice compress. (3) Use chlorpromazine (Thorazine) or other phenothiazides to control nausea and sodium pentobarbital (Nembutal) to produce sedation. (4) Notify physician of any side effect. Discontinue the drug and use supportive therapy, including blood transfusion, as necessary to sustain the patient in toxicity.

MENADIOL SODIUM
DIPHOSPHATE

(Kappadione, Synkayvite, vitamin K₄)

Usual dose: 5 to 15 mg once or twice every 24 hours.

Pediatric dose: 5 to 10 mg once or twice every 24 hours.

Infant dose: 1 to 5 mg for one dose only (phytonadione is preferred).

Dilution: May be given undiluted or added to most infusion solutions.

Rate of administration: Each dose over 1 minute in undiluted form.

Actions: Menadiol is a synthetic, water-soluble vitamin essential for the production of prothrombin by the liver. Hemorrhage will occur in its absence. Rapidly absorbed and utilized; prothrombin time should be elevated within 12 to 18 hours. One third as potent as menadione. Metabolized completely by the body.

Indications and uses: (1) Prevention and treatment of hypoprothrombinemia secondary to deficient absorption from biliary disease, intestinal disease, surgical resection, or after large doses or long-term use of some medications such as salicylates, quinine, sulfonamides, arsenicals, barbiturates, antibiotics, and dicumarol; (2) liver function test.

Precautions: (1) Phytonadione is the drug of choice for impending or actual hemorrhage because of its rapid action. (2) Menadiol is not commonly administered by the IV route. IM or subcutaneous administration provides adequate absorption at a slower rate. (3) Dosage and effects are determined by prothrombin times. Keep physician informed. (4) Use with caution in premature infants; excessive bilirubin levels have occurred. (5) Supplement with whole blood transfusion if necessary. (6) Protect from light. (7) May promote temporary resistance to prothrombin-depressing anticoagulants.

Contraindications: Hemorrhagic disease not caused by prothrombin deficiency and severe nonfunctioning liver disease; last trimester of pregnancy.

Incompatible with: Alkaloids, codeine, levarterenol (Levophed), levorphanol (Levo-Dromoran), meperidine

295

(Demerol), metals, methadone, mineral acids, procaine (Novocain).

Side effects: Rare when used as recommended: allergic reactions such as skin rash; anaphylaxis; cyanosis; depressed liver function; diaphoresis; dizziness; dyspnea; erythrocyte hemolysis; flushing sensation; hypotension; shock; tachycardia.

Antidote: Discontinue the drug and notify the physician of any side effects. Physician may choose to continue drug at as decreased rate of administration. Treat allergic reactions as necessary.

MEPERIDINE HYDROCHLORIDE   pH 3.5 to 6.0
(Demerol)

Usual dose: 10 to 50 mg. Repeat every 2 to 4 hours as necessary.

Pediatric dose: Not recommended for IV use in children.

Dilution: Must be diluted. Use at least 5 ml of sterile water or normal saline for injection or other IV solutions. Sometimes diluted in IV fluids to a dilution of 1 mg/ml and given as a continuous infusion under the direct observation and control of the anesthesiologist.

Rate of administration: 25 mg or fraction thereof over 1 minute. Frequently titrated according to symptom relief and respiratory rate.

Actions: A synthetic narcotic analgesic and descending CNS depressant, similar to but slightly less potent than morphine. Onset of action occurs in about 5 minutes and lasts for about 2 hours. Pain threshold is elevated, and the reaction of the individual to the painful experience is altered. Crosses the placental barrier. Readily absorbed and distributed throughout the body, metabolized in the liver, and excreted in the urine.

Indications and uses: (1) Relief of most moderate to severe pain, (2) preoperative medication, (3) support of anesthesia, (4) obstetrical analgesia.

Precautions: (1) Oxygen and controlled respiratory equipment must always be available. (2) Observe patient frequently and monitor vital signs. (3) Use with caution in glaucoma, head injuries, increased intracranial pressure (elevates spinal fluid pressure), asthma, chronic obstructive pulmonary disease, decreased respiratory reserve or respiratory depression, supraventricular tachycardia, convulsions, acute abdominal conditions previous to diagnosis, the elderly and debilitated, and hepatic or renal insufficiency. (4) Morphine is usually preferred for pain during cardiac arrhythmias. (5) Physical dependence can develop with abuse. (6) IM route frequently used. (7) Potentiated by antacids, anticholinergics, cimetidine (Tagamet), tricyclic antidepressants (amitriptyline [Elavil], etc.), MAO inhibitors (isocarboxazid [Marplan], etc.), isoniazid, neostigmine (Prostigmin), neuromuscular blocking agents, (tubocurarine etc.), oral contraceptives, phenothiazines (promazine [Sparine], etc.), general anesthetics, other narcotic analgesics, and CNS depressants including alcohol. Reduced dosage of both drugs may be indicated.

Contraindications: Hypersensitivity to merperidine; do *not* use for patients who have received MAO inhibitors (isocarboxazid [Marplan], etc.) in the previous 2 weeks; pregnancy prior to labor; lactation.

Incompatible with: Aminophylline, amobarbital (Amytal), furosemide (Lasix), heparin, hydrocortisone sodium succinate (Solu-Cortef), methicillin (Staphcillin), methylprednisolone (Solu-Medrol), morphine, nitrofurantoin (Ivadantin), pentobarbital (Nembutal), phenobarbital (Luminal), phenytoin (Dilantin), secobarbital (Seconal), sodium bicarbonate, sodium iodide, sulfisoxazole (Gantrisin), thiopental (Pentothal).

Side effects: *Minor:* dizziness, flushing, light-headedness, nausea, postural hypotension, rash, restlessness, sedation, sweating, syncope, vomiting. *Major:* allergic reactions, apnea, cardiac arrest, cardiovascular collapse, cold and clammy skin, convulsions, dilated pupils, respiratory depression, shock, tremor.

Antidote: With increasing severity of minor side effects or onset of any major side effect, discontinue the drug and notify the physician. Naloxone hydrochloride (Narcan) or levallorphan tartrate (Lorfan) will reverse serious respiratory depression. A patent airway, artificial ventilation, oxygen therapy, and other symptomatic treatment must be instituted promptly. Resuscitate as necessary.

(Wyamine)

Usual dose: 15 to 60 mg as the initial dose. May be followed by repeat doses of 15 to 45 mg as indicated. At
the same time a continuous infusion of 1 mg/ml may
be given. Dosage requirements are dependent on patient response. 0.5 to 1 mg/kg of body weight should
effect response in most hypotensive states. Up to 3
mg/kg of body weight may be required.

Dilution: May be given undiluted or may be diluted in
5% dextrose in water and given as an infusion. Add
600 mg to 500 ml of diluent to deliver approximately
1 mg/ml.

Rate of administration: Undiluted, each 30 mg or fraction
thereof over 1 minute. Infusion rate is more easily
regulated with a microdrip (60 gtt/ml) or an infusion
pump. Rate will be determined by patient response.

Actions: A potent vasopressor similar to ephedrine. Has
positive inotropic and chronotropic effects. Initial
pressor effect results from increased mycardial contractility and enhancement by increased peripheral
vasoconstriction and resistance. Its use in cardiac arrhythmias results from a decreased atrioventricular
conduction time, a decreased refractory period of the
atrium, and a decreased conduction time in ventricular muscle. It has some CNS stimulation similar to
that of amphetamines and increases cerebral oxygen
utilization. Effective within 1 to 2 minutes for a period
of 1 to 2 hours. After metabolism, it is excreted in the
urine.

Indications and uses: (1) May be used prophylactically
or as a treatment for hypotensive states not associated
with hemorrhage, such as myocardial infarction; (2)
surgical, postoperative, obstetrical, and spinal anesthesia; (3) hypotension secondary to ganglionic blockade.

Precautions: (1) Check blood pressure every 2 minutes
until stabilized at the desired level. Check every 5
minutes thereafter during therapy. (2) Discontinue the
medication temporarily after patient's condition and
blood pressure are stabilized. Restart as necessary un-

til stabilization occurs. (3) If pressor action is not effective, short-term therapy with levarterenol (norepinephrine) may restore the catecholamine sites necessary to make it effective. (4) Diluted infusion may be used to maintain blood pressure in shock caused by hemorrhage until whole blood replacement is begun. (5) Use with care in known hypertensive patients and with cyclopropane or halothane anesthesia. (6) Potentiated or inhibited depending on timing of interaction by guanethidine (Ismelin), methyldopa (Aldomet), rauwolfia alkaloids (Reserpine, etc.), and others. (7) Potentiated by MAO inhibitors (pargyline [Eutonyl], etc.). Hypertensive crisis may result. (8) May cause severe hypertension or stroke with ergot alkaloids. (9) May cause hypotension and bradycardia with hydantoins (phenytoin [Dilantin], etc.).

Contraindications: Do not use to treat overdosage of phenothiazines (chlorpromazine [Thorazine], etc.). A further drop in blood pressure will occur, and irreversible shock may result. Known sensitivity to mephentermine.

Incompatible with: Epinephrine (Adrenalin), hydralazine (Apresoline).

Side effects: Usually minimal: anorexia, anxiety, hypertension, nervousness. Cardiac arrhythmias are possible.

Antidote: No reports of toxic reactions. Notify the physician if CNS stimulation seems excessive. Discontinue drug and notify the physician for hypertension.

MERSALYL AND THEOPHYLLINE

(Foyuretic, Mercutheolin, Mersa, Mersalyn, Theo-Syl-R)

Usual dose: 0.5 ml as initial dose. If no side effects occur and some diuresis is effected, 0.5 to 1.0 ml may be given every 24 hours or every other day. 1 to 2 ml twice weekly is preferred.

Pediatric dose: One half the recommended adult dose.

Dilution: Dilute with 5 to 10 ml of sterile water for injection. Do not add to IV solutions. May be given through Y tube or three-way stopcock of infusion set.

Rate of administration: 0.5 ml of actual medication or fraction thereof over 2 minutes. To deliver a small dose over an extended period of time, use of a small-gauge needle is recommended.

Actions: A potent mercurial diuretic combined with theophylline for prompt absorption. Release of mercury ions irritates renal tubular cells, preventing reabsorption of sodium, chlorides, and water. Effectiveness is enhanced by an acid pH. Edema is relieved. Potassium loss does occur but to a lesser degree than with some other diuretics. 95% is excreted in the urine in 24 hours. Urine output in 24 hours may reach 8 or 9 liters after the initial effective dose.

Indications and uses: Treatment of edema and ascites in (1) cardiac and cardiorenal diseases, (2) nephrosis, (3) cirrhosis of the liver, (4) thrombophlebitic and thyrocardiac edema.

Precautions: (1) Monitor the patient's EKG; IV administration will cause severe cardiac reactions and sudden death. IM route is preferred unless absorption capacity will be severely inhibited. (2) Discontinue use of drug if diuresis is not effected by a dose of 2 ml. (3) Routine checks on electrolyte panel, CO_2, BUN, and urine specific gravity are necessary during therapy. Sodium and potassium chloride replacement may be required. (4) May cause cardiac arrhythmias with digitalis because of potassium depletion. (5) Use extreme care and smaller doses for patients with myocardial infarction and for the elderly, especially those with any urological disease or renal or hepatic insufficiency. (6) Prevent extravasation into surrounding tissue. Sloughing and necrosis will occur. An IV site at or below the bend of the elbow is preferred. (7) Potentiated by urinary acidifying agents (ammonium chloride, etc.) and ethacrynic acid (Edecrin). (8) Inhibited by analgesics and alkalinizing agents.

Contraindications: Acute nephritis; chronic kidney disease with nitrogen retention or urine of fixed specific gravity; known hypersensitivity to mercury; pregnancy and lactation; severe liver disease, ulcerative colitis.

Incompatible with: Any other medication in a syringe because of the potential for toxicity.

Side effects: *Minor:* cutaneous eruptions, dehydration, diarrhea, fever, flushing, gingivitis, hematuria, increased salivation, muscle cramps, nausea, stomatitis, vertigo, vomiting. *Major:* alkalosis, blood volume reduction, circulatory collapse, cyanosis, dyspnea, excessive diuresis, hypokalemia, nephrotoxicity, sudden hypotension, thrombophlebitis, vascular thrombosis, ventricular arrhythmias, death.

Antidote: If any side effects occur, discontinue drug and notify physician. Treat emergency situations symptomatically and resuscitate as necessary. Dimercaprol (BAL) given IM will help to reduce acute toxicity.

METARAMINOL BITARTRATE

pH 3.5 to 4.5

(Aramine)

Usual dose: 0.5 to 5.0 mg direct IV only in an extreme emergency. 15 to 100 mg in 500 ml of specific infusion solution. 150 to 500 mg/500 ml of infusion solution has been used at an extremely slow rate. Adjust to desired clinical fluid volume.

Pediatric dose: 0.01 mg/kg of body weight as a single dose or as a solution of 1 mg/25 ml in dextrose or saline for infusion.

Dilution: Single dose up to 5 mg may be given undiluted. Should be diluted in at least 500 ml of sodium chloride or 5% dextrose and administered as an IV infusion.

Rate of administration: Direct IV administration, 5 mg or fraction thereof over 1 minute. In solution use slowest possible flow rate to correct hypotension gradually and maintain adequate or preset blood pressure. Use of a microdrip (60 gtt/ml) or an infusion pump is helpful.

Actions: A potent vasopressor but less potent than levarterenol. Produces gradual action with long effect. It constricts blood vessels, increases peripheral resistance, and elevates systolic and diastolic pressure. Increases cardiac contractility and cerebral, coronary, and renal blood flow. Inactivated in the body and excreted in the urine. Effective within 1 to 2 minutes. Maximum effect may take 10 minutes and last 20 minutes to 1 hour.

Indications and uses: Acute hypotensive states resulting from anesthesia, hemorrhage, medication reaction, cardiogenic shock, surgical complications, trauma, septicemia, and shock, with brain damage owing to trauma or tumor.

Precautions: (1) Check blood pressure every 5 minutes until stabilized at the desired level. Check every 15 minutes thereafter throughout therapy. (2) Hypovolemia must be corrected to receive adequate response. (3) Whole blood or plasma should be given in a separate IV site. (4) Avoid hypertension; cardiac arrest may result. (5) Discontinue IV administration if vein infiltrates or is thrombosed; can result in tissue necrosis and sloughing. (6) Cumulative effect is possible. Hypertension may remain even after drug is discontinued. (7) MAO inhibitors and tricyclic antidepressants potentiate metaraminol and can cause an acute hypertensive crisis with brain hemorrhage. (8) Use care in liver, heart, and thyroid disease and in hypertension or diabetes. (9) May cause a relapse of malaria. (10) May cause severe hypertension and stroke with ergot alkaloids. (11) May cause arrhythmias with digitalis. (12) May cause hypotension and bradycardia with hydantoins (phenytoin [Dilantin], etc.).

Contraindications: Do not use with cyclopropane or halothane anesthesia.

Incompatible with: Amphotericin B (Fungizone), ampicillin, cephalothin (Keflin), dexamethasone (Decadron), erythromycin (Erythrocin), heparin, hydrocortisone phosphate, hydrocortisone (Solu-Cortef), invert sugar, lactated Ringer's injection, levarterenol (Levophed), methicillin (Staphcillin), methylprednisolone (Solu-Medrol), nitrofurantoin (Ivadantin), oxacillin (Prostaphlin), oxytetracycline (Terramycin), penicillin G potassium or sodium, pentobarbital (Nembutal), phenytoin (Dilantin), prednisolone (Hydeltrasol), Ringer's injection, sodium bicarbonate, sodium lactate injection, sulfisoxazole (Gantrisin), thiopental (Pentothal, warfarin (Coumadin), whole blood.

Side effects: May occur with average doses in some persons: cardiac arrest, cardiac arrhythmias, dizziness, headache, hypertension, nervousness, tachycardia.

Antidote: Notify the physician of any side effects. Most will be treated symptomatically, or dosage of metaraminol will be decreased. Should a sudden or uncontrolled hypertensive state occur, discontinue metarminol, notify the physician, and treat with antihypertensive agents such as nitroprusside (Nipride) or phentolamine (Regitine). Resuscitate as necessary. To prevent sloughing and necrosis in areas where extravasation has occurred, inject 5 to 10 mg of phentolamine diluted in 10 to 15 ml of normal saline liberally throughout the tissue in the extravasated area with a fine hypodermic needle.

METHICILLIN SODIUM

(Celbenin, Staphcillin)

Usual dose: Over 40 kg: 1 Gm every 4 to 6 hours. Under 40 kg: 25 mg/kg of body weight every 4 to 6 hours. Do not exceed adult dose.

Dilution: Each 1 Gm vial is diluted with 1.8 ml of sterile water for injection (4 Gm vial with 5.7 ml, 6 Gm vial with 8.6 ml). Each 1 ml equals 500 mg. Further dilute each 500 mg (1 ml) with a minimum of 25 ml of sodium chloride for injection. May be administered directly IV, through an additive infusion set, or added to specific IV solutions such as isotonic sodium chloride, 5% dextrose in water or normal saline, lactated Ringer's injection, and others (see literature) and given as an infusion over not more than 8 hours. Diluted concentrations of 2 mg/ml are stable for 4 hours, 10 to 30 mg/ml for 8 hours.

Rate of administration: Each 10 ml of properly diluted medication or fraction thereof over 1 minute or longer to avoid vein irritation. Infusion rate of a single dose can be from 30 minutes to 8 hours.

Actions: A semisynthetic penicillin primarily used for its bactericidal action against penicillinase-producing staphylococci. Appears in all body fluids. Absorption into spinal fluid is minimal unless inflammation is present. Excreted in the urine. Excreted in breast milk.

Indications and uses: Severe infections caused by penicillinase-producing staphylococci.

Precautions: (1) Sensitivity studies are necessary to determine the susceptibility of the causative organism to methicillin sodium. Sometimes difficult to determine accurately. (2) Watch for early symptoms of allergic reaction. Individuals with a history of allergic problems are more susceptible to untoward reactions. (3) Avoid prolonged use of this drug; superinfection caused by overgrowth of nonsusceptible organisms may result. (4) Initial solution is stable for 24 hours; stable for 4 days if refrigerated. (5) Renal, hepatic, and hematopoietic function should be checked during long-term therapy. (6) Use caution for infants. Abnormal blood levels may appear because of undeveloped renal function. (7) Inhibited by chloramphenicol, erythromycin, and tetracyclines. Bactericidal action is actually negated by these drugs. (8) Potentiated by aminohippuric acid and probenecid (Benemid). Toxicity may result. (9) May cause thrombophlebitis, especially with too-rapid injection. (10) Inhibits aminoglycosides (gentamicin, etc.).

Contraindications: Known hypersensitivity to any penicillin or cephalothin, and pregnancy.

Incompatible with: Manufacturer recommends: do not use as an additive with any other drug. Do not mix in any solutions other than those specifically recommended. Do not administer into IV tubing if solution is not recommended. Aminophylline, ascorbic acid, cephalothin (Keflin), chloramphenicol, chlorpromazine (Thorazine), codeine, hydrocortisone sodium succinate (Solu-Cortef), levorphanol (Levo-Dromoran), lincomycin (Lincocin), metaraminol (Aramine), methadone, methohexital (Brevital), morphine, oxytetracycline (Terramycin), promethazine (Phenergan), sodium bicarbonate, sulfisoxazole, tetracycline (Achromycin), vancomycin, vitamin B complex.

Side effects: Primarily hypersensitivity reactions such as anaphylaxis, serum sickness, skin rashes, urticaria. Anemia, eosinophilia, fever, glossitis, monilia (oral and rectal), neutropenia, nephrotoxicity, and stomatitis have been reported.

Antidote: Notify the physician of any side effect. For allergic symptoms, discontinue the drug, treat allergic reaction as indicated or resuscitate as necessary, and notify the physician.

METHOCARBAMOL

(Robaxin)

Usual dose: 1 Gm (10 ml) every 8 hours for no more than 3 days. Not recommended for children under 12 years of age except in tetanus. In tetanus treatment, dosage may be as high as 3 Gm every 6 hours.

Pediatric dose: *In tetanus:* 15 mg/kg of body weight initially. Repeat every 6 hours as indicated.

Dilution: May be given undiluted, or a single dose may be given as an IV infusion diluted in no more than 250 ml of isotonic sodium chloride or 5% dextrose solution.

Rate of administration: 300 mg (3 ml) or fraction thereof over 1 minute.

Actions: A skeletal muscle depressant that acts as an interneuronal blocking agent. Diminishes skeletal muscle hyperactivity without altering normal muscle tone. Well absorbed and distributed throughout the body. Concentration of the drug is higher in the brain than in plasma. Metabolized in the liver and excreted in the urine.

Indications and uses: (1) Acute neuromusculoskeletal injury; (2) acute exacerbation of chronic musculoskeletal disorders; (3) acute exacerbations of chronic neurological disorders; (4) orthopedic, gynecological, and dental surgery; (5) convulsive states caused by strychnine poisoning, tetanus, black widow spider bite, lead poisoning, opiate withdrawal, acute alcoholism, and phenothiazine reactions.

Precautions: (1) Observe site of injection continuously. A hypertonic solution; extravasation may cause thrombophlebitis or sloughing. (2) Blood aspirated into syringe will not mix with medication—an expected phenomenon. (3) Keep patient in recumbent position for at least 15 minutes to avoid postural hypotension. (4) Do not refrigerate after dilution. (5) Use caution in known or suspected epileptic patients. (6) Maintenance doses should be oral even if the pills are crushed and given through a nasogastric tube. (7) Potentiated by alcohol, CNS depressants, MAO inhibitors (paragyline [Eutonyl], etc.), and phenothiazines (chlorpromazine [Thorazine], etc.). (8) May interfere with some laboratory tests (5HIAA, VMA).

Contraindications: Hypersensitivity to methocarbamol, known or suspected renal pathology, pregnancy, and lactation. Do not use in conjunction with propoxyphene (Darvon).

Incompatible with: Physically compatible with many drugs. Sufficient information not available. Note precautions and contraindications.

Side effects: Infrequent but more often associated with too-rapid injection or an acute alcoholic state. *Minor:* blurred vision, conjunctivitis, diplopia, dizziness, drowsiness, fainting, fever, flushing, headache, hypotension, gastrointestinal upset, light-headedness, metallic taste, muscular incoordination, nystagmus, pruritus, rash, urticaria, vertigo. *Major:* anaphylactic reaction, bradycardia, convulsions, pain at injection site, sloughing at injection site, syncope, thrombophlebitis.

Antidote: Notify the physician of minor side effects. If these side effects progress or major side effects occur, discontinue the drug, notify the physician, and treat symptomatically. Epinephrine, steroids, and antihistamines should be readily available. Resuscitate as necessary.

METHOTREXATE

(Amethopterin)

Usual dose: *Choriocarcinoma:* 15 to 30 mg/24 hr for 5 days. Repeat course of therapy after 7 to 12 days unless toxicity contraindicates it.

Leukemia: 3.3 mg/M² daily with prednisone 60 mg/M². Give three to six times weekly if tolerated, and continue for up to 8 weeks or until satisfactory response. Dosage range varies, depending on the malignancy being treated, age of the patient, toxicity, and response, Massive doses (3 to 7.5 Gm/M²) are being used more frequently with leucovorin rescue. Highly individualized, requires exacting calculations. Maintenance dose also individualized; 2.5 mg/kg of body weight every 14 days has been utilized.

Psoriasis: 10 to 25 mg once a week. Do not exceed 50 mg. Use smallest effective dose.

Dilution: *Specific techniques required, see precautions.* Reconstitute each 5 mg with 2 ml of sterile water for injection. Each milliliter will equal 2.5 mg of methotrexate. Do not add to IV solutions. May be given through Y tube or three-way stopcock of a free-flowing IV.

Rate of administration: Each 10 mg or fraction thereof over 1 minute.

Actions: An antimetabolite and folic acid antagonist. Cell cycle specific for the S phase, it interrupts the mitotic process during nucleic acid synthesis. Rapidly proliferating malignant cells are inhibited by a cytostatic effect. Readily absorbed and widely distributed, methotrexate is excreted unchanged in the urine within 6 hours.

Indications and uses: (1) To suppress or retard neoplastic growth in uterine choriocarcinoma, acute lymphocytic leukemia, mycosis fungoides, osteogenic sarcoma, and malignancies of the breast, testis, head, neck, and lung; (2) mycosis fungoides; (3) psoriasis.

Precautions: (1) Follow guidelines for handling cytotoxic agents recommended by the National Study Commission on Cytotoxic Exposure (see Appendix, p. 528).

(2) Usually administered in the hospital by or under the direction of the physician specialist. Close patient observation is mandatory. Course of therapy is not repeated until all signs of toxicity from the previous course subside. (3) Discard solution if a precipitate forms. (4) Stable at room temperature for 2 weeks. (5) Complete blood cell counts and bone marrow biopsies are essential to comprehensive treatment. (6) Use with caution during infection or impaired renal or liver function. (7) Often used with other antineoplastic drugs in reduced doses to achieve tumor remission. (8) Methotrexate interacts with numerous drugs such as antidiabetics, barbiturates, corticosteroids, other antineoplastics, and others to produce potentially serious reactions. (9) The following drugs may be toxic when administered concomitantly with methotrexate: alcohol, antibacterials, probenecid, salicylates, barbiturates, any hepatotoxic drug, sulfonamides, tranquilizers, para-aminobenzoic acid (PABA), and phenytoin (Dilantin). Vitamins with folic acid may alter response to methotrexate. (10) May produce teratogenic effects on the fetus. Has mutagenic potential. (11) Maintain adequate hydration. (12) Do not administer any vaccine or chloroquine to patients receiving antineoplastic drugs. (13) Utilize prophylactic antiemetics to reduce nausea and vomiting and increase patient comfort.

Contraindications: Not absolute, but methotrexate is not recommended during pregnancy or with hepatic, renal, or bone marrow damage.

Incompatible with: Limited information available. Note precautions and contraindications. Fluorouracil, prednisolone (Hydeltrasol).

Side effects: Acne, alopecia (occasional), chills, cystitis, depigmentation, diabetes, diarrhea, enteritis, fever, gastrointestinal ulceration, gingivitis, hematological depression, hemorrhage from any site, hepatotoxicity, menstrual dysfunction, nausea, oral ulceration, pharyngitis, pruritus, rash, septicemia, stomatitis, urticaria, vomiting.

Antidote: *Citrovorum factor, folinic acid (leucovorin)* may be given **IM** or **IV** promptly to counteract inadvertent overdosage (IV route is not FDA approved but in common use). Doses equal to dose of methotrexate are frequently required. Should be given within 1 hour. Repeat every 4 to 6 hours four times. Citrovorum factor IV and IM is also indicated as a planned rescue mechanism for large doses of methotrexate required to treat some malignancies. Discontinue methotrexate and notify the physician of any side effects. Death may occur from the progression of most of these side effects. Symptomatic and supportive therapy is indicated.

METHOXAMINE
HYDROCHLORIDE pH 3.0 to 5.0

(Vasoxyl)

Usual dose: 3 to 5 mg initially. May repeat after at least 15 minutes. Follow with continuous or intermittent IV drip or administer IM. One dose of 10 mg is indicated in paroxysmal supraventricular tachycardia.

Dilution: May be given undiluted or may be given as IV infusion by diluting 40 mg of methoxamine in 250 ml of 5% dextrose in water.

Rate of administration: Each 5 mg or fraction thereof over 1 minute. Begin with 5 ml of infusion/min (approximately 1 mg of methoxamine/6 ml). Use the slowest possible flow rate to correct hypotension gradually and maintain adequate or preset blood pressure. Use of a microdrip (60 gtt/ml) or an infusion pump will aid correct evaluation of dosage.

Actions: A potent vasopressor because of peripheral vasoconstriction. Unique in that it does not produce undesired cardiac or CNS stimulation. Cardiac output is slightly reduced because of reflex bradycardia, but central venous pressure and both systolic and diastolic blood pressure are elevated. Renal vessels will be constricted. Onset of action of a single dose is instantaneous and lasts about 1 hour. Widely distributed in body fluids, excreted in the urine.

Indications and uses: (1) Prevention and treatment of hypotension during anesthesia. May be used during most anesthesia including inhalant anesthesia (cyclopropane, etc.) and spinal anesthesia. (2) Shock caused by traumatic, surgical, or medical conditions including myocardial infarction, and drug reactions when cardiac stimulus is contraindicated. (3) Prompt termination of episodes of paroxysmal supraventricular tachycardia.

Precautions: (1) IM injection is preferred. IV administration is for emergencies only and indicated only if systolic blood pressure is 60 mm Hg or less. (2) Discontinue IV administration if vein infiltrates or is thrombosed; can result in tissue necrosis and sloughing. (3) Keep in refrigerator. (4) Check blood pressure every

2 minutes until stabilized at the desired level. Check every 5 minutes thereafter during therapy. Avoid hypertension. (5) Replace blood, plasma, fluids, and electrolytes as necessary in hypovolemic shock. Use Y tube or three-way stopcock with blood. (6) May cause severe hypertension after administration of ergot alkaloids. (7) Use care in hyperthyroidism, with known hypertensive patients, and during halothane anesthesia. (8) Potentiated by MAO inhibitors (isocarboxazid [Marplan], etc.), thyroid preparations, and tricyclic antidepressants. (9) Capable of many interactions with other drugs; however, these may be slightly less serious because of lack of myocardial stimulation.

Contraindications: Do not use in combination with local anesthetics for tissue infiltration to prolong action.

Incompatible with: Limited information available. Note precautions and contraindications. Chemical composition is similar to that of ephedrine, metaraminol, and mephentermine. Alkaline compounds.

Side effects: Rare unless very high dosage is used: bradycardia, headache, hypertension, projectile vomiting, urinary urgency.

Antidote: Atropine may be used to counteract the bradycardia. Notify the physician of any side effect. Should a sudden or uncontrolled hypertensive state occur, discontinue methoxamine, notify the physician, and treat with antihypertensive agents such as nitroprusside (Nipride) or phentolamine (Regitine). Resuscitate as necessary. To prevent sloughing and necrosis in areas where extravasation has occurred, inject 5 to 10 mg of phentolamine diluted in 10 to 15 ml of normal saline liberally throughout the tissue in the extravasated area with a fine hypodermic needle.

METHYLDOPATE
HYDROCHLORIDE

pH 3.5 to 4.2

(Aldomet)

Usual dose: 250 to 500 mg every 6 hours. Up to 1 Gm every 6 hours is acceptable. Maintain with oral medication in same dosage as soon as practical.

Pediatric dose: 20 to 40 mg/kg of body weight/24 hr in divided doses every 6 hours. Maximum dose is 65 mg/kg or 3 Gm, whichever is less.

Dilution: Single dose is diluted in 100 to 200 ml of 5% dextrose in water and given as an infusion.

Actions: A moderate antihypertensive drug, it lowers the blood pressure by replacing norepinephrine in the body with methylnorepinephrine, producing decreased sympathetic activity. Lowers peripheral and renal vascular resistance. Readily permeates brain tissue but does not affect cardiac output. Maximum action does not occur for 2 to 3 hours but lasts 10 hours. Some excretion through the urine. Crosses placental barrier and is excreted in breast milk.

Indications and uses: Hypertensive crises, especially for patients with renal or coronary insufficiency.

Precautions: (1) Check blood pressure every 30 minutes until stabilized at desired level. Slow response lessens usefulness. (2) More effective when combined with diuretics. (3) Liver function tests and complete blood cell count are indicated. (4) Causes false elevated urinary catecholamine response. (5) Observe for adequate urine output. Use caution in impaired liver and renal function, pregnancy, and lactation. (6) Potentiated by MAO inhibitors, CNS depressants (alcohol, anesthesia, narcotics, etc.). Combination may cause death. (7) Inhibited by tricyclic antidepressants (amitriptyline [Elavil], etc.), amphetamines, and others. (8) Potentiates oral anticoagulants, levarterenol (Levophed), and all antihypertensive drugs (hydralazine [Apresoline], etc.). (9) Inhibits levodopa. (10) Capable of paradoxical reactions with adrenergics, amphetamines, antidepressants, and sympathomimetics. Severe hypertension can occur.

Contraindications: Eclampsia, liver disease, mental depression (past or present).

Incompatible with: Amphotericin B (Fungizone), methohexital (Brevital), tetracycline (Achromycin). Physically compatible with many drugs. Consider specific use and precautions above.

Side effects: Apprehension, depression, dizziness, dry mouth, edema, elevated alkaline phosphatase, elevated SGOT, fever, hemolytic anemia, nasal congestion, nightmares, paradoxical hypertension, positive Coombs' test, postural hypotension (mild), sedation.

Antidote: Notify the physician of all side effects. Most can be decreased in severity by reducing dosage. Drug may be discontinued. Dopamine (Intropin) or levarterenol (Levophed) should reverse hypotension of overdose. Hemodialysis may be used in acute overdose.

METHYLERGONOVINE MALEATE   pH 2.7 to 3.5

(Methergine)

Usual dose: 1 ml (0.2 mg or gr $\frac{1}{320}$) may be repeated in 2 to 4 hours as necessary.

Dilution: May be given undiluted. Do not add to IV solutions. May be given through Y tube or three-way stopcock of infusion set.

Rate of administration: 0.2 mg or fraction thereof over 1 minute.

Actions: A synthetic oxytocic, more potent and with a more prolonged action than ergonovine. It exerts a direct stimulation on the smooth muscle of the uterus, causing contraction of the uterus itself and vasoconstriction of uterine vessels. In therapeutic doses the prolonged initial contraction is followed by periods of relaxation and contraction. Preferred because it is less likely to cause hypertension. Effective within 1 minute for up to 3 hours. It is probably detoxified in the liver and excreted in bile and urine.

Indications and uses: (1) Routine management after delivery of the placenta, (2) postpartum atony, (3) hemorrhage, (4) subinvolution.

Precautions: (1) Occasionally given after the anterior shoulder is delivered if the obstetrician directs and is present. (2) IV administration is for emergency use only. IM or oral routes are preferred and should be used after the initial IV dose. Monitor the blood pressure. (3) Should be refrigerated; may not be stored at room temperature more than 60 days. (4) Check expiration date on vial; methylergonovine deteriorates with age. (5) Uterine response may be poor in calcium-deficient patients; calcium replacement may be required for effective response. (6) Use caution in presence of sepsis, obliterative vascular disease, and cardiac, hepatic, or renal involvement. (7) Severe hypertension and cerebrovascular accidents can result in the presence of regional anesthesia (caudal or spinal) and with ephedrine, methoxamine (Vasoxyl), and other vasopressors. Chlorpromazine (Thorazine) IV will reduce this hypertension.

Contraindications: Hypersensitivity, hypertension, pregnancy prior to third stage of labor, toxemia.

Incompatible with: Specific information not available. Do not mix in a syringe with any other drug.

Side effects: Rare in therapeutic doses but may include the following. *Average dose:* allergic phenomena, chest pain (temporary), diaphoresis, dilated pupils, dizziness, dyspnea, headache, hypertension (transient), hypotension, nausea, tinnitus, vomiting, weakness. *Overdose:* abortion, blindness, cerebral vascular accident, convulsions, excitement, gangrene, hypercoagulability, palpitations, shock, tachycardia, thirst, tremor, uterine bleeding.

Antidote: Discontinue the drug immediately at the onset of any side effect and notify the physician. Most side effects are transient, unless there is severe toxicity, and will be treated symptomatically. Severe poisoning is treated with vasodilator drugs, sedatives, and calcium gluconate to relieve muscular pain, as well as other supportive treatment. Heparin is used to control hypercoagulability.

METHYLPREDNISOLONE
SODIUM SUCCINATE

pH 7.0 to 8.0

(Solu-Medrol, A-methaPred)

Usual dose: 10 to 125 mg initially. May be repeated every 2 to 6 hours as necessary. In acute conditions such as severe shock, doses up to 1,000 mg or more every 4 hours have been given. These massive doses should not be used longer than 48 to 72 hours. Dosage is individualized according to the severity of the disease and the response of the patient and is not necessarily reduced for children. Do not give less than 0.5 mg/kg of body weight every 24 hours.

Dilution: Available in a Mix-O-Vial, which is reconstituted by removing the protective cap, turning the rubber stopper a quarter turn, and pressing down, allowing the diluent into the lower chamber. Agitate gently. Using sterile technique, insert a needle through the center of the rubber stopper to withdraw diluted solution. To be diluted only with diluent supplied in Mix-O-Vial. May be given direct IV or further diluted in desired amounts of 5% dextrose in water or normal saline and isotonic saline solution.

Rate of administration: Direct IV administration, each 500 mg or fraction thereof over 1 minute or longer. Direct IV administration is usually the route of choice and eliminates the possibility of overloading the patient with IV fluids. At the discretion of the physician, a continuous infusion may be given, properly diluted, over a specified time.

Actions: An adrenocortical steroid with potent metabolic, antiinflammatory actions and innumerable other effects. Has a greater antiinflammatory potency than prednisolone and less tendency to cause excessive potassium and calcium excretion and sodium and water retention. Has four times the potency of hydrocortisone sodium succinate. May be used in conjunction with other forms of therapy, such as epinephrine for acute allergic reactions or antibiotics in acute infections. Primarily excreted in the urine and feces. 75% excretion occurs within 24 hours, allowing use of very large doses with reasonable safety. Will appear in breast milk.

Indications and uses: (1) Hypersensitivity and dermatological conditions; (2) supplementary therapy for severe allergic reaction (use epinephrine first); (3) to initiate therapy in acute gout, acute systemic lupus erythematosus, and acute rheumatic fever; (4) severe shock, whether hemorrhagic, traumatic, surgical, or septic; (5) overwhelming infections with severe toxicity; (6) ulcerative colitis; (7) esophageal burns; (8) adjunctive therapy in croup, etc.; (9) chemotherapy.

Precautions: (1) Discard unused solutions after 48 hours. (2) May cause elevated blood pressure and salt and water retention. (3) Salt restriction and potassium and calcium replacement are necessary. (4) May mask signs of infection. (5) To avoid relative adrenocortical insufficiency, do not stop therapy abruptly; taper off. Patient is observed carefully, especially under stress, for up to 2 years; exception is very short-term therapy. (6) Maintain on ulcer regime and antacid prophylactically. (7) May increase insulin needs in diabetics. (8) Inhibited by anticonvulsants, some antihistamines, barbiturates, propanolol (Inderal), phenylbutazone (Butazolidin). (9) Not the drug of choice to treat acute adrenocortical insufficiency. (10) Use caution in patients with renal transplants; large doses may cause circulatory collapse. (11) Do not vaccinate for smallpox during therapy.

Contraindications: None in short-term therapy. *Absolute contraindications* in long-term therapy, except in life-threatening situations: tuberculosis (active or healed), ocular herpes simplex, acute psychoses. *Relative contraindications*: active or latent peptic ulcer, chickenpox, congestive heart failure, diabetes mellitus, diverticulitis, fresh intestinal anastomoses, hypertension, myasthenia gravis, osteoporosis, pregnancy, psychotic tendencies, renal insufficiency, thromboembolic tendencies, vaccinia.

Incompatible with: Aminophylline, calcium gluconate, cephalothin (Keflin), chlorpromazine (Thorazine), cytarabine (ARA-C), digitoxin (Crystodigin), diphenhydramine (Benadryl), glycopyrrolate (Robinul), insulin, meperidine (Demerol), metaraminol (Aramine), nafcillin (Unipen), penicillin G sodium and potassium, promethazine (Phenergan), tetracycline, thiamylal (Surital), thiopental (Pentothal), tolazoline (Priscoline), vitamin B complex, and vitamin B complex with C.

Side effects: Do occur but are usually reversible: Cushing's syndrome; electrolyte and calcium imbalance; euphoria; glycosuria; hyperglycemia; hypersensitivity reactions, including anaphylaxis; hypertension; increased intracranial pressure; menstrual irregularities; peptic ulcer perforation and hemorrhage; protein catabolism; spontaneous fractures; transitory burning or tingling, sweating, headache, or weakness, thromboembolism; and many others.

Antidote: Notify the physician of any side effect. Will probably treat the side effect if necessary. Resuscitate as necessary for anaphylaxis and notify physician. Keep epinephrine immediately available.

METHYLTHIONINE CHLORIDE

(Methylene blue)

Usual dose: 1% methylene blue, 1 ml equals 10 mg. 0.1 to 0.2 ml/kg of body weight is recommended dose.

Dilution: Usually given undiluted.

Rate of administration: 1 ml (10 mg) or fraction thereof over 5 minutes.

Actions: Low concentrations will convert methemoglobin to hemoglobin (methemoglobin is toxic and gives the blood a chocolate brown color; it does not carry oxygen). High concentrations convert ferrous iron of hemoglobin to ferric iron and forms methemoglobin. Will stain tissue and turn urine or feces blue or green. Excreted in urine and bile.

Indications and uses: (1) Drug-induced methemoglobinemia, (2) antidote for cyanide poisoning, (3) diagnostic dye, (4) to identify body structures and fistulas.

Precautions: (1) Inject very slowly over several minutes to prevent local high concentration of the compound with toxic effects. (2) Do not exceed recommended dosage. (3) May cause cyanosis or cardiac irregularities.

Contraindications: Intraspinal injection.

Incompatible with: Do not mix with any other drug.

Side effects: *Minor:* bladder irritation, dizziness, headache, nausea, vomiting. *Major:* abdominal pain, anemia, mental confusion, methemoglobin, precordial pain, profuse diaphoresis.

Antidote: Discontinue the drug upon appearance of any side effect. Remove skin stains with hypochlorite solution.

METOCLOPRAMIDE
HYDROCHLORIDE

(Reglan)

Usual dose: 10 mg (2 ml) as a single dose.
Antiemetic: 2 mg/kg of body weight initially 30 minutes before giving cisplatin. Repeat in 2 hours. May be repeated every 3 hours as necessary. Dose may be reduced to 1 mg/kg if initial doses suppress vomiting.

Pediatric dose: *6 to 14 years;* 2.5 to 5 mg. *Under 6 years;* 0.1 mg/kg of body weight.

Dilution: May be given undiluted except when used as an antiemetic for cisplatin chemotherapy.
Antiemetic: Dilute in at least 50 ml of 5% dextrose in water, sodium chloride, Ringer's injection, or lactated Ringer's injection and give as an infusion.

Rate of administration: 10 mg or fraction thereof over 2 minutes.
Infusion: Administer over a minimum of 15 minutes.

Actions: A dopamine antagonist that stimulates tone and amplitude of gastric contractions and increases peristalsis of the duodenum and jejunum. It relaxes the lower esophageal sphincter, pyloric sphincter, and duodenal bulb. Does not stimulate gastric, biliary, or pancreatic secretions. Acts even if vagal innervation is not present. Action is negated by anticholinergic drugs. Onset of action occurs in 1 to 3 minutes and lasts 1 to 2 hours.

Indications and uses: (1) Facilitate small bowel intubation. (2) Stimulate gastric and intestinal emptying of barium to permit radiological examination of the stomach and small intestine. (3) Antiemetic with cisplatin chemotherapy. (4) Acute and recurrent diabetic gastroparesis.

Precautions: (1) A phenothiazine-related drug; may produce sedation and extrapyramidal symptoms. (2) Use caution in pregnancy and lactation. May increase milk production during lactation. (3) Antagonized by anticholinergic drugs (atropine) and narcotic analgesics (morphine). (4) Potentiated by alcohol, sedatives, hypnotics, narcotics, and tranquilizers. (5) Drugs ingested orally may be absorbed more slowly or more rapidly depending on the absorption site. (6) A prolactin-elevating compound; may be carcinogenic. Risk with a single dose almost nonexistent. (7) Too-rapid IV injection will cause intense anxiety, restlessness, and then drowsiness.

Contraindications: Situations in which gastric motility is contraindicated, i.e., gastric hemorrhage, obstructions, or perforation; known hypersensitivity to metoclopramide; patients with epilepsy or patients taking drugs that may also cause extrapyramidal reactions; and pheochromocytoma.

Incompatible with: Specific information not available.

Side effects: *Average dose* bowel disturbances, dizziness, drowsiness, fatigue, headache, insomnia, nausea, restlessness. *Overdose:* disorientation, drowsiness, and extrapyramidal reactions.

Antidote: Notify physician of all side effects. Treat overdose or extrapyramidal reactions with diphenhydramine (Benadryl). Symptoms should disappear within 24 hours. Resuscitate as necessary.

METRONIDAZOLE HYDROCHLORIDE

pH 5.0 to 7.0

(Flagyl IV, Flagyl IV RTU)

Usual dose: Begin with an initial loading dose of 15 mg/kg of body weight. Follow with 7.5 mg/kg in 6 hours and every 6 hours thereafter for 7 to 10 days or longer if indicated. Do not exceed 4 Gm in 24 hours.

Dilution: Flagyl IV RTU is prediluted and ready to use (5 mg/ml). Do not use plastic containers in series connections. Risk of air embolism is present. Flagyl IV requires a specific dilution process. Avoid all contact with aluminum in needles and syringes in initial dilution. Color change will occur. Initially add 4.4 ml of sterile water or 0.9% sodium chloride for injection (100 mg/ml). Solution must be clear. Will be yellow to yellow-green in color with a pH of 0.5 to 2.0. Must be further diluted to at least 8 mg/ml with 0.9% sodium chloride, 5% dextrose in water, or lactated Ringer's for infusion. Must be neutralized before infusion with 5 mEq of sodium bicarbonate per 500 mg. Carbon dioxide gas will be generated and may require venting.

Rate of administration: Must be given as a slow IV infusion, each single dose over 1 hour. Discontinue primary IV during administration.

Actions: A bactericidal agent with cytotoxic effects, active against specific anaerobic bacteria and protozoa. Widely distributed in therapeutic levels to all body fluids (including abscesses). Levels are directly proportional to dose given. Onset of action is prompt and lasts about 8 hours. Crosses placental and blood-brain barriers. Most is excreted in urine, some in feces. Excreted in breast milk.

Indications and uses: (1) Treatment of serious intraabdominal, skin and skin structure, gynecological, bone and joint, central nervous system, and lower respiratory tract infections, bacterial septicemia, and endocarditis caused by susceptible anaerobic bacteria; (2) prophylaxis to reduce infection rates in gynecological, abdominal, and colonic surgery; (3) hepatic encephalopathy; (4) as a radiosensitizer to make resistant tumors more susceptible to radiation therapy.

Precautions: (1) A mixed (anaerobic/aerobic) infection will require use of additional appropriate antibiotics. (2) Sensitivity studies are indicated to determine the susceptibility of the causative organism to metronidazole. (3) Avoid prolonged use of the drug; superinfection caused by overgrowth of nonsusceptible organisms may result. (4) Rotate IV site frequently to avoid thrombophlebitis. Avoid extravasation. (5) Store at room temperature before and after dilution. Discard diluted and neutralized solutions in 24 hours. Do not refrigerate; a precipitate will result. Protect from light when storing. (6) Symptoms of candidosis may be exacerbated and require treatment. (7) May cause decreased SGOT levels. (8) Use caution in hepatic disease, patients predisposed to edema and/or taking corticosteroids, impaired cardiac function (contains 5 to 14 mEq/ml sodium), CNS disease, history of blood dyscrasias, children, and neonates. (9) Avoid alcohol and disulfiram; toxic reactions will occur. (10) Inhibited by barbiturates (phenobarbital, etc.), and hydantoins (phenytoin [Dilantin], etc.). (11) Carcinogenic in rodents; use only when necessary. (12) Potentiates oral anticoagulants (warfarin, etc.).

Contraindications: Hypersensitivity to metronidazole or nitroimidazole derivatives, first trimester of pregnancy.

Incompatible with: Administer separately per manufacturer's recommendation. Discontinue primary infusion during administration.

Side effects: Abdominal discomfort, convulsions, diarrhea, dizziness, fever, headache, metallic taste (expected), nausea, neutropenia (reversible), peripheral neuropathy, pruritus, rash, syncope, thrombophlebitis, vomiting.

Antidote: Notify physician of all side effects. Treatment will be symptomatic and supportive. Benefit/risk of therapy must be reconsidered with onset of convulsions or peripheral neuropathy. Rapidly removed by hemodialysis. Treat anaphylaxis and resuscitate as necessary.

MEZLOCILLIN

(Mezlin)

Usual dose: 200 to 300 mg/kg of body weight/24 hr equally divided in 4 to 6 doses (3 Gm every 4 hours = 18 Gm/24 hr). Do not exceed 24 Gm/24 hr.

Pediatric dose: *Infants 1 month to children 12 years:* 50 mg/kg of body weight every 4 hours (300 mg/kg/24 hr). Limited data available on use in children.

Dilution: Each 1 Gm or fraction thereof should be diluted with at least 10 ml of sterile water, 5% dextrose, or 0.9% sodium chloride for injection. Shake vigorously to dissolve. Must be diluted to a minimum 10% concentration for direct IV use. Should be further diluted to the desired volume (50 to 100 ml) with 5% dextrose in water or 0.45 normal saline or other compatible infusion solutions (see literature) and given as an intermittent infusion.

Rate of administration: *Direct IV:* a single dose properly diluted over 3 to 5 minutes. *Intermittent infusion:* a single dose properly diluted over 30 minutes. Discontinue primary IV infusion during administration. Pediatric dose must be given over 30 minutes.

Actions: An extended-spectrum penicillin. Bactericidal against a variety of gram-negative and gram-positive bacteria including aerobic and anaerobic strains. Especially effective against *Klebsiella* and *Pseudomonas*. Well distributed in all body fluids, tissue, bone, and through inflamed meninges. Onset of action is prompt. Excreted in the urine. Crosses placental barrier. Excreted in breast milk.

Indications and uses: Treatment of serious lower respiratory tract, intraabdominal, urinary tract, gynecological, and skin and skin structure infections and septicemia caused by susceptible organisms.

Precautions: (1) Stable at room temperature for up to 72 hours depending on solution used for admixture. (2) Warm to 37° C (98.6° F) in a water bath for 20 minutes if precipitation occurs on refrigeration. Shake vigorously. (3) Slightly darkened color does not affect potency. (4) Frequently used concurrently with aminoglycosides (gentamicin [Garamycin], etc.), but must

326

be administered in separate infusions. Inactivated by tetracyclines. (5) Sensitivity studies are indicated to determine the susceptibility of the causative organism to mezlocillin. (6) Oral probenecid is indicated to achieve higher and more prolonged blood levels. (7) Watch for early symptoms of allergic reaction. (8) Avoid prolonged use of drug; superinfection caused by overgrowth of nonsusceptible organisms may result. (9) Periodic evaluation of renal, hepatic, and hematopoietic systems and serum potassium is recommended in prolonged therapy. (10) Electrolyte imbalance and cardiac irregularities resulting from high sodium content are very possible. Contains 1.85 mEq sodium/Gm. (11) Confirm patency of vein; avoid extravasation or intraarterial injection. Slow infusion rate for pain along venipuncture site. (12) Usual duration of therapy is 7 to 10 days. Continue at least 2 days after symptoms of infection disappear. (13) Reduce dose only in severe renal impairment with creatinine clearance temporarily below 30 ml/min. May be given to patients undergoing hemodialysis and peritoneal dialysis (see literature for dose). (14) Test for syphilis also before treating gonorrhea.

Contraindications: History of sensitivity to multiple allergens, penicillin sensitivity.

Incompatible with: Aminoglycosides (amikacin, colistimethate, gentamicin, kanamycin, streptomycin, tobramycin), amphotericin B (Fungizone), chloramphenicol, lincomycin, oxytetracycline, polymyxin B, promethazine (Phenergan), tetracycline (Achromycin), vitamin B with C.

Side effects: Anaphylaxis; bleeding abnormalities (with severe renal impairment); convulsions; decreased hemoglobin or hematocrit; diarrhea; elevated SGOT, SGPT, and BUN; eosinophilia; fever; hypokalemia; interstitial nephritis; leukopenia; nausea; neuromuscular excitability; neutropenia; pruritus; psuedoproteinuria; skin rash; taste sensation (abnormal); thrombocytopenia; thrombophlebitis; urticaria; vomiting.

Antidote: Notify the physician immediately of any adverse symptoms. For severe symptoms, discontinue the drug, treat allergic reaction (antihistamines, epinephrine, and corticosteroids), and resuscitate as necessary. Hemodialysis or peritoneal dialysis are effective in overdose.

(Monistat IV)

Usual dose: Initial dose of 200 mg with the physician in attendance, then 600 to 3,600 mg/24 hr equally divided into three infusions and given every 8 hours.

Pediatric dose: 20 to 40 mg/kg of body weight as a total daily dose equally divided into three infusions. Do not exceed 15 mg/kg/infusion.

Dilution: A single dose (200 to 1,200 mg in the adult) must be diluted in 200 ml of normal saline. May use 5% dextrose in water if necessary.

Rate of administration: A single dose over 30 to 60 minutes.

Actions: An antifungal agent. Alters the permeability of the fungal cell membrane. Only effective against specific organisms. Metabolized in the liver with some excretion in the urine.

Indications and uses: Severe systemic fungal infections such as coccidioidomycosis, candidosis, cryptococcosis, paracoccidioidomycosis, and chronic mucocutaneous candidosis.

Precautions: (1) Hospitalize patients for at least several days to initiate treatment. (2) Monitor blood counts, electrolytes, and lipids during therapy. (3) Rapid injection may produce tachycardia or arrhythmias. (4) Supplemented in some situations with intrathecal injection and bladder irrigation. (5) Potentiates coumarin drugs; reduction of anticoagulant dose may be indicated. (6) Antagonizes amphotericin B; neither drug will be effective. (7) Use caution in pregnancy. (8) Lengthy treatment (up to 20 weeks) may be required for cure. (9) Antiemetics previous to each dose will reduce nausea and vomiting. (10) Pruritus is a common side effect and is most uncomfortable. (11) Discard solution that darkens in color.

Contraindications: Known sensitivity to miconazole. Safety for children under 1 year not established.

Incompatible with: Specific information not available. Should be considered incompatible in syringe or solution with any other drug.

Side effects: Allergic reactions including anaphylaxis;

anorexia; cardiac arrhythmias; diarrhea; drowsiness; fever; flushing; nausea; phlebitis; pruritus; rash; tachycardia; and vomiting.

Antidote: Notify the physician of all side effects. Most will respond to symptomatic treatment or reduction of infusion rate and are reversible when the drug is discontinued. Treat allergic reaction as necessary and resuscitate as indicated.

MINOCYCLINE HYDROCHLORIDE   pH 2.0 to 2.8

(Minocin)

Usual dose: 200 mg initially, then 100 mg every 12 hours. Maximum dose is 400 mg/24 hr. Normal renal function is required.

Pediatric dose: 4 mg/kg of body weight as initial dose, followed by 2 mg/kg every 12 hours.

Dilution: Reconstitute each 100 mg vial with 5 ml of sterile water for injection. Must be further diluted in 500 to 1,000 ml of compatible infusion fluids such as sodium chloride or dextrose solutions, Ringer's injection, or lactated Ringer's injection.

Rate of administration: Each 100 mg properly diluted at prescribed rate of infusion (e.g., 500 ml every 6 hours).

Actions: A broad-spectrum antibiotic that is bacteriostatic against many gram-positive and gram-negative organisms. Well distributed in most body tissues, tetracyclines are concentrated in the liver and excreted through bile to urine and feces in a biologically active state. Minocycline may penetrate normal meninges more easily than other tetracyclines. Crosses the placental barrier. Excreted in breast milk.

Indications and uses: (1) Infections caused by susceptible organisms, (2) to substitute for contraindicated penicillin or sulfonamide therapy.

Precautions: (1) Stable at room temperature for 24 hours. (2) Sensitivity studies are necessary to determine the susceptibility of the causative organism to minocycline. (3) Avoid prolonged use; superinfection due to overgrowth of nonsusceptible organisms may result. (4) Use extreme caution in impaired liver or renal function, pregnancy, postpartum, and lactation. Minocycline serum concentrations and liver and kidney function tests are indicated. (5) May cause skeletal retardation in the fetus and infants and permanent tooth discoloration in children under 8 years of age, either by direct administration or by transmission through placenta or breast milk. (6) Inhibits bactericidal action of penicillin, ampicillins, oxacillin, methicillin, etc. May be toxic with sulfonamides. (7)

Potentiates digoxin and anticoagulants; reduced dosage of these drugs may be necessary. (8) Inhibited by alkalinizing agents, barbiturates, calcium, cimetidine (Tagamet), iron and magnesium salts, phenytoin (Dilantin), riboflavin, sodium bicarbonate, and others. (9) Alert patient to the possibility of a photosensitive skin reaction. (10) Determine absolute patency of vein and avoid extravasation; thrombophlebitis is not infrequent. (11) Organisms resistant to one tetracycline are usually resistant to others. (12) Check expiration date. Outdated ampoules may cause nephrotoxicity.

Contraindications: Known hypersensitivity to tetracyclines.

Incompatible with: Sufficient information not available. See tetracycline hydrochloride; same incompatibilities may exist. Forms a precipitate with calcium.

Side effects: Relatively nontoxic in average doses, more toxic in larger doses or if given too rapidly. *Minor:* anogenital lesions, anorexia, blood dyscrasias, diarrhea, dizziness, dysphagia, enterocolitis, nausea, skin rashes, vertigo, vomiting. *Major:* hypersensitivity reactions, including anaphylaxis; liver damage; photosensitivity; systemic moniliasis; thrombophlebitis.

Antidote: Notify the physician of all side effects. If minor side effects are progressive or any major side effect occurs, discontinue drug, treat allergic reactions, or resuscitate as necessary.

(Mithracin)

Usual dose: *Testicular tumors:* 25 to 30 μg/kg of body weight/24 hr. Repeat daily for 8 to 10 days unless significant side effects or toxicity occur. Repeat at monthly intervals if indicated.
Hypercalcemia and hypercalciuria: 25 μg/kg of body weight/24 hr for 3 or 4 days. Repeat weekly as required to maintain normal calcium levels.

Dilution: *Specific techniques required, see precautions.* Each 2.5 mg vial must be initially diluted with 4.9 ml of sterile water for injection (1 ml equals 500 μg). A single daily dose must be further diluted in 1,000 ml of 5% dextrose in water and given as an infusion. Do not use a filter smaller than 5 μm. Loss of potency will occur.

Rate of administration: A single dose every 24 hours over 4 to 6 hours.

Actions: A potent antibiotic, antineoplastic agent. Interferes with cell division by binding with DNA to inhibit and slow production of RNA. Exact mechanism unknown. Cytotoxic to HeLa cell tissue culture and some animal tumors. Will produce hypocalcemia in patients with cancer.

Indications and uses: (1) Testicular tumors not treatable with surgery and/or radiation, (2) hypercalcemia and hypercalciuria associated with many advanced neoplasms.

Precautions: (1) Follow guidelines for handling cytotoxic agents recommended by the National Study Commission on Cytotoxic Exposure (see Appendix, p. 528). (2) Administered only to hospitalized patients by or under the direction of the physician specialist. (3) Determine absolute patency of vein; cellulitis and tissue necrosis may result from extravasation. Discontinue injection, use another vein. Apply heat to the extravasated area. (4) Store in refrigerator before dilution. Prepare fresh daily and discard any unused portion. (5) Dosage based on average weight in presence of edema or ascites. (6) Severe sudden onset of hemorrhage and even death can result from use. (7) Maintain hydration and correct electrolyte imbalance prior to treatment. (8) Use extreme caution in impaired renal or hepatic function. (9) Monitor platelet count, prothrombin time, and bleeding time during and after therapy. (10) Safety for use in pregnancy, lactation, and men and women capable of conception not documented. (11) Many drug interactions are possible; observe patient closely. (12) Do not administer vaccines or chloroquine to patients receiving antineoplastic drugs. (13) Observe closely for all signs of infection. (14) Prophylactic antiemetics may reduce nausea and vomiting and increase patient comfort.

Contraindications: Thrombocytopenia; thrombocytopathy; coagulation disorders or any susceptibility to bleeding; impairment of bone marrow function; lack of hospital and laboratory facilities.

Incompatible with: Specific information not available Should be considered incompatible with any other drug due to toxicity and specific use.

Side effects: *Minor:* anorexia, depression, diarrhea, drowsiness, fever, flushing, headache, nausea, skin rash, stomatitis, vomiting. *Major:* abnormal clot retraction, abnormal liver function tests, abnormal renal function tests, elevation of bleeding and clotting time, epistaxis (severe), hematemesis, hemoglobin depression, leukopenia (unusual), platelet count depression, prothrombin content depression, serum calcium, phosphorus, and potassium depression.

Antidote: Minor side effects will be treated symptomatically. Discontinue the drug and notify the physician immediately of any major side effects. Platelet-rich plasma may help to elevate platelet count. Provide immediate treatment or supportive therapy as indicated; bleeding episodes can be fatal. If extravasation has occured, LA dexamethasone injected into the indurated area with a fine hypodermic needle may be helpful.

MITOMYCIN

(Mutamycin)

Usual dose: 20 mg/M² as a single dose or 2 mg/M² daily for 5 days. After 2-day rest period, repeat 2 mg/M² daily for 5 additional days (total dose equals 20 mg/M²). Entire schedule may be repeated in 6 to 8 weeks if no bone marrow toxicity occurs.

Dilution: *Specific techniques required, see precautions.* Each 5 mg must be diluted with 10 ml of sterile water for injection. Allow to stand at room temperature until completely in solution. May be given through the Y tube or three-way stopcock of a free-flowing infusion of normal saline or 5% dextrose or further diluted in either of the same solutions and given as an infusion.

Rate of administration: A single dose over 5 to 10 minutes. Infusion rate determined by amount and type of solution. Will maintain potency in 5% dextrose in water for 3 hours.

Actions: A highly toxic antibiotic, antineoplastic agent. Cell cycle phase nonspecific, it is most useful in G and S phases, Interferes with cell division by binding with DNA to slow production of RNA. Metabolized in the liver. Some excreted in urine.

Indications and uses: A palliative treatment, adjunct to surgery, radiation, or patients resistant to other chemotherapeutic agents. May be useful in pancreatic, gastric, cervical, breast, bronchogenic, and head and neck carcinoma; malignant melanoma.

Precautions: (1) Follow guidelines for handling cytotoxic agents recommended by the National Study Commission on Cytotoxic Exposure (see Appendix, p. 528). (2) Usually administered in the hospital by or under the direction of the physician specialist. (3) Determine absolute patency of vein; use of an IV catheter is preferred because severe cellulitis and tissue necrosis will result from extravasation. If extravasation occurs, discontinue injection and use another vein. Apply heat to extravasated area. (4) Monitor white blood cells, red blood cells, platelet count, prothrombin time, bleeding time, differential, and hemoglobin before, during, and 7 to 10 weeks after therapy. (5) Use extreme caution in impaired renal function. (6) Dosage based on average weight in presence of edema or ascites. (7) May produce teratogenic effects on the fetus; use caution in men and women capable of conception. (8) Do not administer vaccines or chloroquine to patients receiving antineoplastic drugs. (9) Be alert for signs of bone marrow depression or infection. (10) Commonly used with other antineoplastic drugs and radiation in reduced doses to achieve tumor remission. (11) Prophylactic antiemetics may reduce nausea and vomiting and increase patient comfort.

Contraindications: Known hypersensitivity to mitomycin; thrombocytopenia; coagulation disorders; increased bleeding from other causes; WBC below 4,000; platelet count below 75,000; potentially serious infections; serum creatinine above 1.7 mg%.

Side effects: Alopecia, anaphylaxis, anemia, anorexia, bleeding, blurring of vision, confusion, coughing, dyspnea, edema, elevated BUN, fatigue, fever, headache, hematemesis, hemoptysis, leukopenia, mouth ulcers, nausea, paresthesias, pneumonia, pruritus, skin toxicity, thrombocytopenia, thrombophlebitis, vomiting.

Antidote: Most side effects will be treated symptomatically. Keep the physician informed. All are potentially serious. Hematopoietic depression requires cessation of therapy until recovery occurs. There is no specific antidote. Supportive therapy as indicated will help sustain the patient in toxicity. If extravasation has occurred, LA dexamethasone injected into the indurated area with a fine hypodermic needle may be helpful.

Usual dose: 2.5 to 15 mg (gr ¹⁄₁₆ to ¼). Repeat every 2 to 4 hours as necessary. 10 mg (gr ⅙) is adequate for all but exceptional needs.

Dilution: Should be diluted. Use at least 5 ml of sterile water or normal saline for injection or other IV solutions. Is sometimes added to IV solutions in selected situations (requires close titration). May be given through Y tube or three-way stopcock of infusion set.

Rate of administration: 15 mg or fraction thereof of properly diluted medication over 3 to 5 minutes. Frequently titrated according to symptom relief and respiratory rate.

Actions: An opium derivative, narcotic analgesic, which is a descending CNS depressant. It has definite respiratory depressant actions. Pain relief is effected almost immediately and lasts about 2 hours. Morphine induces sleep while it inhibits perception of pain by binding to opiate receptors decreasing sodium permeability and inhibiting transmission of pain impulses. Depresses many other senses or reflexes. Readily absorbed, detoxified in the liver, and excreted in the urine. Crosses the placental barrier. Excreted in breast milk.

Indications and uses: (1) Relief of severe to excruciating pain and apprehension from coronary occlusion, malignancies, traumatic injury, renal or biliary colic, and painful manipulation or instrumentation such as cystoscopy, burn dressing changes, fracture reduction, dyspnea, seizures of acute left ventricular failure, and pulmonary edema. (2) Postoperative relief of severe pain.

Precautions: (1) Physical dependence can develop with abuse. (2) Oxygen and controlled respiratory equipment must always be available. (3) Observe patient frequently and monitor vital signs. (4) Use caution in the elderly and in patients with impaired hepatic or renal function, emphysema, and anticoagulation therapy. (5) Tolerance for the drug gradually increases, but abstinence for 1 to 2 weeks will restore effectiveness. (6) Potentiated by phenothiazines (chlorpromazine [Thorazine], etc.); other CNS depressants such as narcotic analgesics, general anesthetics, alcohol, anticholinergics, antihistamines, barbiturates, cimetidine (Tagamet), hypnotics, sedatives, and psychotropic agents; MAO inhibitors (isocarboxazid [Marplan], etc.); neuromuscular blocking agents (tubocurarine, etc.); and adrenergic blocking agents (propranolol [Inderal], etc.). Reduced dosage of both drugs may be indicated.

Contraindications: Acute alcoholism, benign prostatic hypertrophy, bronchial asthma, convulsive disorders, craniotomy, head injuries, hypersensitivity to opiates, increased intracranial pressure, premature infants, respiratory depression.

Incompatible with: Aminophylline, amorbarbital (Amytal), chlorothiazide (Diuril), heparin, meperidine (Demerol), methicillin (Staphcillin), nitrofurantoin (Ivadantin), pentobarbital (Nembutal), phenobarbital (Luminal), phenytoin (Dilantin), sodium bicarbonate, sodium iodide, sulfisoxazole (Gantrisin), thiopental (Pentothal).

Side effects: *Average dose:* constipation, delayed absorption of oral medications, hypersensitivity reactions, hypothermia, increased intracranial pressure, nausea, neonatal apnea, orthostatic hypotension, respiratory depression (slight), urinary retention, vomiting. *Overdose:* anaphylaxis, Cheyne-Stokes respiration, coma, excitation, hypotension (severe), inserted T wave on EKG, myocardial depression (severe), pinpoint pupils, respiratory depression (severe), tachycardia, death.

Antidote: With increasing severity of any side effect or onset of symptoms of overdose, discontinue the drug and notify the physician. Naloxone (Narcan) or levallorphan (Lorfan), will reverse serious respiratory depression. A patent airway, artificial ventilation, oxygen therapy, and other symptomatic treatment must be instituted promptly. Resuscitate as necessary.

MOXALACTAM DISODIUM

(Moxam)

Usual dose: 2 to 6 Gm/24 hr in equally divided doses every 8 hours for 5 to 10 days. Range is 250 mg every 12 hours to 4 Gm every 8 hours.

Pediatric dose: *0 to 1 week:* 50 mg/kg of body weight every 12 hours.

1 week to 4 weeks: 50 mg/kg every 8 hours.

Infants: 50 mg/kg every 6 hours.

Children: 50 mg/kg every 6 or 8 hours; up to 200 mg/kg/24 hr may be needed. In gram-negative meningitis use an initial loading dose of 100 mg/kg.

Dilution: Each 1 Gm must be diluted with 10 ml of sterile water, 5% dextrose, or 0.9% sodium chloride. *Direct IV:* may be given through tubing port of free-flowing IV solutions of compatible fluid (see literature). *Intermittent IV:* Must be further diluted to at least 20 ml/Gm with 5% dextrose, 0.9% saline, or other compatible infusion solutions. May be added to 500 to 1000 ml compatible infusion fluids and given as a continuous infusion.

Rate of administration: *Direct IV:* a single dose equally distributed over 3 to 5 minutes. May be given through Y tube or three-way stopcock of infusion set. *Intermittent IV:* a single dose over 30 minutes. Discontinue primary infusion during administration. *Continuous infusion:* 500 to 1,000 ml over 6 to 24 hours, depending on total dose and concentration.

Actions: A broad-spectrum cephalosporin antibiotic similar to cefamandole. Bactericidal to many gram-negative and gram-positive organisms. Effective against many otherwise resistant organisms. Absorbed by most body fluids including inflamed meninges. Excreted in the urine. Crosses placental barrier. Excreted in breast milk.

Indications and uses: Treatment of serious lower respiratory tract, urinary tract, intraabdominal, CNS, skin and skin structure, and bone and joint infections and bacterial septicemia.

Precautions: (1) Sensitivity studies are indicated to determine the susceptibility of the causative organism

339

to moxalactam. (2) Watch for early symptoms of allergic reaction. (3) Reduce total daily dose if renal function is impaired. Calculated according to degree of impairment. (4) Avoid prolonged use of drug; superinfection caused by overgrowth of nonsusceptible organisms may result. (5) Administer within 24 hours of preparation. Selected solutions may be preserved 96 hours with refrigeration. (6) Use extreme caution in the penicillin-sensitive patient; cross-sensitivity may occur. (7) Adverse interaction may occur with promethazine (Phenergan), procainamide (Pronestyl), quinidine, muscle relaxants, potent diuretics, and aminoglycosides. Will produce symptoms of acute alcohol intolerance with alcohol. (8) Frequently used concomitantly with aminoglycosides in severe infections, but these drugs must never be mixed in the same infusion or given concurrently. Nephrotoxicity is markedly increased when both drugs are utilized. (9) Use only if absolutely necessary in pregnancy. (10) Use caution in patients with liver impairment. (11) *Pseudomonas* infections may require higher doses. Choose another drug if response is not prompt. (12) Avoid concurrent administration of bacteriostatic agents. (13) May cause thrombophlebitis. Use small needles and large veins and rotate infusion sites. (14) Electrolyte imbalance and cardiac irregularities resulting from high sodium content are very possible. Contains 3.8 mEq of sodium/Gm. (15) Will cause hypoprothrombinemia; 10 mg/week of prophylactic vitamin K is recommended. Platelet dysfunction can be avoided by limiting dose to 4 Gm/24 hr and using vitamin K.

Contraindications: Known sensitivity to cephalosporins or related antibiotics (penicillins).

Incompatible with: Specific information is not available. Should be considered incompatible in syringe or solution with any other bacteriostatic agent. All aminoglycosides (kanamycin [Kantrex], etc.).

Side effects: Full scope of allergic reactions including anaphylaxis. Bleeding episodes (severe); decreased hemoglobin, hematocrit, prothrombin time, and platelet functions; diarrhea; dyspnea; eosinophilia; elevation of SGOT, SGPT, total bilirubin, alkaline phosphatase, LDH, and BUN (transient); false positive reaction for urine glucose except with Tes-Tape or Keto-Diastix; fever; leukopenia; local site pain; platelet dysfunction; pseudomembranous colitis; thrombocytopenia; thrombophlebitis; transient neutropenia; vaginitis; vomiting.

Antidote: Notify the physician of any side effect. Discontinue the drug if indicated. Treat allergic reaction as indicated and resuscitate as necessary. Hemodialysis may be useful in overdose. Vitamin K, fresh frozen plasma, packed red cells, or platelet concentrates may be indicated in abnormal bleeding tendencies confirmed by lab evaluations. If bleeding is due to platelet dysfunction, discontinue and use cefamandole or cefoperazone with caution.

MULTI-VITAMIN INFUSION

(M.V.I., M.V.I. concentrate)

Usual dose: One 5 to 10 ml dose every 24 hours.

Dilution: Each dose must be diluted in at least 500 ml but preferably 1,000 ml of IV fluids. Soluble in all commonly used infusion fluids, including dextrose, saline, electrolyte replacement fluids, plasma, and protein hydrolysates.

Rate of administration: Give at prescribed rate of infusion fluids.

Actions: A multiple vitamin solution containing fat-soluble and water-soluble vitamins in an aqueous solution. Provides B complex as well as vitamins A, D, and E. Readily absorbable, it provides daily requirements or corrects an existing deficiency.

Indications and uses: Need of optimum vitamin intake to maintain the body's normal resistance and repair processes, such as after surgery, extensive burns, trauma, severe infectious diseases, comatose states.

Precautions: (1) Never used undiluted. (2) Do not use if any crystals have formed. (3) Should be refrigerated.

Contraindications: Known hypersensitivity to thiamine hydrochloride.

Incompatible with: Alkaline solutions, bleomycin (Blenoxane), cephaloridine (Loridine), doxycycline (Vibramycin), erythromycin (Erythrocin), kanamycin (Kantrex), lincomycin (Lincocin), oxytetracycline (Terramycin), tetracycline (Achromycin).

Side effects: Rare when administered as recommended: anaphylaxis, dizziness, fainting.

Antidote: With onset of any side effect, discontinue administration immediately and notify the physician. Treat anaphylaxis or resuscitate as necessary.

(Nafcill, Unipen)

Usual dose: 500 mg every 4 hours. Up to 1 Gm every 4 hours has been given in severe infections.

Pediatric dose: 10 to 40 mg/kg of body weight every 4 to 8 hours. 200 mg/kg/24 hr has been used in serious infections.

Dilution: Each 500 mg vial is diluted with 1.7 ml of sterile water for injection (1 Gm vial with 3.4 ml, 2 Gm vial with 6.8 ml). Each 1 ml equals 250 mg. Further dilute each 500 mg with a minimum of 15 to 30 ml of 5% dextrose in water, isotonic sodium chloride, or other compatible IV solutions (see literature). May be given through Y tube, three-way stopcock, or with additive tubing or may be added to larger volume of compatible solutions and given over 24 hours or less.

Rate of administration: Each 500 mg or fraction thereof properly diluted over 5 to 10 minutes. When diluted in large volumes of infusion fluids, give at rate prescribed.

Actions: A semisynthetic penicillin, bactericidal against penicillin G–sensitive and resistant strains of *Staphylococcus aureus* as well as other specific gram-positive organisms. Readily absorbed into most body fluids and tissues except spinal fluid. Primarily excreted through bile, a small amount is excreted in the urine. Excreted in breast milk.

Indications and uses: Treatment of infections caused by penicillinase-producing staphylococci.

Precautions: (1) Refrigerate unused medication after initial dilution, and discard after 7 days. (2) Sensitivity studies are necessary to determine the susceptibility of the causative organism to nafcillin; sometimes difficult to determine accurately. (3) Watch for early symptoms of allergic reaction. Individuals with a history of allergic problems are more susceptible to untoward reactions. (4) Avoid prolonged use of the drug; superinfection caused by overgrowth of nonsusceptible organisms may result. (5) Renal, hepatic, and hematopoietic function should be checked during long-term therapy. (6) Inhibited by chloramphenicol,

343

erythromycin, and tetracyclines. Bactericidal action may be negated by these drugs. (7) Potentiated by aminohippuric acid and probenecid (Benemid); toxicity may result. (8) May cause thrombophlebitis, especially in the elderly or with too-rapid injection. (9) Inhibits aminoglycosides (gentamicin, etc.). Do not mix in same IV container.

Contraindications: Known hypersensitivity to any penicillin.

Incompatible with: Aminoglycosides (gentamicin, kanamycin, etc.), aminophylline, ascorbic acid, hydrocortisone sodium succinate (Solu-Cortef), methylprednisolone (Solu-Medrol), oxytetracycline (Terramycin), promazine (Sparine), solutions with a pH below 5.0, vitamin B complex with C.

Side effects: Relatively infrequent except for sensitivity reactions such as anaphylaxis, skin rashes, and urticaria. Diarrhea, nausea, pruritus, and vomiting have been reported.

Antidote: Notify the physician of any side effect. For allergic symptoms, discontinue drug, treat allergic reaction as indicated or resuscitate as necessary, and notify the physician.

NALBUPHINE HYDROCHLORIDE

(Nubain)

Usual dose: 10 mg. Repeat every 3 to 6 hours as necessary. Up to 20 mg can be given in a single dose if required. Maximum total daily dose is 160 mg.

Dilution: May be given undiluted.

Rate of administration: Each 10 mg or fraction thereof over 3 to 5 minutes. Frequently titrated according to symptom relief and respiratory rate.

Actions: A synthetic narcotic agonist-antagonist analgesic. It equals morphine in analgesic effect and has one fourth of the antagonist effect of naloxone. Does produce respiratory depression, but this does not increase markedly with increased doses. Pain relief is effected in 2 to 3 minutes and last about 3 to 5 hours.

Indications and uses: Relief of moderate to severe pain, preoperative analgesia, surgical anesthesia supplement, and obstetrical analgesia during labor.

Precautions: (1) May precipitate withdrawal symptoms if stopped too quickly after prolonged use or if patient has been taking opiates. (2) Oxygen and controlled respiratory equipment must be available. (3) Observe patient frequently and monitor vital signs. (4) Physical dependence can develop with abuse. (5) Potentiated by phenothiazines (chlorpromazine [Thorazine], etc.), by other CNS depressants such as narcotic analgesics, general anesthetics, alcohol, anticholinergics, antihistamines, barbiturates, cimetidine (Tagamet), hypnotics, neuromuscular blocking agents (tubocurarine, etc.), psychotropic agents, and sedatives. Reduced doses of both drugs may be indicated. (6) Use caution in respiratory depression or difficulty from any source, impaired renal or hepatic function, and myocardial infarction with nausea and vomiting.

Contraindications: Hypersensitivity to nalbuphine. Biliary surgery, head injury, pregnancy, lactation, and children under 18 years are probable contraindications.

Incompatible with: Specific information not available.

Side effects: Anaphylaxis, blurred vision, bradycardia, clammy skin, dizziness, dry mouth, headache, hypertension, hypotension, nausea, respiratory depression, sedation, tachycardia, urinary urgency, vertigo, vomiting.

Antidote: With increasing severity of any side effect or onset of symptoms of overdose, discontinue the drug and notify the physician. Naloxone hydrochloride (Narcan) will reverse respiratory depression. A patent airway, artificial ventilation, oxygen therapy, and other symptomatic treatment must be instituted promptly.

(Narcan)

Usual dose: *Narcotic overdose:* 0.4 to 2 mg. Repeat in 2 to 3 minutes for three doses if indicated. If effective, dosage may be repeated as necessary for recurrence of symptoms.

Postoperative narcotic depression: 0.1 to 0.2 mg at 2- to 3-minute intervals to desired response. Titrate to avoid excess reduction of narcotic analgesic action.

Pediatric dose: *Ampoules containing 0.02 mg/ml are available.*

Narcotic overdose: 0.01 mg/kg of body weight initially. May repeat as an adult dose. May dilute with sterile water for injection. A single dose of 0.1 mg/kg may be indicated if above dose is ineffective.

Postoperative narcotic depression: 0.005 to 0.01 mg IV at 2- to 3-minute intervals to desired response.

Neonatal dose: 0.01 mg/kg of body weight into umbilical vein.

Dilution: May be given undiluted, diluted with sterile water for injeciton, or further diluted with normal saline or 5% dextrose solution and given as an infusion (2 mg in 500 ml equals a concentration of 0.004 mg/ml).

Rate of administration: Each 0.4 mg or fraction thereof over 15 seconds. Titrate infusion to patient response.

Actions: A potent narcotic antagonist. Overcomes narcotic-induced respiratory depression, as well as other effects of narcotic overdose. Unlike other narcotic antagonists, it does not have any narcotic effect itself. Onset of action is prompt and lasts 3 to 5 hours. Excreted in urine.

Indications and uses: (1) Reversal of narcotic depression; (2) antidote for natural and synthetic narcotics, butorphanol, methadone, nalbuphine, pentazocine, and propoxyphene; (3) diagnosis of acute opiate overdose. (4) *Investigational uses:* reversal of alcoholic coma and improvement of circulation in refractory shock.

Precautions: (1) Does not produce respiratory depression with nonnarcotic drug overdose, a beneficial action.

(2) It is ineffective against respiratory depression caused by barbiturates, anesthetics, other nonnarcotic agents, or pathological conditions. (3) Symptomatic treatment with oxygen and artificial respiration as necessary should be continued until naloxone is effective. Observe patient continuously. Duration of narcotic action may exceed that of naloxone. (4) Will precipitate acute withdrawal symptoms in narcotic addicts; use caution, especially with newborns of narcotic-dependent mothers.

Contraindications: Known hypersensitivity to naloxone, pregnancy (except during labor).

Incompatible with: Limited information available. Preparations containing bisulfite, sulfite, long-chain or high–molecular weight anions, solutions with an alkaline pH.

Side effects: Elevated partial thromboplastin time (occasional), hypertension, irritability and increased crying in the newborn, nausea and vomiting, sweating, tachycardia, tremulousness. Overdose postoperatively may result in excitement, hypertension, hypotension, reversal of analgesia, pulmonary edema, ventricular tachycardia and fibrillation.

Antidote: Notify the physician of any side effect. Treatment will probably be symptomatic. Resuscitate as necessary.

NEOSTIGMINE METHYLSULFATE   pH 5.9

(Prostigmin)

Usual dose: 0.5 to 2 mg as antidote for tubocurarine, etc. Repeat as required to restore voluntary respiration. 5 mg is the normal maximum total dose. *Myasthenia gravis:* 0.5 mg, titrate carefully; usually given IM.

Pediatric dose: 40 μg (0.04 mg)/kg of body weight with 20 μg (0.02 mg)/kg of atropine as antidote for tubocurarine, etc.

Dilution: May be given undiluted. Do not add to IV solutions. May be given through Y tube or three-way stopcock of infusion set.

Rate of administration: 0.5 mg or fraction thereof over 1 minute.

Actions: An anticholinesterase and antagonist of skeletal muscle relaxants. Inhibits the enzyme cholinesterase, allowing acetylcholine to accumulate at the myoneural junction. Restores normal transmission of nerve impulses and makes muscle contraction stronger and more prolonged.

Indications and uses: (1) Antidote for tubocurarine, atropine, hyoscine; (2) treatment of myasthenia gravis.

Precautions: (1) A physician should be present when this drug is used IV. (2) A peripheral nerve stimulator device should be used to monitor effectiveness. (3) Has many additional uses given IM or orally. (4) When used as an antidote for tubocurarine, administer atropine sulfate, 0.6 to 1.2 mg, before IV neostigmine. Pulse rate must be at least 80 beats/min. *Caution:* atropine may mask symptoms of neostigmine overdose. (5) Epinephrine should always be available. (6) Hyperventilate the patient. (7) Use extreme caution and minimal effective dose with small children, cardiac cases, severely ill patients, and asthmatic patients. Titrate exact dose, evaluate response with a peripheral stimulator device. (8) Edrophonium (Tensilon) can differentiate between increased symptoms of myasthenia and cholinergic crisis. (9) Potentiates morphine, codeine, meperidine, etc., and succinylcholine (Anectine). (10) Antagonizes ganglionic blocking agents (trimethaphan [Arfonad], etc.), and amino-

349

glycoside antibiotics (gentamicin [Garamycin], etc.). (11) Potentiated by colistimethate (Coly-Mycin); neuromuscular block may be accentuated.

Contraindications: High concentrations of inhalant anesthesia (halothane or cyclopropane, etc.); known sensitivity to bromides and neostigmine; mechanical intestinal or urinary obstruction; patients taking mecamylamine, peritonitis.

Incompatible with: Limited information available. Because of specific use and potential toxicity, neostigmine should not be mixed with any other drug.

Side effects: Usually caused by overdosage: abdominal cramps, anorexia, anxiety, bradycardia, cardiac arrhythmias and arrest, cholinergic crises, cold moist skin, convulsion, diaphoresis, diarrhea, hypotension, increased bronchial secretions, increased lacrimation, increased salivation, miosis, muscle cramps, muscle weakness, nausea, pulmonary edema, vomiting.

Antidote: *Atropine sulfate.* If side effects occur, discontinue drug and notify the physician. Atropine sulfate in doses of 0.6 mg IV will counteract most side effects and may be repeated every 3 to 10 minutes. Endotracheal intubation or tracheostomy is considered prophylactic in anesthesia or crises. Artificial ventilation, oxygen therapy, cardiac monitoring, adequate suctioning, and treatment of shock or convulsions must be instituted and maintained as necessary. Pralidoxime chloride (PAM) 1 to 2 gm IV followed by 250 mg every 5 minutes may be required to reactivate cholinesterase and reverse paralysis.

(Netromycin)

Usual dose: 1.5 to 3.25 mg/kg of body weight every 12 hours. 1.3 to 2.2 mg/kg every 8 hours in serious systemic infections. Adjust according to severity of infection and to peak and trough concentrations. Normal renal function is necessary.

Pediatric dose: *6 weeks to 12 years:* 1.8 to 2.7 mg/kg of body weight every 8 hours or 2.7 to 4 mg/kg every 12 hours.

Neonatal dose: 2 to 3.25 mg/kg of body weight every 12 hours.

Dilution: Begin with 100 mg/ml concentration for adults, 25 mg/ml concentration for pediatric range, and 10 mg/ml concentration for neonates. Further dilute each single dose in 50 to 200 ml of 0.9% normal saline, 5% dextrose in water, saline, or other compatible solutions (see literature). Decrease volume of diluent for neonates and children based on fluid requirements. Concentrations of 2 to 3 mg/ml are acceptable.

Rate of administration: Each single dose over 30 minutes to 2 hours.

Actions: An aminoglycoside antibiotic with neuromuscular blocking action. Bactericidal against specific gram-positive and gram-negative bacilli. Well distributed throughout all body fluids. Usual half-life is 2 to 2½ hours; half-life is prolonged in infants and the elderly, shorter in severe burns. Crosses the placental barrier. Excreted through the kidneys. Excreted in breast milk.

Indications and uses: (1) Short-term treatment of serious infections caused by specific organisms, (2) primarily used when penicillin and other less toxic antibiotics are ineffective or contraindicated, (3) to treat suspected infection in the immunosuppressive patient.

Precautions: (1) Narrow range between toxic and therapeutic levels. Monitor peak and trough concentrations to avoid peak serum concentrations above 16 μg/ml and trough concentrations above 4 μg/ml. Desired range is 6 to 10 and 0.5 to 2 μg/ml respectively. (2) Synergistic when used in combination with penicillins and cephalosporins. Dose adjustment and appropriate spacing are required due to physical incompatibilities. (3) Use extreme caution if therapy is required over 7 to 10 days. (4) Sensitivity studies are indicated to determine the susceptibility of the causative organism to netilmicin. (5) Reduce daily dose commensurate with amount of renal impairment. Intervals between injections should also be increased. See manufacturer's specific recommendations. (6) Watch for decrease in urine output and rising BUN and serum creatinine. Dosage may require decreasing. Routine serum levels and evaluation of hearing are recommended. (7) Use caution in infants, children, the elderly, and severly burned patients. (8) Potentiated by anesthetics, other neuromuscular blocking antibiotics (kanamycin, streptomycin, etc.), anticholinesterases (edrophonium [Tensilon], etc.), antineoplastics (nitrogen mustard, cisplatin, etc.), barbiturates, muscle relaxants (tubocurarine, etc.), phenothiazines (promethazine [Phenergan], etc.), procainamide, quinidine, and sodium citrate. *Apnea can occur.* (9) Also potentiated by other ototoxic drugs (ethacrynic acid [Edecrin], etc.) and all potent diuretics. An elevated serum level of netilmicin may occur, increasing nephrotoxicity and neurotoxicity. (10) Superinfection may occur from overgrowth of nonsusceptible organisms. (11) Maintain good hydration. (12) Stable for up to 72 hours.

Contraindications: Known netilmicin sensitivity, pregnancy, renal failure.

Incompatible with: Inactivated in solution with carbenicillin, other penicillins, and most cephalosporins. Amphotericin B, cefamandole (Mandol), cephalothin (Keflin), dopamine (Intropin), heparin. Administer separately.

Side effects: Occur more frequently with impaired renal function, higher doses, or prolonged administration. *Minor:* anorexia, burning, dizziness, fever, headache, hypertension, hypotension, itching, lethargy, muscle twitching, nausea, numbness, rash, roaring in ears, tingling sensation, tinnitus, urticaria, vomiting, and weight loss. *Major:* blood dyscrasias; convulsions; elevated bilirubin, BUN, serum creatinine, SGOT, and SGPT; hearing loss; laryngeal edema; and oliguria.

Antidote: Notify the physician of all side effects. If minor side effects persist or any major symptom appears, discontinue the drug and notify the physician. Treatment is symptomatic. Hemodialysis may be indicated.

NICOTINIC ACID AND NICOTINAMIDE

pH 6.0 to 6.5

(Niacin, niacinamide, Vasotherm)

Usual dose: 25 to 100 mg two or more times in 24 hours may be given. Up to 3 Gm/24 hr is unusual but acceptable. Dosage is determined by response. Maintain with oral dosage as soon as feasible.

Dilution: 50 to 100 mg or more may be diluted in 500 ml of isotonic sodium chloride. May be given undiluted.

Rate of administration: IV infusion may be given at a prescribed rate not to exceed the recommended rate for undiluted solution. Larger doses may extend over 12 to 24 hours. Undiluted nicotonic acid should be given at a rate not to exceed 2 mg or fraction thereof over 1 minute.

Actions: Nicotinic acid is a water-soluble vitamin that is converted to niacinamide in the body. It is essential to the metabolic activity of all living cells. Nicotinic acid produces marked peripheral vasodilation, nicotinamide does not. Metabolized in the liver, excess is excreted in the urine.

Indications and uses: (1) Treatment of acute pellagra, which usually occurs secondary to an underlying disease; (2) improvement of deficient peripheral circulation.

Precautions: (1) Other B vitamins are also indicated. (2) Use caution in patients with severe diabetes, history of peptic ulcer, impaired liver function, gallbladder disease, gout, pregnancy, lactation, women of childbearing age, and aspirin sensitivity. (3) Large doses may increase blood glucose levels. (4) Begin therapy with small doses and increase gradually. (5) Potentiates some antihypertensive drugs.

Contraindications: Active acute peptic ulcer, arterial bleeding, hemorrhage, hepatic dysfunction, hypersensitivity, serious hypotension.

Incompatible with: Alkalies, kanamycin (Kantrex).

Side effects: Expected to occur with nicotinic acid but not with nicotinamide; sometimes violent flushing with tingling, burning, and itching of the skin accompanied by an overwhelming sensation of heat is most uncomfortable for the patient. Occasionally dizziness, faintness, nausea, and vomiting occur. These symptoms are transient and subside without ill effects. With large doses, activation of peptic ulcer, abnormal liver function tests, hyperuricemia, hypotension, skin rash, or dryness may occur. Anaphylaxis is rare but may occur.

Antidote: Discontinue the drug and notify the physician of severe side effects. Treat anaphylaxis and resuscitate as necessary.

NIKETHAMIDE

pH 6.5 to 7.5

(Coramine)

Usual dose: 1 to 20 ml of a 25% solution (250 mg to 5 Gm). 5 to 10 ml is most common, and 5 ml may be repeated as necessary every 5 minutes for 1 hour and every 30 to 60 minutes thereafter as needed.

Newborn dose: *Asphyxia neonatorum:* 1.5 ml of a 25% solution may be given into the umbilical vein. *Cardiac arrest:* 0.5 ml of a 25% solution may be injected by intracardiac route.

Dilution: May be given undiluted or diluted with an equal volume of sterile water for injection.

Rate of administration: 10 ml (2.5 Gm) or fraction thereof over 1 minute.

Actions: An analeptic CNS stimulant. In respiratory depression it affects the medullary respiratory center to increase the rate and depth of respiration. It is a peripheral vasoconstrictor and produces some rise in blood pressure. A relatively safe drug with low toxicity, it converts to the vitamin nicotinamide in the body.

Indications and uses: (1) Treatment of respiratory depression secondary to anesthesia overdose, acute alcoholism, and narcotic, hypnotic, or carbon dioxide poisoning; (2) cardiac decompensation, coronary occlusion, shock and collapse; (3) sometimes used in conjunction with electroshock therapy.

Precautions: (1) Used for adjunctive therapy only. Should be supplemented by other standard emergency measures as indicated, such as artificial respiration, gastric lavage, oxygen, additional stimulants and vasopressors, etc. (2) Monitor vital signs. (3) A clear airway is essential to effectiveness of therapy. (4) Not felt to be the drug of choice for barbiturate overdose. (5) Antagonized by phenothiazines (chlorpromazine [Thorazine], etc.), but these drugs will not prevent convulsions caused by overdose. (6) Arterial injection will cause spasm and thrombosis. (7) Safety for use in pregnancy not established. (8) Rarely used; analeptic action of doxapram is more effective.

Contraindications: None is specific, except known sensitivity to nikethamide or related compounds. Not useful for chronic respiratory failure.

Incompatible with: Alkalies, dimenhydrinate (Dramamine), pentobarbital (Nembutal).

Side effects: Anxiety, burning and itching of the nose, convulsions, coughing, hypertension, muscular twitching, nausea, sneezing, tachycardia, tremor, vomiting.

Antidote: Notify the physician of side effects. Depending on severity and depth of respiratory depression, the physician may elect to continue the drug and treat the symptoms or to discontinue the drug. Diazepam (Valium) or a short-acting barbiturate (pentobarbital [Nembutal], etc.) will quiet CNS stimulation. Resuscitate as necessary.

NITROFURANTOIN SODIUM   pH 7.7 to 9.8

(Ivadantin)

Usual dose: *Over 60 kg:* 180 mg (larger doses have been used) twice every 24 hours. *Under 60 kg:* 3 mg/kg of body weight twice every 24 hours.

Dilution: Dissolve crystals immediately before use with 20 ml of 5% dextrose or sterile water for injection without bacteriostatic agent. Shake well, Must be further diluted and given as an infusion. Do not wipe vials with alcohol sponges. Use a sterile needle at each step of the dilution. Maintain aseptic technique. May be diluted only in 5% dextrose in water or saline, normal saline, or ⅙ molar sodium lactate. *Over 60 kg:* each 20 ml (180 mg) to 500 ml of IV solution. *Under 60 kg:* each 1 ml (9 mg) in at least 25 ml of IV solution.

Rate of administration: *Over 60 kg:* 1 mg (approximately 3 ml) over 1 minute. *Under 60 kg:* 0.5 mg (approximately 1.5 ml) over 1 minute. Rate may be decreased depending on patient reaction.

Actions: A urinary antiseptic most effective in acid urine, it is bacteriostatic and bactericidal toward a wide range of gram-negative and gram-positive organisms occurring in the urinary tract. It is rapidly absorbed, and up to 50% of this drug is excreted unchanged in the urine. Urine may have a brownish discoloration.

Indications and uses: Genitourinary infections due to susceptible organisms.

Precautions: (1) Sensitive to sunlight and ultraviolet light. Protect diluted IV solutions by wrapping with foil. (2) For IV use only. (3) Dilute immediately before using and discard any remaining diluted solution after 24 hours. (4) Comprehensive blood testing should be done previous to and during therapy. Patients of Mediterranean and Near Eastern origin and black patients are especially susceptible to hemolysis with nitrofurantoin. (5) Use caution in anemia, avitaminosis, debilitating disease, diabetes, electrolyte imbalance, and impaired renal function. (6) Institute therapy with oral nitrofurantoin as soon as feasible. (7) Not effective in viral or fungal infections. (8) Antibacterial activity may be increased by probenecid and acid-producing agents or decreased by phenobarbital and alkali-producing agents. (9) Alters some clinical laboratory values.

Contraindications: Anuria, children under 12 years, hypersensitivity, oliguria, pregnancy, severe renal damage.

Incompatible with: Do not mix in syringe or solution with any other antibacterials. Ammonium chloride, amphotericin B (Fungizone), calcium chloride, cephalothin (Keflin), codeine, insulin, kanamycin (Kantrex), levarterenol (Levophed), levorphanol (Levo-Dromoran), meperidine (Demerol), metaraminol (Aramine), methadone, morphine, oxacillin (Prostaphlin), oxytetracycline (Terramycin), paraaminobenzoic acid, parabens, phenols, polymyxin B (Aerosporin), procaine (Novocin), prochlorperazine (Compazine), promethazine (Phenergan), streptomycin, sulfisoxazole (Gantrisin), tetracaine (Pontocaine), tetracycline (Achromycin), vancomycin (Vancocin), vitamin B complex. Compatible only in IV solutions listed under Dilution.

Side effects: Asthma, chest pain, cough, fever, headache, hemolytic anemia, hypersensitive skin reactions, hypotension, hypothermia, insomnia, jaundice, lethargy, muscle aching, nausea, numbness, peripheral neuritis, pneumonitis (chemical), tingling, vomiting.

Antidote: Notify the physician of all side effects. Nausea and vomiting are the most common and can usually be alleviated by decreasing either the dose or the rate of administration. For any side effect the physician may treat symptomatically or discontinue the drug in favor of an alternate. Discontinue the drug immediately if numbness, tingling, asthmatic symptoms, or pneumonitis occur.

NITROGLYCERIN IV

(Nitro-Bid IV, Nitrostat IV, Tridil)

Usual dose: 5 μg/min initially. Increase by 5 μg/min increments every 3 to 5 minutes until some blood pressure response is noted. Reduce increments and/or increase time to fine tune to desired hemodynamic response. If no response at 20 μg/min, 10 μg/min increases may be used. No fixed optimum dose.

Dilution: Must be diluted and administered as an infusion. Use only glass infusion bottles and specific (non-polyvinyl chloride) infusion tubing (provided by manufacturer). Do not use filters. Dilute in a given amount of 5% dextrose or 0.9% normal saline for infusion. Concentration dependent on initial preparation (0.8 mg/ml or 5 mg/ml) and patient fluid tolerances. 10 ml of 0.8 mg/ml in 250 ml of diluent equals 32 μg/ml (in 1,000 ml, 8 μg/ml). 10 ml of 5 mg/ml in 250 ml diluent equals 200 μg/ml (in 1,000 ml, 50 μg/ml). May be used in dilutions from 25 to 400 μg/ml.

Rate of administration: Dependent on patient response and effective dose. Specific adjustments required, see under Usual dose. Use extreme caution in patients responsive to initial 5 μg/min dose. Decrease adjustments and increase intervals between as patient begins to respond. Use of an infusion pump or microdrip (60 gtt/ml) is required. Exact and constant delivery is mandatory.

Actions: A smooth muscle relaxant and vasodilator. Affects arterial and venous beds. Reduces myocardial oxygen consumption, preload and afterload by reducing systolic, diastolic and mean arterial blood pressure, central venous and pulmonary capillary wedge pressures, and pulmonary and systemic vascular resistance. Effective coronary perfusion is usually maintained. Widely distributed throughout the body. Onset of action in 1 to 2 minutes and lasts 3 to 5 minutes. Some excretion in urine.

Indications and uses: (1) Control of blood pressure in perioperative hypertension (especially cardiovascular procedures), (2) congestive heart failure in presence of acute myocardial infarction, (3) treatment of angina pectoris if patient is unresponsive to therapeutic doses of organic nitrates and/or a beta blocker, (4) controlled hypertension during surgical procedures.

Precautions: (1) Special tubing causes problems with infusion pump control. Patient may still be receiving nitroglycerin even though pump is off or tubing clamped. Low flow rates may not deliver accurate dosage. (2) Plastic (polyvinyl chloride) tubing or containers will absorb up to 80% of diluted nitroglycerin. Use extreme caution and adjust dosage if changing tubing, using extension tubings, etc. (3) If changing preparations from 0.8 mg/ml to 5.0 mg/ml, use new tubing or clear tubing with a minimum of 15 ml, adjust dosage carefully, and observe effects. (4) Protect vials from light. Solution is stable for up to 48 hours. (5) Maintain adequate systemic blood pressure and coronary perfusion pressure. Heart rate and blood pressure measurements are mandatory, pulmonary wedge pressure is recommended. (6) Observe for fall in pulmonary wedge pressure. Precedes arterial hypotension and impending shock. Reduce or discontinue drug temporarily. (7) Reduce dose gradually to prevent rebound symptoms. (8) Potentiated by alcohol, antihypertensives, other vasodilators, and tricyclic antidepressants. (9) Inhibited by sympathomimetics (phenylephrine, epinephrine). (10) Inhibits acetylcholine, histamine, norepinephrine, dopamine (Intropin), etc. (11) Potentiates nondepolarizing muscle relaxants (tubocurarine [Curare], etc.); may cause apnea. (12) Use caution in hepatic or renal disease.

Contraindications: Hypersensitivity to nitrates, hypotension or uncorrected hypovolemia, cerebral hemorrhage, head trauma, increased intracranial pressure, pericardial tamponade, pericarditis or constrictive pericarditis, and postural hypotension. Safety for use in pregnancy, lactation, and children not established.

Incompatible with: Manufacturer states, "Do not admix with any other drug."

Side effects: Abdominal pain, apprehension, dizziness, headache, hypotension, muscle twitching, nausea, palpitations, postural hypotension, restlessness, retrosternal discomfort, tachycardia, vomiting. Severe hypotension may result in shock, inadequate cerebral circulation, constrictive pericarditis, and pericardial tamponade.

Antidote: Notify physician of all side effects. For accidental overdose with severe hypotension and reflex tachycardia and/or fall in pulmonary wedge pressure, reduce rate or temporarily discontinue until condition stabilizes. Lower head of bed (Trendelenburg). An alphaadrenergic agonist (methoxamine [Vasoxyl] or phenylephrine [Neo-Synephrine]) is rarely required. Treat anaphylaxis and resuscitate as necessary.

NITROPRUSSIDE SODIUM

(Nipride, Nitropress)

Usual dose: 3 μ/kg of body weight/min. Reduce dose to as little as 0.5 μ/kg/min in patients who are receiving other antihypertensive agents by any route. Do not exceed 8 μ/kg/min. If 8 μ/kg/min does not promote adequate blood pressure reduction in 10 minutes, discontinue administration and use another antihypertensive agent.

Pediatric dose: 1.4 μg (0.0014 mg)/kg of body weight/min, adjusted slowly to individual response.

Dilution: Each 50 mg must be dissolved with 2 to 3 ml of 5% dextrose in water. Further dilute this stock solution in a minimum of 250 ml of 5% dextrose in water. Must be administered as an infusion. Larger amounts of solution may be used. 50 mg in 250 ml equals 200 μ/ml. 50 mg in 500 ml equals 100 μ/ml. No other diluent may be used. Immediately after mixing, wrap infusion bottle in aluminum foil to protect from light.

Rate of administration: Use flow rate required to reduce blood pressure gradually to preset or desired levels. Do not exceed maximum dose. Response should be noted almost immediately. Use an infusion pump or a microdrip (60 gtt/ml) to regulate dosage accurately.

Actions: A potent, rapid-acting antihypertensive agent. Produces peripheral vasodilation through direct action on smooth muscle of the blood vessels. Effective almost immediately. Will lower diastolic blood pressure 30% to 40% or more below pretreatment levels. Increases cardiac output. Effectiveness ends when IV infusion is stopped. Blood pressure will return to pretreatment levels in 1 to 10 minutes. Rapidly converted to thiocyanate and eventually excreted in the urine.

Indications and uses: Drug of choice for hypertensive emergencies, cardiogenic shock, controlled hypotension during anesthesia. *Investigational uses:* (1) Alone or in combination with dopamine to reduce afterload in hypertensive patient with myocardial infarction, persistent chest pain, or left ventricular failure. (2) In severe refractory congestive heart failure. (3) To treat lactic acidosis due to impaired peripheral perfusion. (4) To attenuate vasoconstrictor effects of dopamine and levarterenol.

Precautions: (1) Use only freshly prepared solutions; usually discard infusion within 4 hours of mixing. (Literature now states "stable to 24 hours.") (2) Solution has a faint brownish tint; discard immediately if highly colored, blue, green, or dark red. (3) Determine patency of vein, avoid extravasation. (4) Check blood pressure every 1 minute until stabilized at the desired level and every 5 to 15 minutes thereafter during therapy. Continuous monitoring is preferred. (5) Monitor pulmonary wedge pressure in patients with myocardial infarction or severe congestive heart failure. (6) Oral hypertensive agents may be given concomitantly to maintain ongoing blood pressure regulation. Reduced nitroprusside dosage may be indicated. (7) Use caution in hypothyroidism, liver or renal impairment, and the elderly. (8) Safety for use in pregnancy and children not yet established. (9) In long-term use, measure blood thiocyanate levels daily. Must not exceed 10 mg/100 ml. Potentiated by ganglionic blocking agents (pentolinium [Ansolysen], etc.) and halothane anesthesia.

Contraindications: Compensatory hypertension, for example, arteriovenous shunt or coarctation of the aorta; known inadequate cerebral circulation; or emergency surgery on moribund patients.

Incompatible with: Do not use as an additive with any other drug.

Side effects: Usually occur with too-rapid rate of infusion and are reversible: abdominal pain, apprehension, coma, diaphoresis, dizziness, dyspnea, headache, muscle twitching, nausea, palpitations, profound hypotension, restlessness, retching, retrosternal discomfort. With prolonged therapy or overdose, hypothyroidism and/or cyanide intoxication can occur.

Antidote: At first sign of side effects, decrease rate of administration. If blood pressure begins to rise or side effects persist, notify the physician. Hemodialysis or peritoneal dialysis may be indicated for thiocyanate levels over 10 mg/100 ml. For massive overdose with signs of cyanide toxicity, discontinue nitroprusside. Administer amyl nitrate inhalations for 15 to 30 seconds each minute until 3% sodium nitrite solution can be initiated as an IV injection. Do not exceed a rate of 2.5 to 5.0 ml 3% sodium nitrite solution/min to a total dose of 10 to 15 ml. Monitor blood pressure carefully. Next, inject sodium thiosulfate 12.5 Gm in 50 ml of 5% dextrose in water intravenously over 10 minutes. Observe patient. If signs of overdosage reappear, repeat the above process but use one half the dosage. Correct hypotension with vasopressors (dopamine [Intropin]).

NORMAL SERUM ALBUMIN (HUMAN)

pH 6.4 to 7.4

(Albuminar-5, Albutein, Buminate, Plasbumin)

Usual dose: Variable, depending on hemoglobin and hematocrit and amount of pulmonary or venous congestion present. Range is from 5 to 75 Gm/24 hr. Available as 5% solution (5 Gm/100 ml) in 50 ml, 250 ml, 500 ml, and 1,000 ml vials or 25% solution (25 Gm/100 ml) in 20 ml, 50 ml, and 100 ml vials. Maximum dose is 250 Gm in 48 hours.

Hypoproteinemia: 1 ml/pound of body weight/24 hr of 25% solution.

Burns: Maintain albumin level just below 4 Gm/100 ml.

Shock: Initial dose determined by patient's condition.

Pediatric dose: 5 to 25 Gm/24 hr.

Erythroblastosis fetalis: 1 Gm/kg of body weight 1 to 2 hours before blood transfusion or with transfusion.

Hypoproteinemia in premature infants: 3 to 4 ml/pound of body weight.

Dilution: May be given undiluted in solution (preferred) or further diluted with normal saline or 5% glucose for infusion.

Rate of administration: Variable, depending on indication, present blood volume, patient response, and concentration of solution. Any rate greater than 10 ml/minute may cause hypotension. Averages are:

Normal blood volume: 2 ml/min.

Deficient blood volume: 25 to 50 Gm as rapidly as tolerated. 25 Gm may be repeated in 15 to 30 minutes.

Hypoproteinemia: 2 to 3 ml/min.

Shock: 1 ml/min if normal blood volume is present. A more rapid rate may be utilized in hypovolemia.

Rate of administration in infants and children should be about one fourth to one half the adult rate.

Actions: A sterile natural plasma protein substance prepared by a specific process, which makes it free from the danger of serum hepatitis. Expands blood volume proportionately to amount of circulating blood, prevents marked hemoconcentration, aids in reduction of edema, and raises serum protein levels. Low sodium content helps to maintain electrolyte balance and should promote diuresis in presence of edema.

Indications and uses: (1) Shock, actual or impending; (2) burns; (3) hypoproteinemia with or without edema; (4) nephrosis; (5) hepatic cirrhosis; (6) cerebral edema; (7) hyperbilirubinemia or erythroblastosis fetalis as adjunct to exchange transfusion.

Precautions: (1) Use only clear solutions. (2) Store at room temperature below 37° C (98.6° F). Use promptly after opening. (3) Whole blood or packed cells are adjunctive to use of large amounts of serum albumin to prevent anemia. (4) Monitor blood pressure. (5) Hemoglobin, hematocrit, electrolyte, and serum protein evaluations are mandatory during therapy. Alkaline phosphatase may be elevated. (6) Observe patient carefully for increased bleeding resulting from more normal blood pressure, circulatory embarrassment, pulmonary edema, or lack of diuresis. Central venous pressure readings are most helpful. (7) Use caution in hypertension, low cardiac reserve, hepatic or renal failure, or lack of albumin deficiency. (8) The 5% product is isotonic and osmotically approximates human plasma. One volume of 25% to four volumes of diluent is isotonic. 25 Gm of albumin is the osmotic equivalent of 2 units of fresh frozen plasma. (9) Maintain hydration with additional fluids.

Contraindications: Anemia (severe), cardiac failure, history of allergic reaction to albumin, normal or increased intravascular volume.

Incompatible with: Ionosol D-CM, Ionosol G with dextrose 10%.

Side effects: *Minor:* fever, nausea, salivation, vomiting. *Major:* circulatory failure, dyspnea, elevated central venous pressure, precipitous hypotension, pulmonary edema.

Antidote: Notify the physician of all side effects. Minor side effects are generally tolerated and treated symptomatically. For major side effects, discontinue albumin and treat symptomatically. Resuscitate as necessary.

ORPHENADRINE CITRATE

(Banflex, Flexoject, Flexon, K-Flex, Myolin, Norflex, O-Flex, X-Otag)

Usual dose: 60 mg (2 ml) every 12 hours.

Dilution: May be given undiluted, or a single dose may be diluted in 5 to 10 ml of sterile water for injection.

Rate of administration: Equivalent of 30 mg or fraction thereof over 1 minute.

Actions: A diphenhydramine derivative with anticholinergic effects. Produces long-acting muscle relaxation, through interneuronal blocking activity, with minimal toxic effects.

Indications and uses: (1) Acute spasm of voluntary muscle, especially posttraumatic, discogenic, and tension spasms; (2) treatment of nicotine-induced convulsions.

Precautions: (1) Equal effectiveness produced by IM or oral route. Use IV only when necessary for rapid onset of action. (2) Use caution in tachycardia, cardiac arrhythmias, cardiac decompensation, coronary insufficiency. (3) Not recommended for concomitant use with propoxyphene (Darvon) or perphenazine (Trilafon). (4) Potentiates anticholinergic drugs. (5) Not recommended for children.

Contraindications: Bladder neck obstruction, cardiospasm, glaucoma, hypersensitivity to orphenadrine citrate, myasthenia gravis, pregnancy and lactation, prostatic hypertrophy, pyloric or duodenal obstruction, stenosing peptic ulcer.

Incompatible with: No specific information available. Note precautions and contraindications.

Side effects: Usually associated with higher doses or too-rapid administration: blurred vision, dizziness, drowsiness, dryness of mouth, excitation, headache, light-headedness, nausea, palpitations, pupil dilation, tachycardia, urinary retention, urticaria, vomiting, weakness.

Antidote: Notify the physician of any side effects. Reduction of dosage will probably relieve them. For symptoms of hypersensitivity, discontinue the drug, notify the physician, and treat symptomatically. Resuscitate as necessary.

(Bactocil, Prostaphlin)

Usual dose: Over 40 kg: 250 mg to 1 Gm or more every 4 to 6 hours. Under 40 kg: 50 to 100 mg/kg of body weight/24 hr in equally divided doses every 6 hours.

Infant dose: Prematures and neonates: 25 mg/kg of body weight/24 hr in equally divided doses every 6 hours.

Dilution: Each 500 mg or fraction thereof should be diluted in 5 ml of sterile water or sodium chloride for injection. May be further diluted in 5% dextrose in water or saline, normal saline, lactated Ringer's solution, or other compatible IV solutions (see literature).

Rate of administration: 1 Gm (10 ml) or fraction thereof slowly over 10 minutes. May be administered in specific IV solutions (check literature) over a 6-hour period. Concentration should be about 2 mg/ml.

Actions: A semisynthetic penicillin with bactericidal effect against penicillinase-producing organisms, gram-positive cocci, beta hemolytic streptococci, and others. Easily absorbed. Evidenced in most body fluids including trace amounts in spinal fluid. Excreted primarily in the urine. Crosses placental barrier.

Indications and uses: Infection caused by penicillinase-producing staphylococci.

Precautions: (1) Sensitivity studies are necessary to determine the susceptibility of the causative organism to oxacillin. (2) Superinfection caused by overgrowth of nonsusceptible organisms is a possibility. (3) Periodic liver, kidney, and hematopoietic studies are advised. (4) Limited experience in use on prematures and neonates. Use with caution. (5) Diluted solution is stable for no more than 6 hours. (6) Penicillins interact with many drugs and some of these, such as antibiotics (chloramphenicol, erythromycins, and tetracyclines), can inhibit the bactericidal activity of the penicillins. (7) Inhibits aminoglycosides (gentamicin, kanamycin, etc.). Do not mix in same IV container.

Contraindications: Known sensitivity to any penicillin or cephalothin; pregnancy.

Incompatible with: Amikacin (Amikin), levarterenol (Levophed), metaraminol (Aramine), oxytetracycline (Terramycin).

Side effects: Relatively infrequent: diarrhea, elevated SGOT, hypersensitivity with anaphylaxis, nausea, pruritus, skin rash, thrombophlebitis, transient hematuria in newborns, urticaria, vomiting.

Antidote: Notify the physician of early symptoms. For severe symptoms discontinue drug, treat allergic reaction or resuscitate as necessary, and notify the physician.

OXYMORPHONE HYDROCHLORIDE

pH 2.7 to 4.5

(Numorphan)

Usual dose: 0.5 mg initially. May repeat every 2 to 4 hours. Up to 1.5 mg may be required.

Dilution: Each dose should be diluted with 5 ml of sterile water or normal saline for injection. May give through Y tube or three-way stopcock of infusion set.

Rate of administration: A single dose properly diluted over 3 to 5 minutes. Usually titrated according to symptom relief and respiratory rate.

Actions: An opium derivative and CNS depressant closely related to morphine. Ten times more potent than morphine milligram for milligram. Onset of action is prompt and lasts 3 to 4 hours. Detoxified in the liver and excreted in the urine. Crosses placental barrier. Excreted in breast milk.

Indications and uses: (1) Relief of moderate to severe pain, (2) support of anesthesia, (3) obstetrical analgesia, (4) relief of anxiety in dyspnea of acute left ventricular failure and pulmonary edema.

Precautions: (1) Oxygen and controlled respiratory equipment must be available. (2) Observe patient frequently and monitor vital signs. (3) Physical dependence can develop with abuse. (4) Use caution in the elderly and in patients with impaired hepatic or renal function and emphysema. (5) Potentiated by phenothiazines and other CNS depressants, such as narcotic analgesics, alcohol, antihistamines, barbiturates, cimetidine (Tagamet), hypnotics, sedatives, MAO inhibitors (isocarboxazid [Marplan], etc.), neuromuscular blocking agents (tubocurarine, etc.), and psychotropic agents. Reduced dosages of both drugs may be indicated. (6) Tolerance to oxymorphone gradually increases.

Contraindications: Bronchial asthma, children under 12 years of age, increased intracranial pressure, known hypersensitivity to opiates.

Incompatible with: Specific information not available (consider similarity to morphine).

Side effects: Nausea, vomiting, and drowsiness are less

frequent than with morphine. *Minor:* anorexia, constipation, dizziness, skin rash, urinary retention, and urticaria. *Major:* anaphylaxis, hypotension, respiratory depression, somnolence.

Antidote: Notify the physician of any side effect. If minor side effects progress or any major side effect occurs, discontinue the drug and notify the physician. Treat anaphylaxis as indicated or resuscitate as necessary. Naloxone hydrochloride (Narcan) or levallorphan tartrate (Lorfan) will reverse serious respiratory depression.

OXYTETRACYCLINE
HYDROCHLORIDE IV

pH 1.8 to 2.8

(Terramycin IV)

Usual dose: 250 to 500 mg every 6 to 12 hours. Maximum dose in 24 hours is 500 mg every 6 hours. Normal renal function is required.

Pediatric dose: 12 mg/kg of body weight/24 hr in two equal doses. May vary from 10 to 20 mg/kg/24 hr.

Dilution: Each 250 mg or fraction thereof is diluted with 10 ml of sterile water for injection. Each 500 mg or fraction thereof must be further diluted with a minimum of 100 ml of 5% dextrose in water or isotonic saline for injection or preferably added to some standard infusion solutions such as normal saline, dextrose in water or saline, or Ringer's solution.

Rate of administration: Each 100 mg or fraction thereof over a minimum of 5 minutes. Never exceed this rate. Must be completed within 12 hours of dilution.

Actions: A broad-spectrum antibiotic that is bacteriostatic against many gram-positive and gram-negative organisms. Thought to interfere with the protein synthesis of microorganisms. Well distributed in most body tissues and often bound to plasma protein, tetracyclines are concentrated in the liver and excreted through the bile to urine and feces in a biologically active state. Crosses the placental barrier. Excreted in breast milk.

Indications and uses: (1) Infections caused by susceptible strains or organisms, such as rickettsiae, spirochetal agents, viruses, and many other gram-negative and gram-positive bacteria; (2) to substitute for contraindicated penicillin or sulfonamide therapy.

Precautions: (1) Must be stored away from heat and light. (2) Check expiration date; outdated ampoules may cause nephrotoxicity. (3) After reconstitution store at 2° to 8° C (36° to 46° F) and use within 48 hours. (4) Buffered with ascorbic acid. (5) Sensitivity studies are necessary to determine the susceptibility of the causative organism to oxytetracycline. (6) Avoid prolonged use of drug. Superinfection caused by overgrowth of nonsusceptible organisms may result. (7)

Use caution in impaired liver or renal function, pregnancy, postpartum, and lactation. Tetracycline serum concentrations and liver and kidney function tests are indicated. (8) May cause skeletal retardation in the fetus and infants and permanent tooth discoloration in children under 8 years of age, including in utero or through mother's milk. (9) Inhibits bactericidal action of penicillin, ampicillin, oxacillin, methicillin, etc. May be toxic with sulfonamides. (10) May potentiate digoxin and anticoagulants. Reduced dosage of these drugs may be necessary. (11) Potentiated by alcohol barbiturates, cimetidine (Tagamet), phenytoin (Dilantin), and other hepatotoxic drugs; severe liver damage may result. (12) Inhibited by alkalinizing agents, calcium, iron, and magnesium salts, riboflavin, sodium bicarbonate, and others. (13) Alert patient to photosensitive skin reaction. (14) Determine patency of vein, avoid extravasation. (15) Organisms resistant to one tetracycline are usually resistant to others.

Contraindications: Known hypersensitivity to tetracyclines.

Incompatible with: Any solution with a pH above 6.0. Aminophylline, amikacin (Amikin), amobarbital (Amytal), amphotericin B (Fungizone), ampicillin, calcium chloride, calcium gluconate, carbenicillin (Geopen), cephapirin (Cefadyl), cefazolin, cephalothin (Keflin), chloramphenicol (Chloromycetin), colistimethate (Coly-Mycin M), cloxacillin, erythromycin (Ilotycin, Erythrocin), heparin, hydrocortisone phosphate, hydrocortisone sodium succinate (Solu-Cortef), iron dextran, lactated Ringer's injection with 5% dextrose, lactated Ringer's injection, metaraminol (Aramine), methicillin (Staphcillin), nafcillin (Unipen), nitrofurantoin (Ivadantin), oxacillin (Prostaphlin), potassium penicillin G, pentobarbital (Nembutal), phenobarbital (Luminal), phenytoin (Dilantin), phytonadione (Aquamephyton), polymyxin B (Aerosporin), prochlorerazine (Compazine), sodium bicarbonate, sodium lactate, succinylcholine (Anectine), sulfisoxazole (Gantrisin), tetracycline (Achromycin), thiopental (Pentothal), trifluoperazine, vancomycin (Vancocin), vitamin B complex with C, warfarin (Coumadin).

Side effects: Relatively nontoxic in average doses, more toxic in large doses or if given too rapidly. *Minor:* anogenital lesions, anorexia, blood dyscrasias, diarrhea, dysphagia, enterocolitis, nausea, skin rashes, vomiting. *Major:* hypersensitivity reactions including anaphylaxis; liver damage; photosensitivity; systemic moniliasis; thrombophlebitis.

Antidote: Notify the physician of all side effects. If minor side effects are progressive or any major side effect occurs, discontinue the drug, treat the allergic reaction, or resuscitate as necessary.

(Pitocin, Syntocinon)

Usual dose: Determined by intended use, dilution, and rate of administration.

Dilution: *Induction of labor:* dilute 1 ml (10 units) in 1 liter of 0.9% normal saline or 5% dextrose in normal saline for infusion (10 mU/ml).

Control of postpartum bleeding: dilute 1 to 4 ml (10 to 40 units) in 1 liter of above infusion fluids (10 to 40 mU/ml).

Incomplete or inevitable abortion: dilute 1 ml (10 units) to 500 ml of above infusion fluids (20 mU/ml).

Rotate gently to distribute medication through solution in all situations.

Rate of administration: Given only as an intravenous infusion. Use of an infusion pump or other accurate control device is required. In all situations, use the minimal effective rate and monitor strength, frequency, and duration of contractions, resting uterine tone, fetal heart rate, and maternal blood pressure at least every 15 minutes or more often if indicated.

Induction of labor: begin with 1 to 2 mU/min (0.1 to 0.2 ml), increase in increments of 1 to 2 mU/min at 15- to 30-minute intervals until contractions simulate normal labor. Maximum dose rarely exceeds 20 mU/min.

Control of postpartum bleeding: rate of infusion must control uterine atony. Begin with 10 to 20 mU/min. Increase or decrease rate as indicated. Proceed quickly but with caution due to strength of solution.

Incomplete or inevitable abortion: 10 to 20 mU/min.

Actions: A synthetic posterior pituitary derivative that will produce rhythmic contraction of uterine smooth muscle. Its effectiveness depends on the level of uterine excitability, which usually increases as a pregnancy progresses. Very rapid acting, it has a shorter duration of action than ergot derivatives and is the drug of choice for induction of delivery. Probably detoxified in the liver and excreted in the urine. Has a weak antidiuretic effect.

Indications and uses: (1) After selective patient evaluation by the physician, it is used to induce or stimulate labor at term or before. (2) To control postpartum bleeding. (3) Treatment of incomplete or inevitable abortion.

Precautions: (1) An IV of 0.9% normal saline without oxytocins must be hung, connected by Y tube or three-way stopcock, and ready for use in adverse reactions. (2) Should be administered only in the hospital, and the physician must be immediately available. (3) Monitor blood pressure, fetal heart tones, strength and timing of contractions, and resting uterine tone at least every 15 minutes or more often if indicated. Continuous observation of the patient is required. (4) Monitor oral fluid intake and observe for signs of fluid retention. Water intoxication has caused maternal death. (5) Oxytocins must be administered by only one route at a time. Do not combine oral and IV routes, etc. (6) Severe hypertension can result in the presence of local anesthesia and regional anesthesia (caudal or spinal) and with dopamine (Intropin), ephedrine, epinephrine, methoxamine (Vasoxyl), and other vasopressors. Chlorpromazine (Thorazine) IV will reduce this hypertension. (7) Refrigerate to store for long periods.

Contraindications: Abruptio placentae, cephalopelvic disproportion, cesarean section (previous) or uterine surgery, dead fetus, fetal distress, fetal malpresentation, hypersensitivity, hypertonic uterine contractions, serious medical or obstetrical conditions (past or present), toxemia (severe).

Incompatible with: Levarterenol (Levophed), prochlorperazine (Compazine), warfarin (Coumadin).

Side effects: Afibrinogenemia, anaphylaxis, cardiac arrhythmias, fetal bradycardia, fetal death, fluid retention leading to coma and convulsion, hypertension, nausea, pelvic hematoma, postpartum hemorrhage, severe uterine spasm or contraction, subarachnoid hemorrhage, uterine rupture, vomiting.

Antidote: Nausea and vomiting are tolerable and can be treated symptomatically. Call the physician's attention immediately to any side effect noted or suspected.

Discontinue the drug immediately for uterine hyperactivity or fetal distress. Administer oxygen to the mother. Use of a Y connection or three-way stopcock, allowing the oxytocin drip to be discontinued while the vein is kept open, is required. These side effects can occur during labor and delivery and into the postpartum period. Careful evaluation and selection of patients eliminate many hazards, but the nurse must be prepared for an emergency.

PANCURONIUM BROMIDE

(Pavulon)

Usual dose: Must be individualized, depending on previous drugs administered and degree and length of muscle relaxation required. 0.04 to 0.1 mg/kg of body weight initially. 0.01 mg/kg in increments as required to maintain muscle relaxation.

Dilution: May be given undiluted.

Rate of administration: A single dose over 60 to 90 seconds.

Actions: A skeletal muscle relaxant five times as potent as tubocurarine chloride (curare). Causes paralysis by interfering with neural transmission at the myoneural junction. Onset of action is dose dependent. May occur in 30 seconds and lasts about 25 minutes. It may take another 30 minutes before complete recovery occurs. Excreted in the urine.

Indications and uses: (1) Adjunctive to general anesthesia, (2) in management of patients undergoing mechanical ventilation.

Precautions: Should be stored in refrigerator. (2) Administered only by or under the direct observation of the anesthesiologist. (3) This drug produces apnea. Controlled artificial ventilation with oxygen must be continuous and under direct observation at all times. Maintain a patent airway. (4) Use a peripheral nerve stimulator to monitor response to pancuronium and avoid overdosage. (5) Repeated doses may produce a cumulative effect. (6) Impaired pulmonary function or respiratory deficiencies can cause critical reactions. Use caution in impaired liver or kidney function. (7) Myasthenia gravis increases sensitivity to drug. (8) Potentiated by hypokalemia, some carcinomas, inhalant anesthetics (ether, etc.), neuromuscular blocking antibiotics (clindamycin [Cleocin]), kanamycin [Kantrex], gentamicin [Garamycin], etc.), carbon dioxide, diuretics, diazepam (Valium) and other muscle relaxants, digitalis, magnesium sulfate, MAO inhibitors, quinidine, morphine, lidocaine, meperidine, propranalol (Inderal), and others. Markedly reduced dose of pancuronium must be used with caution. (9) Antagonized by anticholinesterases, aminophylline, and potassium ions. Hyperkalemia may cause cardiac arrhythmias. (10) Succinylcholine must show signs of wearing off before pancuronium is given. Use caution. (11) Patient may be conscious and completely unable to communicate by any means. Pancuronium has no analgesic properties. Respiratory depression with morphine may be preferred in some patients requiring mechanical ventilation. (12) Action is altered by dehydration, electrolyte imbalance, body temperatures, and acid-base imbalance.

Contraindications: Known hypersensitivity to pancuronium or bromides.

Incompatible with: Specific information not available. Note precautions.

Side effects: Prolonged action resulting in respiratory insufficiency or apnea. Airway closure caused by relaxation of epiglottis, pharynx, and tongue muscles. Hypersensitivity reactions are possible. Anaphylaxis, histamine release, hypotension, and shock may occur.

Antidote: All side effects are medical emergencies. Treat symptomatically. Controlled artificial ventilation must be continuous. Pyridostigmine (Mestinon) or neostigmine (Prostigmin) given with atropine will probably reverse the muscle relaxation. Not effective in all situations. Resuscitate as necessary.

PAPAVERINE HYDROCHLORIDE   pH 3.0 to 4.5

Usual dose: 1 to 4 ml (30 to 120 mg) every 3 to 6 hours if indicated. Second dose may be given in 10 minutes only when treating extrasystoles.

Dilution: May be given undiluted or may be diluted in an equal amount of sterile water for injection. Usually not added to IV solutions. May be given through Y tube or three-way stopcock of infusion set.

Rate of administration: 1 ml (30 mg) or fraction thereof over 2 minutes.

Actions: An opium alkaloid, nonnarcotic and nonaddictive, it is an excellent direct smooth muscle relaxant and antispasmodic. More effective on muscle in spasm, it has a particular affinity for the smooth muscle of blood vessels. Affects cardiac muscle to depress conduction and increase refractory period. Improved circulation and muscle relaxation decrease pain. Metabolized in the liver and excreted in the urine.

Indications and uses: (1) Vascular spasm associated with an acute myocardial infarction; (2) peripheral or pulmonary embolism; (3) peripheral vascular disease and cerebral angiospastic states; (4) visceral spasm of ureteral, biliary, or gastrointestinal colic; (5) angina pectoris.

Precautions: (1) May be used with narcotics if the relaxant effect is not adequate to relieve discomfort. Narcotic dosage should be reduced. (2) Rapid IV injection may cause death. (3) IM injection is preferred. (4) Use with caution in glaucoma and impaired liver function. (5) Antagonizes effects of levodopa.

Contraindications: Complete AV heart block.

Incompatible with: Alkaline solutions, aminophylline, lactated Ringer's injection.

Side effects: *Minor:* blurred or double vision, diaphoresis, discomfort (generalized), flushing, hypertension (slight), hypotension, respiratory depth increase, scleral jaundice, sedation, tachycardia. *Major:* respiratory depression, ventricular ectopic rhythms (transient), sudden death.

Antidote: Notify the physician of any minor side effects. If minor symptoms progress or any major side effect appears, discontinue the drug immediately and notify the physician. Treatment of toxicity will be symptomatic and supportive. Resuscitate as necessary.

383

PARALDEHYDE

(Paral)

Usual dose: 3 to 5 ml. May repeat in 6 to 8 hours with extreme caution.

Dilution: Each 1 ml should be diluted with at least 2 ml of sodium chloride for injection.

Rate of administration: Each 1 ml or fraction thereof of diluted medication over at least 1 minute. 3 ml of paraldehyde would take 9 minutes.

Actions: A potent CNS depressant. used as a sedative and a hypnotic. Effective within 30 minutes, lasts 6 to 8 hours. Metabolized in the liver and partly excreted in the lungs.

Indications and uses: (1) Delirium tremens, (2) tetanus, (3) eclampsia, (4) status epilepticus, (5) poisoning from convulsant drugs.

Precautions: (1) Use a glass syringe; reacts rapidly with plastics. (2) Use IV route only in an emergency. Oral, rectal, or IM route is as efficient with fewer side effects. (3) Use only fresh, clear solutions. (4) Air exposure converts paraldehyde to toxic acetic acid; discard unused medication carefully. Corrosive to tissues. (5) A lethal and addictive drug. (6) Position patient on side to prevent aspiration of increased bronchial secretions. (7) Breath will have a distinctive odor. (8) Do not use concurrently with sulfonamides or disulfiram (Antabuse). (9) Additive effects with anesthetics, MAO inhibitors (isocarboxazid [Marplan], etc.), and tricyclic antidepressants (amitriptyline [Elavil], etc.). (10) Produces excitement or delirium in presence of pain.

Contraindications: Severe hepatic insufficiency, respiratory disease, gastroenteritis with ulceration.

Incompatible with: Plastics, chlorpromazine (Thorazine), prochlorperazine (Compazine); do not mix in syringe or solution with any other drug.

Side effects: Acidosis, circulatory collapse, cough, cyanosis, dilation of right heart, hypotension, liver damage, pulmonary edema, pulmonary hemorrhage, rapid labored respiration, renal damage, death.

Antidote: Discontinue the drug and notify the physician of any side effects. Symptomatic and supportive treatment is most important in overdosage. Mechanical ventilation may be essential in respiratory depression. Doxapram (Dopram) may be useful.

PENICILLIN G POTASSIUM AND
PENICILLIN G SODIUM   pH 6.0 to 7.0

(Penicillin G, Pfizerpen)

Usual dose: 1 to 20 million units/24 hr equally distributed over 24 hours as a continuous infusion. Doses up to 80 million units/24 hr have been given in life-threatening infections. *(400,000 units equals approximately 250 mg.)*

Pediatric dose: 25,000 units/kg of body weight every 6 hours. Dosage can vary greatly and must be adjusted depending on the severity of the infection.

Neonatal dose: 30,000 units/kg of body weight every 12 hours.

Dilution: Initial dilution must be with sterile water for injection. Direct flow of water against sides of the vial while gently rotating vial. Shake vigorously. Directions on vial should be followed to provide desired number of units per milliliter. Available with 1, 5, 10, and 20 million units per vial. May be added to 0.9% sodium chloride or dextrose solutions for infusion.

Rate of administration: Penicillin is not given by direct IV route. Administer as ordered as continuous IV drip; for example, 5 million units in 1,000 ml of 5% dextrose in water over 12 hours. Is sometimes given by intermittent infusion (a single dose in 100 ml every 2, 4, or 6 hours). Dosage level must be maintained to provide therapeutic serum levels. Too-rapid administration or excessive doses may cause electrolyte imbalance and/or seizures. Stable at room temperature for at least 24 hours.

Actions: Bactericidal against penicillin-sensitive microorganisms during the stage of active multiplication. Excreted in the urine. Excreted in breast milk. Available in a potassium or sodium salt containing 1.7 mEq of the salt in 1,000,000 units (39 to 46 mg).

Indications and uses: (1) Severe infections caused by penicillin G–sensitive microorganisms (e.g., streptococcal, pneumococcal, Vincent's gingivitis, spirochetal infections, meningitis, endocarditis); (2) prophylaxis against bacterial endocarditis in specific situations.

Precautions: (1) Sensitivity studies are necessary to determine the susceptibility of the causative organism to penicillin. (2) Adjust dosage down for individuals with impaired kidney function. (3) Allergic reactions are most likely to occur in patients with a history of sensitivity to multiple allergens. (4) Periodic evaluation of renal and hematopoietic systems is recommended in prolonged therapy. (5) Electrolyte imbalance from potassium or sodium content is very possible. (6) Avoid prolonged use of drug; superinfection caused by overgrowth of nonsusceptible organisms may result. (7) Penicillins interact with many drugs; some of these, such as antibiotics (chloramphenicol, erythromycin, aminoglycosides [kanamycin, etc.], and tetracyclines), will inhibit the bactericidal activity of penicillins. Inactivated by acids, alkalies, oxidizing agents, and carbohydrate solutions with an alkaline pH. (8) Optimal pH range is 6.0 to 7.0. (9) Observe for thrombophlebitis. (10) Potassium penicillin is most frequently used.

Contraindications: Known sensitivity to any penicillin.

Incompatible with: To preserve bactericidal action, do not mix other agents with penicillin in the infusion solution. Acid media, alkaline media, aminophylline, amphotericin B (Fungizone), ascorbic acid, cephalothin (Keflin), chlorpromazine (Thorazine), dopamine (Intropin), heparin, hydroxyzine (Vistaril), lincomycin (Lincocin), metaraminol (Aramine), oxytetracycline (Terramycin), pentobarbital (Nembutal), phenytoin (Dilantin), prochlorperazine (Compazine), promazine (Sparine), promethazine (Phenergan), sodium bicarbonate, tetracycline, thiopental (Pentothal), trifluoperazine (Stelazine), vancomycin (Vancocin), vitamin B complex with C.

Side effects: *Minor:* arthralgia, chills, edema, fever, prostration, skin rash, urticaria. *Major:* anaphylaxis, convulsions, hyperreflexia, potassium poisoning with coma, sodium-induced congestive heart failure.

Antidote: For all side effects, discontinue the drug, treat the allergic reaction or resuscitate as necessary, and notify the physician. Treat minor side effects symptomatically according to physician's order.

PENTAZOCINE (LACTATE)

(Talwin)

Usual dose: 5 to 30 mg. May repeat every 3 to 4 hours or decrease to 5 to 15 mg and repeat every 2 hours. 360 mg equals maximum dose in 24 hours.

Dilution: May be given undiluted. It is preferable to dilute each 5 mg with at least 1 ml of sterile water for injection.

Rate of administration: Each 5 mg or fraction thereof over 1 minute.

Actions: A weak narcotic antagonist with a potent analgesic action, pentazocine is somewhat less effective than morphine and meperidine in equivalent doses. Onset of action is prompt, 2 to 3 minutes, and lasts about 2 hours. Crosses the placental barrier. Excreted in breast milk.

Indications and uses: (1) Relief of moderate to severe pain, (2) preoperative medication, (3) support of anesthesia, (4) obstetrical analgesia.

Precautions: (1) Oxygen and controlled ventilation equipment must always be available. (2) Observe patient continuously during injection and frequently thereafter. Monitor vital signs. (3) Low addictive element. (4) Use with caution in bronchial asthma, relief of biliary pain, history of drug abuse, myocardial infarction (especially if nausea and vomiting are present), during delivery of premature infants, decreased renal or hepatic function, respiratory depression from any cause, and a history of seizures. (5) Mild narcotic antagonist. May precipitate withdrawal symptoms in patients accumstomed to narcotics. (6) May have less effective analgesia in heavy smokers. (7) Use caution with CNS depressants, such as narcotic analgesics, general anesthetics, alcohol, anticholinergics, antihistamines, barbiturates, hypnotics, sedatives, psychotropic agents, MAO inhibitors, and neuromuscular blocking agents (tubocurarine etc.).

Contraindications: Children under 12 years, head injury, hypersensitivity to pentazocine, pathological brain conditions, increased intracranial pressure.

Incompatible with: All barbiturates, aminophylline, glycopyrrolate (Robinul), sodium bicarbonate.

Side effects: Allergic reactions, apprehension, blurred vision, circulatory depression, confusion, constipation, cramps, depression, diarrhea, disorientation, double vision, dreams, drug dependence, dry mouth, dyspnea, facial edema, floating feeling, flushing, hallucinations, headache, hypertension, insomnia, muscle tremor, neonatal apnea, nervousness, nystagmus, paresthesias, perspiration, pruritus, respiratory depression, sedation, seizures, shock, tachycardia, taste alteration, urinary retention, uterine contraction depression.

Antidote: For any side effect, discontinue the drug and notify the physician. Treat side effects symptomatically. For overdose or respiratory depression, naloxone hydrochloride (Narcan) is the antidote of choice. If naloxone is not available, methylphenidate (Ritalin) may be of value in respiratory depression (only available in oral form).

PENTOBARBITAL SODIUM   pH 9.0 to 10.5

(Nembutal sodium)

Usual dose: 100 mg initially. Wait 1 full minute between each dose to determine drug effect. Additional doses in increments of 25 to 50 mg may be given as indicated. Maximum dose ranges from 200 to 500 mg.

Pediatric dose: Initial dose is 50 mg.

Dilution: May be given undiluted or, preferably, may be further diluted in sterile water, sodium chloride for injection, or Ringer's injection. Any desired amount of diluent may be used. 9 ml of diluent with 1 ml of pentobarbital (50 mg) equals 5 mg/ml.

Rate of administration: 50 mg or fraction thereof over 1 minute. Titrate slowly to desired effect.

Actions: A sedative, hypnotic barbiturate of short duration with anticonvulsant effects. Pentobarbital is a CNS depressant. Onset of action is prompt by the IV route and lasts about 3 to 4 hours. Will effectively depress the motor cortex if adequate doses are administered. Pain perception is unimpaired. Detoxified in the liver and excreted fairly quickly in the urine in changed form. Crosses the placental barrier. Excreted in breast milk.

Indications and uses: (1) Preanesthetic sedation, (2) dental and minor surgical sedation, (3) control of convulsions caused by disease and drug poisoning, (4) sedation in psychotic states.

Precautions: (1) Use only absolutely clear solutions. (2) Rapid injection rate may cause symptoms of overdose. (3) Record blood pressure, pulse, and respiration every 3 to 5 minutes. Keep patient under constant observation. (4) Maintain a patent airway. (5) Treat the cause of a convulsion. (6) May be habit forming. (7) Use caution in status asthmaticus, shock, severe liver diseases, uremia, and depressive state after a convulsion. (8) Determine absolute patency of vein; use of large veins is preferred to prevent thrombosis. Avoid extravasation. Intraarterial injection will cause gangrene. (9) Use extreme caution if any other CNS depressants have been given, such as alcohol, narcotic analgesics, anesthetics, antidepressants, sedatives, aminoglycoside antibiotics, tranquilizers, etc.; potentiation with respiratory depression may occur. (10) Inhibits effectiveness of propranolol (Inderal), corticosteroids, doxycycline (Vibramycin), oral anticoagulants, oral contraceptives, quinidine. Capable of innumerable interactions with many drugs. (11) Will cause birth defects. (12) May cause paradoxical excitement in children or the elderly.

Contraindications: Delivery (when maximal drug effect would be at the time of delivery), history of porphyria, known hypersensitivity to barbiturates, pregnancy, premature delivery, severe respiratory depression.

Incompatible with: Brompheniramine (Dimetane-Ten), cefazolin (Kefzol), cephalothin (Keflin), chlordiazepoxide (Librium), chlorpheniramine (Chlor-Trimeton), chlorpromazine (Thorazine), cimetidine (Tagamet), clindamycin (Cleocin), codeine, diphenhydramine (Benadryl), droperidol (Inapsine), ephedrine, erythromycin (Ilotycin), fructose solutions, glycopyrrolate (Robinul), hydrocortisone sodium succinate (Solu-Cortef), hydroxyzine (Vistaril), insulin (aqueous), kanamycin (Kantrex), levarterenol (Levophed), levorphanol (Levo-Dromoran), meperidine (Demerol), methadone, morphine, oxytetracycline (Terramycin), penicillins, pentazocine (Talwin), phenytoin (Dilantin), prochlorperazine (Compazine), promazine (Sparine), promethazine (Phenergan), sodium bicarbonate, streptomycin, succinylcholine (Anectine), tetracycline, triflupromazine (Vesprin), vancomycin (Vancocin).

Side effects: *Average dose:* asthma, bronchospasm, depression, dermatitis, facial edema, fever, hypotension, neonatal apnea, pain at or below injection site, respiratory depression (slight), thrombocytopenic purpura.

Overdose: apnea, coma, cough reflex depression, hypotension, laryngospasm, lowered body temperature, pulmonary edema, reflexes (sluggish or absent), renal shutdown, respiratory depression.

Antidote: Discontinue drug immediately for pain at or below injection site. Notify the physician of any side effects. Symptomatic and supportive treatment are

391

most important in overdosage. Maintain an adequate airway with artificial ventilation if indicated. Keep the patient warm. Intravenous volume expanders (dextran) will help maintain adequate circulation. Diuretics or hemodialysis will promote the elimination of the drug. Vasopressors (dopamine [Intropin]) will maintain blood pressure.

PERPHENAZINE

(Trilafon)

Usual dose: 1 mg, repeat as necessary, allowing 2 to 3 minutes between doses, only until symptoms are controlled. Do not exceed 5 mg.

Dilution: Each 5 mg (1 ml) must be diluted with 9 ml of normal saline for injection. 1 ml will equal 0.5 mg. May be further diluted and given as an infusion under observation of anesthesiologist (use an infusion pump or a microdrip, 60 gtt/ml).

Rate of administration: 0.5 mg or fraction thereof over 1 minute.

Actions: A phenothiazine derivative said to be six times more potent than chlorpromazine (Thorazine) with effects on the central, autonomic, and peripheral nervous systems. Decreases anxiety and tension, relaxes muscle, produces sedation, and tranquilizes. A potent antiemetic. Onset of action is prompt and lasting. Excretion is slow through the kidneys.

Indications and uses: Control of severe vomiting, intractable hiccups, or acute symptoms such as violent retching during surgery.

Precautions: (1) Use IV only when absolutely necessary. (2) Check label on ampoule. Only single-dose, 5 mg ampoules may be given IV. (3) Handle carefully; may cause contact dermatitis. Sensitive to light. Slightly yellow color does not affect potency. Discard if markedly discolored. (4) Keep patient in supine position and monitor blood pressure and pulse between doses. (5) May mask diagnosis of brain tumor, drug intoxication, and intestinal obstruction. (6) Use caution in coronary disease, severe hypertension or hypotension, and epilepsy. (7) Temperature without etiology indicates drug intolerance. (8) Potentiates CNS depressants such as narcotics, barbiturates, alcohol, anesthetics, MAO inhibitors (pargyline [Eutonuyl], etc.), oral antidiabetics, insulin, anticholinergics, antihistamines, antihypertensives, hypnotics, muscle relaxants, and rauwolfia alkaloids. Reduce dosage of any medication potentiated by phenothiazines by one fourth to one half; has less potentiating effect than other phenothiazines. (9) Contraindicated with quinidine, epinephrine, and thiazide diuretics. (10) Capable of innumerable other interactions.

Contraindications: Comatose or severely depressed states and hypersensitivity to phenothiazines.

Incompatible with: Specific information not available. Refer to other phenothiazines such as prochlorperazine (Compazine).

Side effects: Usually transient if drug is discontinued, but may require treatment if severe: anaphylaxis, blurring of vision, cardiac arrest, dermatitis, dizziness, dryness of mouth, dysphagia, extrapyramidal symptoms (such as abnormal positioning, extreme restlessness, pseudoparkinsonism, weakness of extremities), elevated blood pressure, excitement, hypersensitivity reactions, hypotension, slurred speech, spastic movements (especially about the face), tachycardia, temperature without etiology, tightness of the throat, tongue discoloration, tongue protrusion, and many others.

Antidote: Discontinue the drug at onset of any side effect and notify the physician. Counteract hypotension with dopamine (Intropin) or levarterenol (Levophed) and extrapyramidal symptoms with benztropine mesylate (Cogentin) or diphenhydramine (Benadryl). Epinephrine is contraindicated for hypotension; further hypotension will occur. In treating respiratory depression and unconsciousness, avoid analeptics such as doxapram (Dopram); they may cause convulsions. Resuscitate as necessary.

PHENOBARBITAL SODIUM

(Luminal sodium)

Usual dose: 100 to 320 mg. May be repeated in 6 hours. 600 mg is the maximum single dose.

Pediatric dose: 3 t0 6 mg/kg of body weight.

Dilution: Sterile powder must be slowly diluted with sterile water for injection. Use a minimum of 10 ml of diluent regardless of dose desired. Also available in a sterile solution. Further dilute solution up to 10 ml with sterile water for injection.

Rate of administration: gr 1 (65 mg) or fraction thereof over 1 minute. Titrate slowly to desired effect.

Actions: A sedative, hypnotic barbiturate of long duration with potent anticonvulsant effects. Phenobarbital is a CNS depressant. Onset of action is prompt by the IV route and becomes rapidly more intense. Effects last from 6 to 10 hours. Will effectively depress the motor cortex with small doses. Pain perception is unimpaired. Rapidly absorbed by all body tissues and excreted in changed form in the urine. Excreted more readily in alkaline urine. Crosses the placental barrier. Excreted in breast milk.

Indications and uses: (1) Prolonged sedation (medical and psychiatric), (2) anticonvulsant.

Precautions: (1) Solutions from powder form must be freshly prepared. Use only absolutely clear solutions. Discard powder or solution exposed to air for 30 minutes. (2) Use only enough medication to achieve the desired effect. Rapid injection rate may cause symptoms of overdose. (3) IV route is used only if oral or IM route is not feasible. (4) Keep patient under constant observation. Record vital signs every hour, or more often if indicated. (5) Maintain a patent airway. (6) Treat the cause of a convulsion. (7) Keep equipment for artificial ventilation available. (8) Determine absolute patency of vein; use of large veins is preferred to prevent thrombosis. Avoid extravasation. Intraarterial injection with cause gangrene. (9) May be habit forming. (10) Use caution in elderly and debilitated patients and those with pulmonary disease. (11) Use extreme caution if any other CNS depressants have been given, such as alochol, narcotic analgesics, anesthetics, antidepressants, sedatives, aminoglycoside antibiotics, tranquilizers, etc. Potentiation with respiratory depression may occur. (12) Inhibits effectiveness of propranolol (Inderal), corticosteroids, doxycycline (Vibramycin), oral anticoagulants, oral contraceptives, quinidine. Capable of innumerable interactions with many drugs. (13) Will cause birth defects. (14) May cause paradoxical excitement in children or the elderly.

Contraindications: History of porphyria, impaired renal function, known hypersensitivity to barbiturates, previous addiction, severe respiratory depression.

Incompatible with: Acidic solutions, aminophylline, calcium chloride, cephalothin (Keflin), chlorpromazine (Thorazine), cimetidine (Tagamet), clindamycin (Cleocin), codeine, diphenhydramine (Benadryl), droperidol (Inapsine), ephedrine, erythromycin (Ilotycin), hydralazine (Apresoline), hydrocortisone sodium succinate (Solu-Cortef), hydroxyzine (Vistaril), insulin (aqueous), kanamycin (Kantrex), levarterenol (Levophed), levorphanol (Levo-Dromoran), meperidine (Demerol), magnesium sulfate, methadone, morphine, oxytetracycline (Terramycin), parabens, penicillin G potassium, pentazocine (Talwin), phenytoin (Dilantin), phytonadione (Aquamephyton), procaine (Novocain), prochlorperazine (Compazine), promazine (Sparine), promethazine (Phenergan), sodium bicarbonate, streptomycin, succinylcholine (Anectine), tetracycline, thiamine, trifluoperazine (Stelazine), tripelennamine (Pyribenzamine), vancomycin (Vancocin), warfarin (Coumadin).

Side effects: Rarely occur with average doses. *Average dose:* asthma, bronchospasm, depression, dermatitis, facial edema, fever, headache, hypotension, nausea, neonatal apnea, respiratory depresson (slight), thrombocytopenic purpura, vertigo.

Overdose: apnea, coma, cough reflex depression, delirium, hypotension, laryngospasm, lowered body temperature, pulmonary edema, renal shutdown, respiratory depression, sluggish or absent reflexes, stupor.

Antidote: Notify the physician of any side effects. Symptomatic and supportive treatment is most important in overdosage. Maintain an adequate airway with artificial ventilation if indicated. Keep the patient warm. Intravenous volume expanders (dextran) will help maintain adequate circulation. Diuretics or hemodialysis will promote the elimination of the drug. Vasopressors (dopamine [Intropin], etc.) will maintain blood pressure.

PHENOLSULFONPHTHALEIN INJECTION

(P.S.P.)

Usual dose: 1 ml (6 mg) as a single dose.

Dilution: May be given undiluted.

Rate of administration: 1 ml over 1 minute.

Actions: A dye used to determine the excretory function of the kidneys. In the normal kidney the dye appears in the urine within 3 to 5 minutes.

Indications and uses: Kidney function test.

Precautions: (1) Accurate results are not obtained if there is residual urine in the bladder, if there is circulatory inadequacy, if the patient is taking probenecid (Benemid), or if dehydration is present. (2) Have patient empty bladder completely before giving dye. (3) Collect voided specimens of at least 40 ml at exactly 1 hour and 2 hours after injection. (4) Urine will have a reddish orange color.

Contraindications: Known sensitivity to phenolsulfonphthalein.

Incompatible with: Any other drug in syringe.

Side effects: Almost nonexistent, but hypersensitivity reactions including anaphylaxis are possible.

Antidote: For hypersensitivity reactions, discontinue the drug, treat as necessary with antihistamines and/or epinephrine, and notify the physician. Resuscitate as necessary.

(Regitine)

Usual dose: Preoperatively, 5 mg 1 to 2 hours before surgery. May be repeated. During surgery the same doses are used as indicated to control epinephrine intoxication. To prevent necrosis caused by levarterenol, add 10 mg of phentolamine to each 1,000 ml of IV solution containing levarterenol.

Pediatric dose: 1 mg. For preoperative and operative use only.

Dilution: Each 5 mg should be diluted with 1 ml of sterile water for injection. May be further diluted with 5 to 10 ml of sterile water for injection.

Rate of administration: Each 5 mg or fraction thereof over 1 minute.

Indications and uses: (1) Prevention and treatment of hypertensive episodes of pheochromocytoma preoperatively and during surgery, (2) prevention and treatment of necrosis and sloughing occurring with dopamine (Intropin) and levarterenol bitartrate (Levophed), (3) definitive diagnosis of pheochromocytoma. (4) *Investigational use:* hypertensive crisis due to MAO inhibitor/sympathomimetic amine interactions and rebound hypertension after discontinuation of clonidine, propranolol, or other hypertensive agents.

Precautions: (1) Use only freshly prepared solutions. (2) For diagnosis of pheochromocytoma, urinary tests such as VMA are safer. Phentolamine is used only when absolutely necessary. Specific procedure must be followed. Consult with physician and pharmacist. (3) Use care in the presence of any arrhythmia. It is preferable to have a normal sinus rhythm. (4) Monitor vital signs every 2 minutes. (5) May be used concomitantly with propranolol (Inderal).

Contraindications: Coronary artery disease, coronary insufficiency, hypersensitivity to phentolamine, myocardial infarction (previous or present), pregnancy and lactation.

Incompatible with: Iron salts.

Side effects: *Minor:* diarrhea, dizziness, nasal stuffiness, nausea, tachycardia, tingling of skin, weakness, vom-

iting. *Major:* cardiac arrhythmias, cerebrovascular occlusion, cerebrovascular spasm, hypotension (severe),
myocardial infarction, shock, tachycardia, vomiting
under anesthesia.

Antidote: For minor side effects, notify the physician. If
symptoms progress or any major side effect occurs,
discontinue the drug and notify the physician immediately. Administer dopamine (Intropin) for shock
caused by hypotension. Do not use epinephrine. Maintain the patient as indicated. If tachycardia or cardiac
arrhythmias occur, defer use of digitalis derivatives
if possible until rhythm returns to normal.

PHENYLEPHRINE
HYDROCHLORIDE pH 3.0 to 5.5

(Neo-Synephrine)

Usual dose: 0.2 mg. From 0.1 to 0.5 mg may be used initially. May be repeated every 10 to 15 minutes. Never exceed 0.5 mg in a single dose. Highly individualized.

Dilution: *Direct IV:* dilute each 1 mg with 9 ml of sterile water for injection (0.1 mg equals 1 ml).
Infusion: dilute 10 mg in 500 ml of dextrose or sodium chloride for injection to provide a 1:50,000 solution.

Rate of administration: *Direct IV:* single dose over 20 to 30 seconds to treat paroxysmal supraventricular tachycardia; over 1 minute in other situations.
For infusion: regulate drip rate to provide and maintain individual's low normal blood pressure. Use an infusion pump or microdrip (60 gtt/ml) to administer.

Actions: A sympathomimetic, similar to epinephrine. A potent long-lasting vasoconstrictor. Unique in that it slows the heart rate, increases stroke volume, and does not induce any change in rhythm of the pulse. Renal vessel constriction will occur. Repeated injections produce comparable results. Effective within seconds and lasts about 15 minutes.

Indications and uses: (1) To maintain adequate blood pressure in inhalation and spinal anesthesia, shock-like states, drug-induced hypotension, and hypersensitivity reactions; (2) to treat paroxysmal supraventricular tachycardia; (3) to prolong anesthesia; (4) specific antidote for hypotension produced by chlorpromazine hydrochloride (Thorazine).

Precautions: (1) Check blood pressure every 2 minutes until stabilized at the desired level. (2) Start with a small dose, giving only as much of the drug as required to alleviate undesirable symptoms. (3) Blood volume depletion should be corrected. May be administered concurrently with blood volume replacement. (4) Hypotension of powerful peripheral adrenergic blocking agents, chlorpromazine, or pheochromocytomectomy may require carefully calculated increased dosage therapy. (5) Discontinue IV administration if vein infiltrates or is thrombosed; can cause tissue necrosis and sloughing. (6) Use extreme caution in the elderly, hyperthyroidism, bradycardia, partial heart block, myocardial disease, or severe arterio-sclerosis. (7) May cause severe hypertension with er-gonovine or oxytocin. (8) Potentiated by halothane anesthetics, tricyclic antidepressants (desipramine [Norpramin], etc.), guanethidine, MAO inhibitors (iso-carboxazid [Marplan], etc.), other vasopressors (epi-nephrine [Adrenalin]); hypertensive crisis and death can result. (9) Use caution with digitalis; arrhythmias may occur. (10) Will cause bradycardia and hypoten-sion with hydantoins (phenytoin [Dilantin], etc.).

Contraindications: Anesthesia with inhalant anesthetics (halothane, etc.), hypertension, ventricular tachy-cardia.

Incompatible with: Alkaline solutions, iron salts, phe-nytoin (Dilantin).

Side effects: Bradycardia, fullness of head, headache, hy-pertension, tingling of extremities, tremulousness, ventricular extrasystoles, ventricular tachycardia (short paroxysms), vertigo.

Antidote: To prevent sloughing and necrosis in areas where extravasation has occurred, inject 5 to 10 mg of phentolamine (Regitine) diluted in 10 to 15 ml of normal saline liberally throughout the tissue in the extravasated area with a fine hypodermic needle. Treatment should be started as soon as extravasation is recognized. Notify the physician of all side effects. IM injection may be preferable. Treat hypertension with phentolamine (Regitine). Treat cardiac arrhyth-mias as indicated and resuscitate as necessary.

(Dilantin sodium)

Usual dose: *Anticonvulsant:* 100 to 250 mg initially. 100 to 150 mg may be repeated in 30 minutes if indicated. Initial dose may be repeated every 4 hours.

Antiarrhythmic: 50 to 100 mg every 10 to 15 minutes. Do not exceed a total dose of 15 mg/kg of body weight.

Pediatric dose: 250 mg/M^2 as anticonvulsant.

Dilution: Special solvent provided; add 2.2 ml to 100 mg vial and 5.2 ml to 250 mg vial. 1 ml equals 50 mg. Shake to dissolve. Immerse vial in warm water to dissolve phenytoin powder. Do not add to IV solutions. May be injected through Y tube or three-way stopcock of infusion set.

Rate of administration: *Anticonvulsant:* 50 mg or fraction thereof over 1 minute.

Antiarrhythmic: 25 mg or fraction thereof over 1 minute.

Actions: A synthetic anticonvulsant, chemically related to barbiturates. Selectively stabilizes seizure threshold and depresses seizure activity in the motor cortex. Also exerts a depressant effect on the myocardium by selectively elevating the excitability threshold of the cell, reducing the cell's response to stimuli. Readily absorbed, phenytoin is metabolized in the liver and excreted in changed form in the urine. Crosses placental barrier. Excreted in breast milk.

Indications and uses: (1) Treatment of status epilepticus (grand mal seizures), (2) control of seizures in neurosurgery, (3) treatment of supraventricular and ventricular arrhythmias including those caused by digitalis intoxication. Especially useful for patients who are unable to tolerate quinidine or procainamide (not FDA approved, but in common usage).

Precautions: (1) Use solution only when completely dissolved and clear; discard if hazy or if a precipitate forms. May be light yellow in color. (2) Determine absolute patency of vein. Avoid extravasation. Very alkaline; follow each injection with sterile normal saline to reduce local venous irritation. (3) May cause convulsions in hypoglycemia caused by pancreatic tumor. (4) Use caution, lower dosage, and slower rate of administration in the seriously ill, elderly, and those with impaired liver or renal function. (5) Capable of innumerable catastrophic drug interactions, including the following: potentiated by amphetamines, analeptics, anticoagulants, antidepressants, benzodiazepines (diazepam [Valium], etc.), chloramphenicol, digitalis, disulfiram (Antabuse), estrogens, myocardial depressants, phenothiazines, sulfonamides, and others. Toxicity and fatality may result. (6) Inhibited by alcohol, antituberculosis drugs, antihistamines, barbiturates. (7) Potentiates CNS depressants, diuretics, folic acid antagonists, muscle relaxants. (8) Inhibits corticosteroids, quinidine, and others. (9) Alters some clinical laboratory tests. (10) Severe hypotension and bradycardia result with concomitant administration with dopamine (Intropin) and all other sympathomimetic antihypertensive drugs

Contraindications: Bradycardia, complete heart block, known sensitivity to hydantoin derivatives, second-degree heart block.

Incompatible with: Any other drug in syringe or solution. Will precipitate if pH is altered.

Side effects: *Minor:* ataxia, confusion, dizziness, drowsiness, fever, hyperplasia of gums, nervousness, skin eruptions, tremors, visual disturbances. *Major:* bradycardia, cardiac arrest, heart block, hypotension, respiratory arrest, tonic seizures, ventricular fibrillation.

Antidote: Notify the physician of any side effects. If minor symptoms progress or any major side effect occurs, discontinue the drug and notify the physician. Maintain a patent airway and resuscitate as necessary. Symptoms of heart block or bradycardia may be reversed with IV atropine. Epinephrine may be useful. Use with caution. Hemodialysis may be required in overdose.

PHOSPHATE

(Potassium phosphate, sodium phosphate)

Usual dose: Dependent on individual needs of the patient. In total parenteral nutrition, 10 to 15 mM of phosphorus/L of TPN solution should maintain normal serum phosphate. Larger amounts may be required.

Dilution: Must be diluted in 500 to 1,000 ml of suitable IV solution and given as an infusion. Soluble in most commonly used IV solutions. Mix thoroughly.

Rate of administration: Dependent on the individual needs of the patient. Consider sodium/potassium content. Infuse slowly.

Actions: Helps to maintain calcium levels, has a buffering effect on acid-base equilibrium, and influences renal excretion of the hydrogen ion. Normal level in adults is 3.0 to 4.5 mg/100 ml of serum; in children, 4.0 to 7.0 mg/100 ml.

Indications and uses: To prevent or correct hypophosphatemia in patients with restricted or no oral intake.

Precautions: (1) Rapid infusion may cause phosphate or potassium intoxication. Serum calcium may be reduced rapidly, causing hypocalcemic tetany. (2) Monitor serum calcium, potassium, phosphate, chlorides, and sodium. (3) Use sodium phosphate with caution in renal impairment, cirrhosis, cardiac failure, or any edematous, sodium-retaining state. (4) Use potassium phosphate with caution in cardiac disease, renal disease, and digitalized patients.

Contraindications: Any disease with high phosphate or low calcium levels, hyperkalemia, renal or adrenal insufficiency (potassium phosphate), hypernatremia (sodium phosphate).

Incompatible with: Calcium salts, protein hydrolysate (10% or greater solutions), and Ringer's lactate. Mix thoroughly after each addition of supposedly compatible drugs or solutions.

Side effects: Elevated phosphates, reduced calcium levels, and hypocalcemic tetany; elevated potassium levels causing cardiac arrhythmias; flaccid paralysis; heaviness of the legs; hypotension; listlessness; mental confusion; and paresthesia of the extremities.

Antidote: For any side effect discontinue the drug and notify the physician. Restore serum calcium with calcium gluconate or chloride. Shift potassium from serum to cells with 150 ml of ⅙ molar sodium lactate or 10% to 20% dextrose with 10 units of regular insulin for each 20 Gm of dextrose at 300 to 500 ml/hr. Correct acidosis with sodium bicarbonate. Reduce sodium by restriction, diuretics, or hemodialysis. Resuscitate as necessary.

PHYSOSTIGMINE SALICYLATE

(Antilirium)

Usual dose: 0.5 to 2 mg initially. 1 to 4 mg may be repeated as necessary as life-threatening signs recur (arrhythmias, convulsions, deep coma).

Pediatric dose: 0.5 mg initially. May be repeated at 5- to 10-minute intervals only if toxic effects persist and there is no sign of cholinergic effects. Maximum total dose is 2 mg.

Dilution: May be given undiluted. Do not add to IV solutions. May be given through Y tube or three-way stopcock of infusion set.

Rate of administration: 1 mg or fraction thereof over 1 minute.

Actions: An extract of *Physostigma venenosum* seeds. It inhibits the destructive action of cholinesterase and prolongs and exaggerates the effects of acetylcholine. Stimulates parasympathetic nerve stimulation (pupil contraction, increased intestinal musculature tonus, bronchial constriction, and salivary and sweat gland stimulation). Does enter the CNS. Onset of action occurs in 5 minutes and lasts about 1 hour.

Indications and uses: To reverse central nervous system toxic effects caused by drugs capable of producing anticholinergic poisoning including atropine, glycopyrrolate, and other anticholinergics, antispasmodics (Diazepam [Valium], etc.), and tricyclic antidepressants.

Precautions: (1) Rapid IV administration may cause bradycardia, hypersalivation, respiratory distress, and convulsions. (2) Atropine must always be available. (3) Potentiates morphine, codeine, meperidine, etc., and succinylcholine (Anectine). (4) Antagonizes ganglionic blocking agents (trimethaphan [Arfonad], etc.), and aminoglycoside antibiotics (kanamycin [Kantrex], etc.). (5) Potentiated by colistimethate (Coly-Mycin); neuromuscular block may be accentuated.

Contraindications: Asthma, cardiovascular disease, diabetes, gangrene, mechanical obstruction of the intestines or urogenital tract, vagotonic states, and patients receiving choline esters or depolarizing neuromuscular blocking agents (succinylcholine).

Incompatible with: No specific information available. Because of potential toxicity, should not be mixed with any other drug.

Side effects: Anxiety, bradycardia, cholinergic crisis (overdose), coma, defecation, delirium, disorientation, emesis, hallucinations, hyperactivity, hypersensitivity, nausea, salivation, seizures, sweating, urination.

Antidote: Keep physician informed of side effects. For excessive nausea or sweating, reduce dose. Discontinue drug for excessive defecation, emesis, salivation, or urination. Treat cholinergic crisis or hypersensitivity with the specific antagonist atropine sulfate in doses of 0.6 mg IV. May be repeated every 3 to 10 minutes. Endotracheal intubation or tracheostomy are considered prophylactic in anesthesia or crisis. Artifical ventilation, oxygen therapy, cardiac monitoring, adequate suctioning, and treatment of shock or convulsions must be instituted and maintained as necessary.

(Aquamephyton, vitamin K₁)

Usual dose: 2.5 to 25 mg. Up to 50 mg in rare instances. A single dose is preferred, but it may be repeated if clinically indicated.

Newborn dose: 0.5 to 1.0 mg IM or subcutaneous only.

Dilution: May be diluted only with normal saline for injection or 5% dextrose in saline. Dilution with at least 10 ml of diluent is recommended to facilitate prescribed rate of administration.

Rate of administration: Each 1 mg or fraction thereof over 1 minute or longer.

Actions: Vitamin K, a fat-soluble vitamin, is essential for the production of prothrombin by the liver. Hemorrhage will occur in its absence. Fastest-acting vitamin K_1 preparation. Results should be detectable in 1 to 2 hours. Usually controls hemorrhage in 3 to 6 hours, and normal prothrombin levels should be obtained in 12 to 14 hours. Metabolized completely by the body. Excreted as metabolites in the urine.

Indications and uses: (1) Anticoagulant-induced prothrombin deficiency (warfarin or dicumarol); (2) hemorrhagic disease of the newborn; (3) hypoprothrombinemia resulting from antibacterial therapy and salicylates; (4) hypoprothrombinemia resulting from obstructive jaundice, biliary fistula, sprue, ulcerative colitis, celiac disease, intestinal resection, cystic fibrosis of the pancreas, and regional enteritis—these diseases limit the absorption and synthesis of vitamin K.

Precautions: (1) Dosage and effect are determined by prothrombin times. Keep the physician informed. (2) Use the smallest dose that achieves effective results to prevent clotting hazards. (3) Supplement with whole blood transfusion if indicated. (4) Photosensitive; protect from light in all dilutions. (5) Discard after single use. (6) IV is not the route of choice; used only when IM or subcutaneous route cannot be used. (7) May cause temporary resistance to prothrombin-depressing anticoagulants by increasing the amount of phytonadione in the liver and blood. Anticoagulation will require larger doses of same or use of heparin sodium. (8) Pain and swelling at injection site can occur.

Contraindications: Liver disease if the response to an initial dose is not satisfactory; hypersensitivity to components.

Incompatible with: Acid pH barbiturates, ascorbic acid, cyanocobalamin (vitamin B_{12}), dextran, pentobarbital (Nembutal), phenobarbital (Luminal), phenytoin (Dilantin), vancomycin (Vancocin), warfarin (Coumadin).

Side effects: Cyanosis, diaphoresis, dizziness, dyspnea, hypotension, peculiar taste sensations, tachycardia, transient flushing sensations. Anaphylaxis, shock, and death have occurred with IV injection.

Antidote: Should not be necessary if dosage is accurately calculated before administration. Action can be reversed by warfarin or heparin if indicated. Discontinue the drug and notify the physician of any side effects. For most side effects the physician will probably choose to continue the drug at a decreased rate of administration. Treat allergic reactions as necessary.

(Pipracil)

Usual dose: 3 to 4 Gm every 4 to 6 hours. Maximum dose
is usually 24 Gm/24 hr.

Dilution: Each 1 Gm or fraction thereof should be diluted
with at least 5 ml of sterile water or 0.9% sodium
chloride for injection. Shake vigorously to dissolve.
May be further diluted to desired volume (50 to 100
ml) with 5% dextrose in water, 0.9% normal saline,
or other compatible infusion solutions (see literature)
and given as an intermittent infusion.

Rate of administration: *Direct IV:* a single dose over 3 to
5 minutes.
Intermittent infusion: a single dose properly diluted
over 30 minutes. Discontinue primary IV infusion during administration.

Actions: An extended-spectrum penicillin. Bactericidal
against a variety of gram-negative and gram-positive
bacteria including aerobic and anaerobic strains. Especially effective against *Klebsiella* and *Pseudomonas.*
Well distributed in all body fluids, tissue, and bone and
through inflamed meninges. Onset of action is prompt.
Excreted in bile and urine. Crosses the placental barrier. Excreted in breast milk.

Indications and uses: Treatment of serious lower respiratory tract, intraabdominal, urinary tract, gynecological, skin and skin structure, bone and joint, and
gonococcal infections and septicemia caused by susceptible organisms. May be used in either liver or
renal impairment, since excretion occurs in bile and
urine. Frequently used to initiate therapy in serious
infections because of broad spectrum.

Precautions: (1) Stable at room temperature for 24 hours.
(2) Frequently used concurrently with aminoglycosides (kanamycin [Kantrex], etc.), but must be administered in separate infusions. Inactivated by tetracyclines. (3) Sensitivity studies are indicated to determine the susceptibility of the causative organism
to piperacillin. (4) Oral probenecid is indicated to
achieve higher and more prolonged blood levels. (5)
Watch for early symptoms of allergic reaction. (6)

Avoid prolonged use of drug; superinfection caused by overgrowth of nonsusceptible organisms may result. (7) Periodic evaluation of renal, hepatic, and hematopoietic systems and serum potassium is recommended in prolonged therapy. (8) Electrolyte imbalance and cardiac irregularities resulting from high sodium content are very possible. Contains 1.98 mEq of sodium/Gm. (9) Confirm patency of vein; avoid extravasation or intraarterial injection. Slow infusion rate for pain along venipuncture site. (10) Usual duration of therapy is 7 to 10 days. Continue at least 2 days after symptoms of infection disappear. (11) Reduce dose only in severe renal impairment with creatinine clearance temporarily below 40 ml/min. May be given to patients undergoing hemodialysis and peritoneal dialysis (see literature for dose).

Contraindications: History of allergic reaction to any penicillin or cephalosporin.

Incompatible with: Aminoglycosides (amikacin, colistimethate, gentamicin, kanamycin, streptomycin, tobramycin), amphotericin B (Fungizone), chloramphenicol, lincomycin, oxytetracycline, polymyxin B, promethazine (Phenergan), tetracycline (Achromycin), vitamin B with C.

Side effects: Anaphylaxis, convulsions, diarrhea, dizziness, fatigue, headache, increased creatinine or BUN, leukopenia, muscle relaxation (prolonged), nausea, neutropenia, pruritus, thrombocytopenia, thrombophlebitis, skin rash, vomiting.

Antidote: Notify the physician immediately of any adverse symptoms. For severe symptoms, discontinue the drug, treat allergic reacton (antihistamines, epinephrine, and corticosteroids), and resuscitate as necessary. Hemodialysis or peritoneal dialysis are effective in overdose.

PLASMA PROTEIN FRACTION   pH 6.7 to 7.3

(Plasmanate, Plasma-Plex, Plasmatein, Protenate)

Usual dose: Variable, depending on indication for use, condition of patient, and response to therapy. Range is from 250 to 1,500 ml/24 hr. Suggested initial doses are as follows: *shock,* 250 to 1,000 ml; *burns,* 500 to 1,000 ml; *hypoproteinemia,* 1,000 to 1,500 ml/24 hr. Each 500 ml bottle yields 25 Gm of plasma protein. Do not exceed 250 Gm in 48 hours.

Pediatric dose: 20 to 30 ml/kg of body weight to treat acute shock.

Dilution: Available as a 5% solution buffered with saline in 250 and 500 ml bottles with injection sets. Plasmanate is also available in a 50 ml size. No further dilution is required.

Rate of administration: Variable, depending on indication, present blood volume, and patient response. Averages are *normal blood volume:* 1 ml/min; *treatment of shock and burns in the adult:* 5 to 8 ml/min. Higher rates may be tolerated if necessary. Rapid infusion (over 10 ml/min) may cause hypotension. Decrease flow rate as patient improves. *Treatment of shock in infants and children:* 5 to 10 ml/min. Do not exceed 10 ml/min in children. *Treatment of hypoproteinemia:* single 500 ml dose over 1 hour. For larger amounts the maximum rate is 100 ml/hr.

Actions: A sterile natural plasma protein substance containing 88% albumin, 7% alpha globulin, and 5% beta globulin. Contains 130 to 160 mEq sodium/L. It expands intravascular volume, maintains colloid osmotic pressure, prevents marked hemoconcentration, and maintains appropriate electrolyte balance in burns.

Indications and uses: (1) Emergency treatment of shock due to burns, infections, surgery, or trauma; (2) temporary treatment of hemorrhage when whole blood is unavailable; (3) hypoproteinemia.

Precautions: (1) Use immediately after opening and discard any unused portion. Contains no preservatives. (2) Do not use if solution is turbid or a sediment is

413

visible. (3) May be given without regard to blood group or type. (4) Adjust or slow rate according to clinical response and rising blood pressure. (5) Monitor vital signs (including central venous pressure if possible) and urine output every 5 to 15 minutes for 1 hour and hourly thereafter depending on condition. (6) Observe carefully for increased bleeding due to higher than normal blood pressure, circulatory embarrassment, pulmonary edema, or hypervolemia. (7) Whole blood may be indicated for considerable red blood cell loss or anemia due to large amounts of plasma protein. (8) Additional fluids are required for dehydrated patients. Tissue dehydration caused by osmotic action of plasma proteins can be acute. (9) Hemoglobin, hematocrit, electrolyte, and serum protein evaluations are necessary during therapy. May cause an elevated alkaline phosphatase level. (10) Not effective for coagulation mechanism defects. (11) Added protein load requires caution in hepatic or renal impairment. (12) If continuous protein loss occurs or edema is present, normal serum albumin (25%) may be the preferred product.

Contraindications: Cardiac failure; cardiopulmonary bypass; history of allergic reactions to albumin; normal or increased intravascular volume; severe anemia.

Incompatible with: Alcohol, levarterenol (Levophed).

Side effects: Allergic and/or pyrogenic reactions can occur. Incidence of toxicity is low when administered with appropriate caution. Slight nausea does occur. Hypotension can be sudden if administered too rapidly.

Antidote: Notify the physician of all symptoms and side effects. Discontinue infusion for sudden hypotension. Decrease flow rate if indicated and treat symptomatically. Resuscitate as necessary.

POLYMYXIN B SULFATE

(Aerosporin)

Usual dose: 15,000 to 25,000 units/kg of body weight/24 hr. Give one half of total 24 hour dose every 12 hours. Normal renal function is necessary for this dose. In impaired renal function, decrease dose from 15,000 units/kg/24 hr downward.

Infant dose: With normal kidney function, up to 40,000 units/kg of body weight/24 hr.

Dilution: Each 500,000 units of powder must be initially diluted with 5 ml of sterile water or normal saline for injection (100,000 units/ml). Each single dose must be further diluted in 300 to 500 ml of 5% dextrose in water and given as a continuous infusion.

Rate of administration: Each single dose properly diluted over a minimum of 60 to 90 minutes.

Actions: A polypeptide antibiotic with neuromuscular blocking action. Bactericidal against many gram-negative organisms. Poorly absorbed into serum and tissue. Does not pass the blood-brain barrier. Slowly excreted in the urine. Development of resistant strains seldom occurs.

Indications and uses: Treatment of acute infections caused by susceptible gram-negative organisms, especially *Pseudomonas aeruginosa.*

Precautions: (1) Refrigerate unused medication after initial dilution and discard after 72 hours. (2) Sensitivity studies are necessary to determine the susceptibility of the causative organism to polymyxin B. (3) Watch for decrease in urine output, rising BUN, serum creatinine, and declining creatinine clearance levels. Drug may need to be discontinued. Routine serum levels and renal function evaluation are necessary. (4) Potentiated by anesthetics, other neuromuscular blocking antibiotics (kanamycin, streptomycin, etc.), anticholinesterases (edrophonium, [Tensilon], etc.), antineoplastics (nitrogen mustard, etc.), barbiturates, muscle relaxants (tubocurarine, etc.), phenothiazines (promethazine [Phenergan], etc.), procainamide, quinidine, and sodium citrate. *Apnea can occur.* Concurrent use is not recommended. (5) Superinfection may occur from overgrowth of nonsusceptible organisms. (6) Maintain good hydration.

Contraindications: Known polymyxin sensitivity, pregnancy.

Incompatible with: Strong acids or alkalies; cobaltous, ferrous, magnesium or manganous ions. Amphotericin B, cefazolin (Kefzol), cephalothin (Keflin), chloramphenicol (Chloromycetin), chlorothiazide (Diuril), heparin, magnesium sulfate, nitrofurantoin (Ivadantin), prednisolone (Hydeltrasol), tetracycline (Achromycin).

Side effects: Albuminuria; apnea; ataxia; azotemia; cylindruria; dizziness; fever; flushing; increasing blood levels without increased dose; increased BUN, NPN, creatinine; oliguria; peripheral paresthesias; rash; thrombophlebitis.

Antidote: Discontinue the drug and notify the physician of all side effects. Depending on diagnosis, dosage may be reduced or an alternate drug indicated. Nephrotoxicity is reversible. Most treatment will be symptomatic. Maintain an adequate airway and artificial ventilation as indicated. Treat allergic reactions and resuscitate as necessary.

POTASSIUM CHLORIDE AND
POTASSIUM ACETATE

Usual dose: 20 to 60 mEq/24 hr. Up to 400 mEq/24 hr has been given in selected situations with extreme caution.

Dilution: Each individual dose must be diluted in 500 to 1,000 ml of suitable IV solution and given as an infusion. Soluble in all commonly used IV solutions. In severe hypokalemia, solutions without dextrose are preferred (dextrose might decrease serum potassium level).

Rate of administration: A maximum of 10 mEq/hr of potassium chloride in any given amount of infusion fluid should not be exceeded. With serious potassium depletion (under 2.5 mEq/L serum), 40 mEq/hr has been given with extreme caution.

Actions: Helps to maintain osmotic pressure and ion balance. Flow of potassium into the cell (serum deficiency) increases membrane resting potential and decreases membrane permeability. Flow of potassium out of the cell (serum excess) decreases resting membrane potential and increases membrane permeability.

Indications and uses: Prophylaxis or treatment of potassium deficiency (hypokalemia due to diuretic therapy, digitalis intoxication, low dietary potassium intake, vomiting and diarrhea, diabetic acidosis, metabolic alkalosis, corticosteroid therapy, increased renal excretion due to acidosis, hemodialysis, etc.).

Precautions: (1) Use only clear solutions. (2) Normal kidney function is of utmost importance. (3) Routine serum potassium levels, EKGs, and evaluation of adequate urine output are mandatory. Continuous cardiac monitoring is preferable for infusion of over 10 mEq of potassium in 1 hour. (4) Potentiated by spironolactone (Aldactone). (5) Digitalis intoxication may occur with hypokalemia. (6) Thiazide diuretics cause hypokalemia. (7) Potassium phosphate is preferred for specific intracellular deficiency not caused by alkalosis, since phosphate is the usual ion attached

417

to potassium in the body. Not used in the presence of kidney failure. (8) Potassium acetate is preferred for potassium deficiency patients with renal tubular acidosis. Metabolic acidosis and hyperchloremia are most likely present.

Contraindications: Adrenal cortex insufficiency, hyperkalemia, impaired renal function, postoperative oliguria (not absolute), shock with hemolytic reactions and/or dehydration.

Incompatible with: Amphotericin B (Fungizone), mannitol.

Side effects: Bradycardia, cardiac arrest, dysphagia, EKG changes (including increased amplitude of T wave, decreased amplitude of R wave, below baseline depression of S wave, disappearing P wave, PR prolongation), respiratory distress, weakness, ventricular fibrillation, voluntary muscle paralysis, death.

Antidote: For any side effect discontinue the drug and notify the physician. For severe hyperkalemia (over 8 mEq/L plasma) use IV dextrose, 10% to 20%, with 10 units of regular insulin for each 20 Gm of dextrose (give 300 to 500 ml/hr) or 150 ml of ⅙ molar sodium lactate. Use IV sodium bicarbonate to correct acidosis. Eliminate potassium-containing foods and medicines. Monitor EKG continuously. If P waves are absent, give calcium gluconate or chloride (do not use if patient is receiving digitalis). All of these measures cause a shift of potassium into the cells and may be used simultaneously. Sodium polystyrene sulfonate (Kayexalate) orally or as retention enemas is used to actually remove potassium from the body. Resuscitate as necessary.

PRALIDOXIME CHLORIDE

(PAM, Protopam chloride)

Usual dose: *Poisoning:* 1 Gm initially. Repeat in 1 hour if indicated. Double dose for overwhelming toxicity. If symptoms continue, additional doses can be given with extreme caution. Atropine must be given before pralidoxime but after adequate ventilation has been established.
Cholinergic crisis due to overdose of carbamate anticholinesterase drugs (neostigmine, pyridostigmine, etc.): 1 to 2 Gm followed by 250 mg every 5 minutes.

Pediatric dose: 20 to 40 mg/kg of body weight as initial dose in poisoning.

Dilution: Each 1 Gm of sterile powder is diluted with 20 ml of sterile water for injection. Should be further diluted in 100 ml of normal saline and given as an IV infusion.

Rate of administration: Each 1 Gm or fraction thereof over 5 minutes. *Infusion:* given over 15 to 30 minutes.

Actions: An anticholinesterase antagonist that reactivates cholinesterase inhibited by phosphate esters. A chemical reaction with anticholinesterases and depolarization at the neuromuscular junction also takes place. Rapidly absorbed and well dispersed throughout body fluids. Most of a single dose is excreted within 6 hours in the urine.

Indications and uses: (1) Antidote for anticholinesterase drug or chemical overdose or poisoning. Primarily useful for many phosphate ester insecticide poisons with anticholinesterase activity (parathion, etc.). (2) Control of overdose of anticholinesterase drugs used to treat myasthenia gravis. Confirm diagnosis with edrophonium (Tensilon).

Precautions: *In all indications including poisoning:* (1) Establish and maintain an adequate airway and controlled respiration as indicated. (2) Give atropine, 2 to 4 mg IV, after cyanosis disappears. Repeat every 10 minutes until atropine toxicity (pulse 140 beats/min). Ventricular fibrillation can occur if oxygenation is inadequate. Maintain atropinization for up to 48 hours. (3) Monitor vital signs and EKG continuously.

(4) Morphine, theophylline (aminophylline), succinyl-choline, reserpine compounds, and phenothiazines are contraindicated. May defeat effectiveness. Potentiates barbiturates. *In poisoning:* (5) Wear rubber gloves to protect hands. (6) Remove contaminated clothing and cleanse contamined skin surfaces with water, baking soda solution, and alcohol. (7) Thiopental sodium may be required to stop convulsions. Use with extreme caution. May cause additional respiratory depression. (8) Maintain adequate urine output. (9) Use caution in myasthenia gravis; may cause a myasthenic crisis. (10) Toxicity may recur as poison is absorbed from bowel.

Contraindications: None when indicated. Increases toxicity of Sevin (carbamate insecticide).

Incompatible with: Any other drug in syringe or solution because of specific use.

Side effects: Usually minor and transient: blurred vision, diplopia, dizziness, headache, impaired accomodation, laryngospasm, muscle rigidity, nausea, pharyngeal pain, tachycardia.

Antidote: Has not been needed. Patient should be observed for atropine intoxication. Maintain vital signs by any means necessary.

PREDNISOLONE PHOSPHATE   pH 7.0 to 8.0

(Hydeltrasol, Key-Pred SP, PSP-IV, Solu-Predalone)

Usual dose: 4 to 60 mg/24 hr initially. 10 to 20 mg every 3 to 4 hours may be given. Total dose usually does not exceed 400 mg every 24 hours. Dosage is individualized according to the severity of the disease and the response of the patient.

Pediatric dose: Smaller dosage is usually required.

Dilution: May be given without mixing or dilution. Always use a separate syringe for Hydeltrasol. May be added to sodium chloride injection or dextrose injection and given by IV infusion. Use solution within 24 hours of dilution.

Rate of administration: 10 mg or fraction thereof over 1 minute. Decrease rate of injection if any complaints of burning or tingling along injection site.

Actions: Rapidly absorbed synthetic adrenocortical steroid with potent metabolic and antiinflammatory actions. May be used in conjunction with other forms of therapy, such as epinephrine for acute allergic reactions or antibiotics in acute infections. It is three to four times more potent than hydrocortisone. It is absorbed primarily into the lymph stream and probably excreted in the urine. Excreted in breast milk.

Indications and uses: (1) Supplementary therapy for severe allergic reactions (use epinephrine first); (2) adrenocortical insufficiency, total, relative, and operative; (3) shock unresponsive to conventional therapy; (4) acute exacerbations of disease for patients receiving steroid therapy; (5) acute life-threatening infections with massive antibiotic therapy; (6) to induce remission of some malignancies; (7) viral hepatitis; (8) thyroid crisis; (9) diagnostic aid to distinguish between adrenocortical hyperplasia and adrenocortical tumor.

Precautions: (1) Give a single daily dose by 9 AM. (2) Sensitive to heat. (3) May cause elevated blood pressure and salt and water retention. (4) Salt restriction and potassium replacement are necessary. (5) May mask signs of infection. (6) To avoid adrenocortical insufficiency, do not stop therapy abruptly; taper off. Patient is observed carefully, especially under stress, for up to 2 years. (7) Maintain on ulcer regime and antacid prophylactically. (8) May increase insulin needs in diabetes. (9) Caution when used with cyclophosphamide (Cytoxan). (10) Often used in combination with salicylates. (11) Inhibited by barbiturates, hydantoins, rifampin, troleandomycin. (12) Do not vaccinate for smallpox during therapy.

Contraindications: *Absolute contraindications*, except in life-threatening situations: tuberculosis (active or healed), ocular herpes simplex, and acute psychoses. *Relative contraindications:* active or latent peptic ulcer, chickenpox, diabetes mellitus, diverticulitis, fresh intestinal anastomoses, hypertension, myasthenia gravis, osteoporosis, pregnancy, psychotic tendencies, renal insufficiency, thromboembolic tendencies, and vaccinia.

Incompatible with: Calcium glucoheptonate, calcium gluconate, dimenhydrinate (Dramamine), metaraminol (Aramine), methotrexate, polymyxin B (Aerosporin), prochlorperazine (Compazine), promazine (Sparine), promethazine (Phenergan). Not generally mixed with any other drug in a solution.

Side effects: Do occur, but are usually reversible: anaphylaxis, Cushing's syndrome (moon face, fat pads, etc.), decrease in spermatozoa, euphoria, fat emboli, fluid and electrolyte imbalance with edema, increased intracranial pressure, menstrual irregularities, peptic ulcer with perforation and hemorrhage, protein catabolism with negative nitrogen balance, relative adrenocortical insufficiency, spontaneous fractures, suppression of growth, transitory burning or tingling.

Antidote: Notify the physician of any side effect. Will probably treat the side effect. Resuscitate as necessary for anaphylaxis and notify the physician. Keep epinephrine immediately available.

PROCAINAMIDE HYDROCHLORIDE

pH 4.0 to 6.0

(Pronestyl)

Usual dose: 0.2 to 1 Gm (100 mg/ml). 100 mg every 5 minutes (600 mg over 30 minutes) may be given as an infusion until arrhythmia is suppressed or maximum initial dose (1 Gm) is reached. An initial loading dose of 12 mg/kg of body weight (total dose) may also be given by the above method as an alternate dosage regime. Follow either choice of initial dosage with an infusion of 6 mg/kg every 3 hours. Maintain with oral procainamide as soon as possible but at least 4 hours after last IV dose.

Dilution: *Direct IV:* dilute each 100 mg with 10 ml of 5% dextrose in water or sterile water for injection.
Infusion: add 1 Gm of procainamide to 250 to 500 ml of 5% dextrose in water. Solution gives 4 or 2 mg of procainamide for each milliliter.

Rate of administration: 20 mg or fraction thereof over 1 minute. Use an infusion pump or a microdrip (60 gtt/ml) for infusion. Up to 50 mg may be given direct IV over 1 minute with extreme caution.

Actions: A procaine derivative. Exerts a depressing antiarrhythmic action on the heart, slowing the rate, slowing conduction, reducing myocardial irritability, and prolonging the refractory period. Decreases membrane permeability of the cell and prevents loss of sodium and potassium ions. Onset of action should occur in 2 to 3 minutes. Plasma levels decrease slowly; it is excreted in the urine.

Indications and uses: (1) Ventricular and supraventricular arrhythmias, such as extrasystoles and tachycardia; (2) atrial arrhythmias of recent occurrence, such as fibrillation; (3) paroxysmal atrial tachycardia unresponsive to other measures; (4) prophylactically, before or during surgery in patients with known heart conditions and for arrhythmias caused by anesthesia.

Precautions: (1) Photosensitive; protect from light. Store in refrigerator. (2) Solution should be clear, may be light yellow. Discard if darker than light amber. (3) Monitor the patient's EKG and blood pressure con-

423

tinuously. Keep patient in a supine position. (4) Oral or IM administration is the route of choice; IV route is for emergencies only. (5) Discontinue IV use when the cardiac arrhythmia is interrupted or when the ventricular rate slows without regular atrioventricular conduction. (6) Small emboli may be dislodged when atrial fibrillation is corrected. (7) Use extreme caution in first- or second-degree blocks, ventricular tachycardia after a myocardial infarction, digitalis intoxication, and impaired liver and kidney function. (8) Potentiates or is potentiated by neuromuscular blocking antibiotics (kanamycin [Kantrex], etc.), anticholinergics (atropine, etc.), thiazide diuretics, antihypertensive agents, muscle relaxants, succinylcholine (Anectine), cimetidine (Tagamet), and others. (9) Use care with digitalis, lidocaine (Xylocaine), and quinidine. Lower doses of both drugs may be required. (10) May elevate SGOT levels.

Contraindications: Complete atrioventricular heart block, known sensitivity to procainamide or any other local anesthetic of the amide type, myasthenia gravis.

Incompatible with: Phenytoin (Dilantin). Physically compatible with many drugs. However, combination is not practical because of individualized rate adjustments necessary to achieve desired effects.

Side effects: *Minor:* anorexia, chills, fever, flushing, giddiness, hallucinations, mental confusion, nausea, skin rash, vomiting, weakness. *Major:* agranulocytosis, hypotension with a blood pressure drop over 15 mm Hg, lupus erythematosus–like symptoms, PR interval prolongation, QRS complex widening, QT interval prolongation, ventricular asystole, ventricular fibrillation, ventricular tachycardia.

Antidote: Notify the physician of any side effects. If minor symptoms progress or any major side effect appears, discontinue the drug immediately and notify the physician. Use dopamine (Intropin) or phenylephrine hydrochloride (Neo-Synephrine) to correct hypotension. Treatment of toxicity is symptomatic and supportive. Hemodialysis may be indicated. Resusciate as necessary. Depending on arrhythmia, quinidine or lidocaine is effective alternate.

PROCHLORPERAZINE EDISYLATE

pH 4.5 to 5.5

(Compazine)

Usual dose: 5 to 10 mg, may be repeated one time in 1 to 2 hours if indicated. 40 mg/24 hr is the maximum parenteral dose.

Dilution: Each 5 mg (1 ml) should be diluted with 9 ml of normal saline for injection. 1 ml will equal 0.5 mg. Add 10 to 20 mg to 1 liter of isotonic IV solution and give as an infusion. Prochlorperazine may cause the solution to turn a light yellow color.

Rate of administration: Each 5 mg or fraction thereof over 1 minute. Infusion may be given at ordered rate, or rate may be increased or decreased as symptoms indicate. Use an infusion pump or a microdrip (60 gtt/ml) for infusion.

Actions: A phenothiazine derivative said to be four times more potent than chlorpromazine (Thorazine), with effects on the central, autonomic, and peripheral nervous systems. Decreases anxiety and tension, relaxes muscle, produces sedation, and tranquilizes. A potent antiemetic. Onset of action is prompt and lasting. Excretion is slow through the kidneys.

Indications and uses: (1) Control of nausea, vomiting, retching, and hyperexcitability before, during, and after surgery; (2) treatment of withdrawal symptoms from alcohol, barbiturates, or narcotics; (3) antipsychotic drug.

Precautions: (1) Use IV only when absolutely necessary. (2) Sensitive to light. Slightly yellow color does not affect potency. Discard if markedly discolored. (3) Handle carefully; may cause contact dermatitis. (4) Keep patient in supine position and monitor blood pressure and pulse before administration and between doses. (5) May mask diagnosis of brain tumor, drug intoxication, and intestinal obstruction. (6) Use caution in coronary disease, severe hypertension or hypotension, epilepsy, and children. (7) Potentiates CNS depressant effects of narcotics, barbiturates, alcohol, anesthetics. Additive effects with MAO inhibitors (pargyline [Eutonlyl], etc.), oral antidiabetics, insulin, anticholinergics, antihistamines, antihypertensives, hypnotics, muscle relaxants, phenytoin (Dilantin), propranolol (Inderal), and rauwolfia alkaloids. Reduce dosage of any medication potentiated by phenothiazines by one fourth to one half. (8) Contraindicated with quinidine, epinephrine, and thiazide diuretics. (9) Capable of innumerable other interactions. (10) Greater extrapyramidal and antiemetic effects than other phenothiazines with less sedative and hypotensive reactions. (11) May discolor urine pink to reddish brown. (12) Photosensitivity of skin is possible.

Contraindications: Bone marrow depression, children under 2 years of age or 10 kg, comatose or severely depressed states, hypersensitivity to phenothiazines, lactation, pregnancy, except labor and delivery; do not use in pediatric surgery.

Incompatible with: Aminophylline, amobarbital (Amytal), amphotericin B, ampicillin, calcium glucoheptonate, calcium gluconate, cephalothin (Keflin), chloramphenicol (Chloromycetin), chlorothiazide (Diuril), dexamethasone (Decadron), dimenhydrinate (Dramamine), epinephrine (Adrenalin), erythromycin (Ilotycin), heparin, hydrocortisone sodium succinate (Solu-Cortef), kanamycin (Kantrex), levallorphan (Lorfan), methicillin (Staphcillin), methohexital (Brevital), nitrofurantoin (Ivadantin), oxytetracycline (Terramycin), oxytocin, paraldehyde, penicillin G potassium, pentobarbital (Nembutal), phenobarbital (Luminal), phenytoin (Dilantin), prednisolone (Hydeltrasol), secobarbital (Seconal), sulfisoxazole (Gantrisin), tetracycline, thiopental (Pentothal), vancomycin (Vancocin), vitamin B complex with C. *Should be considered incompatible in syringe with any other drug.*

Side effects: Usually transient if drug is discontinued but may require treatment if severe: anaphylaxis, blurring of vision, cardiac arrest, dermatitis, dizziness, dryness of mouth, dysphagia, elevated blood pressure, excitement, extrapyramidal symptoms (such as abnormal positioning, extreme restlessness, pseudoparkinsonism, weakness of extremities), hypersensitivity reactions, hypotension, slurred speech, spastic movements (especially about the face), tachycardia, temperature without etiology, tightness of the throat, tongue discoloration, tongue protrusion, and many others.

Antidote: Discontinue the drug at onset of any side effect and notify the physician. Counteract hypotension with dopamine (Intropin) and extrapyramidal symptoms with benztropine mesylate (Cogentin) or diphenhydramine (Benadryl). Epinephrine is contraindicated for hypotension. Further hypotension will occur. In treating respiratory depression and unconsciousness, avoid analeptics such as doxapram (Dopram); they may cause convulsions. Resuscitate as necessary.

(Norazine, Prozine, Sparine)

Usual dose: 25 to 50 mg. May repeat as indicated by symptoms. If necessary to repeat with 1 hour, use caution.

Dilution: May be given undiluted, but never exceed a concentration of 25 mg/ml. Each 25 to 50 mg (1 ml, depending on initial dilution) should be further diluted with 9 ml of normal saline for injection. 1 ml of diluted solution will equal 2.5 to 5 mg of promazine.

Rate of administration: 25 mg or fraction thereof over 1 minute.

Actions: A phenothiazine derivative, primarily an antianxiety agent, with effects on the central, autonomic, and peripheral nervous systems. Decreases anxiety and tension, relaxes muscle, produces sedation, and tranquilizes. A potent antiemetic. Onset of action is prompt and lasting. Excretion is slow through the kidneys.

Indications and uses: (1) Control of nausea, vomiting, retching, hiccups, and hyperexcitability before, during, and after surgery; (2) treatment of withdrawal symptoms from alcohol, barbiturates, or narcotics; (3) antipsychotic drug.

Precautions: (1) Use IV only when absolutely necessary. Establish unquestionable patency of vein. Avoid extravasation. (2) Intraarterial injection will cause gangrene. (3) Handle carefully; may cause contact dermatitis. (4) Monitor blood pressure and pulse before administration and betwee doses. Keep patient in supine position. (5) Use with caution in the presence of cerebral arteriosclerosis, coronary heart disease, severe hypertension or hypotension, epilepsy, heat exhaustion, liver disease, and respiratory problems. (6) May mask diagnosis of brain tumor, drug intoxication, and intestinal obstruction. (7) Potentiates CNS depressant effects of narcotics, babiturates, alcohol, anesthetics. Additive effects with MAO inhibitors (pargyline [Eutonyl], etc.), oral antidiabetics, insulin, anticholinergics, antihistamines, antihypertensives, hypnotics, muscle relaxants, phenytoin (Dilantin), propranolol (Inderal), and rauwolfia alkaloids. Reduce dosage of any medication potentiated by phenothiazines by one fourth to one half. (8) Contraindicated with quinidine, epinephrine, and thiazide diuretics. (9) Capable of innumerable other interactions. (10) In large doses, extrapyramidal, antiemetic, and sedative effects are moderate. Hypotensive effects are very prominent. (11) May discolor urine pink to reddish brown. (12) Photosensitivity of skin is possible.

Contraindications: Bone marrow depression, children under 12 years, comatose or severely depressed states, hypersensitivity to phenothiazines, lactation, pregnancy except labor and delivery.

Incompatible with: Aminophylline, amobarbital (Amytal), ampicillin (Polycillin), atropine, chloramphenicol (Chloromycetin), chlorothiazide (Diuril), dimenhydrinate (Dramamine), epinephrine (Adrenalin), heparin, hydrocortisone phosphate, hydrocortisone sodium succinate (Solu-Cortef), methicillin (Staphcillin), methohexital (Brevital), nafcillin (Unipen), penicillin G potassium and sodium, pentobarbital (Nembutal), phenobarbital (Luminal), phenytoin (Dilantin), prednisolone (Hydeltrasol), sodium bicarbonate, sulfisoxazole (Gantrisin), thiopental (Pentothal), vitamin B with C (Folbesyn), warfarin (Coumadin).

Side effects: Usually transient if drug is discontinued but may require treatment if severe; considered less toxic than prochlorperazine. Anaphylaxis, blurring of vision, cardiac arrest, cerebral edema, convulsions, dermatitis, dizziness, dryness of mouth, dysphagia, elevated blood pressure, excitement, extrapyramidal symptoms (such as abnormal positioning, extreme restlessness, pseudoparkinsonism, weakness of extremities), hypersensitivity reactions, hypotension, slurred speech, spastic movements (especially about the face), tachycardia, temperature without etiology, tightness of the throat, tongue discoloration, tongue protrusion, and many others.

Antidote: Discontinue the drug at onset of any side effect and notify the physician. Counteract hypotension with dopamine (Intropin) and extrapyramidal symptoms with benztropine mesylate (Cogentin) or diphenhydramine (Benadryl). Epinephrine is contraindicated for hypotension. Further hypotension will occur. In treating respiratory depression and unconciousness, avoid analeptics such as doxapram (Dopram), they may cause convulsions. Resuscitate as necessary.

**(Anergan 25, Phenazine 25, Phenergan,
Prometh-25, Prorex, Prothazine, Provigan,
V-Gan 25, Zipan-25)**

Usual dose: 25 mg. May be repeated in 2 hours if indicated. Up to 50 mg in a single dose may be required.
Maintain with IM or oral medication as soon as feasible.

Pediatric dose: 125 μg to 500 μg/kg of body weight every
4 to 6 hours. IV route is rarely used.

Dilution: Never exceed a concentration of 25 mg/ml. Each
25 to 50 mg (1 ml), depending on initial dilution,
should be diluted with 9 ml or normal saline for injection. 1 ml of diluted solution will equal 2.5 to 5 mg
of promethazine.

Rate of administration: Each 25 mg or fraction thereof
over 1 minute.

Actions: A phenothiazine derivative with effects on the
central, autonomic, and peripheral nervous systems.
It has potent antihistaminic, antiemetic, and amnesic
actions. Potentiates the analgesic and sedative effects
of narcotics and other CNS depressants. Promethazine
relaxes smooth muscle. Onset of action is prompt and
lasts 4 to 6 hours. Readily absorbed, primarily metabolized in the liver, and excreted in the urine.

Indications and uses: (1) Prophylaxis or treatment of minor transfusion reactions; (2) treatment of hypersensitivity reactions; (3) treatment of acute nausea, vomiting, and motion sickness; (4) adjunct to narcotic analgesics, in control of postoperative pain; (5) sedation
to meet surgical and obstetrical needs.

Precautions: (1) Multiple-dose vials or diluted solutions
should be refrigerated. (2) Sensitive to light. Slightly
yellow color does not alter potency. Discard if greatly
discolored. (3) Handle carefully; may cause contact
dermatitis. (4) Determine absolute patency of vein;
extravasation will cause necrosis. (5) Keep patient in
supine position. Monitor blood pressure and pulse before administration and between doses. (6) Potentiates

CNS depressant effects of narcotics, alcohol, anesthetics, and barbiturates. Additive effects with MAO inhibitors (pargyline [Eutonyl], etc.), oral antidiabetics, anticholinergics, antihistamines, antihypertensives, hypnotics, insulin, muscle relaxants, phenytoin (Dilantin), propranolol (Inderal), rauwolfia alkaloids, and sulfonamides. Reduce dosage of any medication potentiated by phenothiazines by one fourth to one half. (7) May produce apnea with neuromuscular blocking antibiotics (gentamicin, etc.). (8) Contraindicated with quinidine, epinephrine, and thiazide diuretics. (9) Capable of innumerable other interactions. (10) Sedative effect may require ambulation to be monitored. (11) Use with extreme caution in children and the elderly.

Contraindications: Bone marrow depression, comatose or severely depressed states, hypersensitivity to phenothiazines, lactation, pregnancy. Never inject into artery.

Incompatible with: Aminophylline, calcium gluconate, carbenicillin (Geopen), chloramphenicol (Chloromycetin), chlordiazepoxide (Librium), chlorothiazide (Diuril), codeine, dextran, dimenhydrinate (Dramamine), heparin, hydrocortisone sodium succinate (Solu-Cortef), methicillin (Staphcillin), methohexital (Brevital), methylprednisolone (Solu-Medrol), morphine, nitrofurantoin (Ivadantin), penicillin G potassium and sodium, pentobarbital (Nembutal), phenobarbital (Luminal), phenytoin (Dilantin), secobarbital (Seconal), sulfioxazole (Gantrisin), thiopental (Pentothal), vitamin B with C.

Side effects: *Average dose:* blurring of vision, dizziness, dryness of mouth, hyperexcitability, hypersensitivity reactions, hypertension (rare), hypotension (mild), nightmares, spastic movements of upper extremities. *Overdose:* anaphylaxis, cardiac arrest, coma, convulsions, deep sedation, repiratory depression. All side effects of phenothiazines are possible, but rarely occur. See prochlorperazine (Compazine).

Antidote: Discontinue the drug at onset of any side effect and notify the physician. Counteract hypotension with dopamine (Intropin) and extrapyramidal symptoms

432

with benztropine mesylate (Congentin) or diphenhydramine (Benadryl). Epinephrine is contraindicated for hypotension. Further hypotension will occur. In treating respiratory depression and unconsciousness, avoid analeptics such as doxapram (Dopram), they may cause convulsions. Resuscitate as necessary.

PROPIOMAZINE HYDOCHLORIDE   pH 4.3 to 5.3

(Largon)

Usual dose: 10 to 40 mg (20 mg average) given alone or in conjunction with one fourth to one half the usual dose of narcotics. May be repeated in 3 to 4 hours as indicated.

Pediatric dose: 0.5 (average dose) to 1 mg/kg of body weight, but do not exceed adult dose.

Dilution: Each 20 mg (1 ml) should be diluted with 9 ml of normal saline for injection. 1 ml will equal 2 mg.

Rate of administration: Each 10 mg or fraction thereof over 1 minute. A slower rate of injection may be indicated by the accompanying narcotic.

Actions: A phenothiazine derivative that potentiates the analgesic and sedative effects of narcotics. Used alone it produces sedation and reduces anxiety. Has some antihistaminic effect and a mild antiemetic effect. Prompt onset of action with a short duration of effect is a desirable action. Slowly excreted through kidneys.

Indications and uses: Sedation and relief of restlessness preoperatively, during surgery, and during labor and delivery.

Precautions: (1) Solution must be clear. Discard if cloudy or if a precipitate is present. (2) Establish unquestionable patency of vein. Avoid extravasation. Intraarterial injection will cause gangrene. (3) Monitor blood pressure and pulse before administration and between doses. Keep patient in supine position. (4) Use with caution in cerebral arteriosclerosis, coronary heart disease, severe hypertension, epilepsy, heat exhaustion, liver disease, and respiratory problems. (5) May mask diagnosis of brain tumor, drug intoxication, and intestinal obstruction. (6) Potentiates CNS depressant effects of narcotics, barbiturates, alcohol, and anesthetics. Additive with MAO inhibitors (pargyline [Eutonyl], etc.), oral antidiabetics, insulin, anticholinergics, antihistamines, antihypertensives, hypnotics, muscle relaxants, phenytoin (Dilantin), propranolol (Inderal), and rauwolfia alkaloids. Reduce dosage of any medication potentiated by phenothiazines by one fourth to one half. (7) Contraindicated with quinidine,

epinephrine, and thiazide diuretics. (8) Capable of innumerable other interactions.

Contraindications: Bone marrow depression, comatose
or severely depressed states, first trimester of pregnancy, hypersensitivity to phenothiazines, lactation.

Incompatible with: Sufficient information not available,
but refer to other phenothiazines such as promazine
(Sparine), etc. Alkaline solutions, barbiturates.

Side effects: Dryness of mouth, hypertension (moderate),
hypotension, tachycardia, thrombophlebitis. All side
effects of phenothiazines could occur, but rarely do.
For additional possible side effects see prochlorperazine (Compazine).

Antidote: Dryness of mouth, moderate hypertension, and
tachycardia are usually tolerable. Notify physician if
excessive. For all other side effects discontinue drug
at onset and notify the physician. Counteract hypotension with dopamine (Intropin) and extrapyramidal
symptoms with benztropine mesylate (Cogentin) or
diphenhydramine (Benadryl). Epinephrine is contraindicated for hypotension. Further hypotension
will occur. Resuscitate as necessary.

PROPRANOLOL HYDROCHLORIDE   pH 2.8 to 3.5

(Inderal)

Usal dose: 0.5 to 3 mg given 1 mg at a time. If there is no change in rhythm for at least 2 minutes after the initial dose, cycle may be repeated one time. *No further propranolol may be given by any route for at least 4 hours.*

Dilution: Each 1 mg can be diluted in 10 ml of 5% dextrose in water for injection or may be given undiluted. May be diluted in 50 ml of normal saline for infusion.

Rate of administration: Each 1 mg or fraction thereof must be given over 1 minute. Give 1 mg as an infusion over 10 to 15 minutes. Allow adequate time for circulation. Observe monitor and discontinue propranolol as soon as rhythm change occurs.

Actions: Propranolol is a beta adrenergic blocker with antiarrhythmic effects. Cardiac response to sympathetic nerve stimulation is inhibited, slowing the heart rate (especially ventricular rate) by inhibiting atrioventricular conduction, decreasing the force of cardiac contractility, and decreasing arterial pressure and cardiac output. Propranolol also decreases the plasma level of free fatty acid and blood glucose. Well distributed throughout the body, the onset of action occurs within 1 to 2 minutes and lasts about 4 hours. Metabolized in the liver. Some excreted in the urine.

Indications and uses: (1) Management of life-threatening cardiac arrhythmias, such as paroxysmal atrial tachycardia, sinus tachycardia, atrial or ventricular extrasystoles, atrial flutter and fibrillation, tachyarrhythmia caused by digitalis intoxication, anesthesia (other than chloroform and ether, etc.), thyrotoxicosis, and catecholamines (epinephrine and norepinephrine); (2) ventricular tachycardia and arrhythmias caused by tumor manipulation during excision of pheochromocytoma; (3) to reduce blood pressue in systolic hypertension caused by hyperdynamic beta adrenergic circulatory state that occurs in younger persons.

Precautions: (1) Continuous EKG and pulmonary wedge or central venous pressure monitoring is mandatory during administration of IV propranolol. Discontinue the drug when a rhythm change is noted and wait to note full effect before giving additional medication if indicated. (2) Oral administration is preferred. Use IV administration only when necessary. (3) Not considered the drug of choice for arrhythmias in myocardial infarction. (4) Antagonizes antihistamines, antiinflammatory agents, isoproterenol (Isuprel), and others. (5) Potentiated by general anesthetics, cimetidine (Tagamet), phenothiazines (promethazine [Phenergan], etc.), phenytoin (Dilantin), and urethane. Death can occur. (6) Potentiates antidiabetics, barbiturates, narcotics, and muscle relaxants. Increased CNS depression may cause death. (7) Used concurrently with digitalis or alpha adrenergic blockers as indicated. (8) Use with extreme caution in asthmatics, diabetics, or patients with a history of hypoglycemia. May cause hypoglycemia and mask the symptoms. (9) Epinephrine concurrently is contraindicated. (10) Use with clonidine may precipitate acute hypertension. (11) Use with verapamil may potentiate both drugs with severe depression of myocardium ad AV conduction. (12) BUN may be elevated in patients with impaired renal function. (13) Should be discontinued 48 hours previous to major surgery (beta blockade interferes with cardiac response to reflex stimuli).

Contraindications: Allergic rhinitis, bronchial asthma, cardiogenic shock, complete heart block, congestive heart failure (unless caused by tachycardia), myocardial-depressing anesthetics (chloroform, ether, etc.), pregnancy and lactation, right ventricular failure caused by pulmonary hypertension, second-degree heart block, sinus bradycardia; contraindicated concurrently with all antihypertensive drugs including diuretics, and may not be given to patients receiving antidepressants or MAO inhibitors (pargyline [Eutonyl], etc.), until after a 2-week withdrawal period.

Incompatible with: Any other drug in syringe because of toxicity. Note precautions and contraindications.

Side effects: Bradycardia, cardiac failure, cardiac standstill, erythematous rash, hallucination, hypotension, laryngospasm, paresthesia of the hands, respiratory distress, syncopal attacks, visual disturbances, vertigo.

Antidote: For any side effect, discontinue the drug and notify the physician immediately. Effects can be reversed by dopamine, isoproterenol, or levarterenol, but protracted severe hypotension may result. Use atropine for bradycardia, digitalis and diuretics for cardiac failure, epinephrine for hypotension, aminophylline and isoproterenol (with extreme care) for bronchospasm, glucagon for hypoglycemia. Treat other side effects symptomatically and resuscitate as necessary.

Usual dose: 1 mg for every 100 USP units of heparin. May be repeated if needed in 10 to 15 minutes. Never exceed 50 mg in any 10-minute period.

Dilution: Each 50 mg of powder is diluted with 5 ml of sterile bacteriostatic water for injection. Shake vigorously. May be further diluted with at least an equal volume of normal saline or 5% dextrose in water. May be given as an infusion by diluting in a given amount of the same infusion solutions.

Rate of administration: 20 mg (2 ml) or fraction thereof over 1 minute. Do not exceed 50 mg in 10 minutes. As an infusion, may be given over 2 to 3 hours with dosage titrated according to coagulation studies. Use infusion pump or microdrip (60 gtt/ml) to administer.

Actios: An anticoagulant if adminstered alone. In the presence of heparin, protamine forms a stable salt, neutralizing the anticoagulant effect of both drugs. Each 1 mg of protamine can neutralize 100 USP units of heparin. It is effective for about 2 hours. The dose of protamine required decreases rapidly with the time elapsed after heparin injection. (30 minutes after IV heparin 0.5 mg of protamine will neutralize 100 USP units of heparin).

Indications and uses: To neutralize the anticoagulant activity of heparin in severe heparin overdosage.

Precautions: (1) Discard after open, or may be refrigerated for up to 24 hours if initial mixture contains a preservative. (2) Prompt administration of protamine sulfate may decrease dosage requirements. (3) Dosage adjusted as indicated by coagulation studies. (4) Facilities to treat shock must be available. (5) After cardiac surgery, even with adequate neutralization, further bleeding may occur any time within 24 hours (heparin "rebound"). Observe the patient continuously. Additional protamine sulfate may be indicated.

Contraindications: None when used as indicated.

Incompatible with: Cephalosporins, penicillins. Should be considered incompatible in syringe or solution with any other drug because of individualized rate adjustment necessary to produce desired effects.

Side effects: Occur more frequently with too-rapid injection; anaphylaxis, bradycardia, dyspnea, feeling of warmth, flushing, severe hypertension or hypotension.

Antidote: Discontinue the drug and notify the physician, who may recommend a decrease in rate of administration or, if side effects are severe, symptomatic treatment such as administraton of whole blood, vasopressors (dopamine [Intropin], etc.) for hypotension, atropine for bradycardia, oxygen for dyspnea, etc. Resuscitate as necessary.

PROTEIN (AMINO ACID) PRODUCTS

pH 5.0 to 7.0

(Aminosyn 3.5% M, 5%, 7%, 8.5%, 10%, 7% and 8.5% with electrolytes, Aminosyn RF, crystalline amino acid infusions, FreAmine III 8.5%, 10%, and 3% with electrolytes, hyperalimentation, Nephramine, protein hydrolysates, total parenteral nutrition, Travasol 5.5%, 8.5%, 10%, 3.5% M with electrolytes, 5.5% and 8.5% with electrolytes, Veinamine)

Usual dose: Based on protein requirements, physical condition, and weight (actual grams of available protein vary with various brands). Consider total body fluid needs. Average adult will require 2 L/24 hr providing 1 to 2 Gm protein/kg of body weight. Glucose supplies nonprotein calories.

Pediatric dose: Sufficient milliliters to provide 2 to 3 Gm protein/kg of body weight/24 hr to meet average needs.

Infant dose: Sufficient milliliters to provide 2 to 3 Gm protein/kg of body weight/24 hr.

Dilution: If required, dilute under strict aseptic techniques according to manufacturer's specific instructions. Various brands supply additional calories with alcohol, fructose, or glucose. These additional calories permit available protein to be used for repair of tissue in addition to meeting basic caloric needs.

Rate of administration: Start with 1 L/24 hr and gradually increase by 1 L/24 hr to desired amount. Begin infusion at a rate of approximately 1 ml/kg of body weight/hr. Gradually increase to 2 ml/kg/hr. *Total daily dose should be evenly distributed over the 24-hour period. Maintain a constant drip rate.* Never exceed 4 ml/kg/hr. Use of infusion pump and microfilter is recommended.

Actions: Supplies essential and nonessential amino acids and calories with the intent of providing nitrogen in a readily assimilable form.

Indications and uses: Maintenance of positive nitrogen balance in severe illness when oral alimentation is not practical for prolonged periods or normal gastrointestinal absorption is impaired.

Precautions: (1) Use promptly after mixing; laminar flow hood preferred; refrigerate briefly if necessary, and discard any unused portion. (2) Use only clear solution; observe against adequate light for particulate matter or evidence of container damage. (3) Catheter insertion for administration is a sterile surgical procedure (must be a large vein [subclavian or superior vena cava preferred]; 50% glucose is a sclerosing solution). (4) Peripheral veins are suitable for specific products, especially when amino acid products are diluted with 5% or 10% dextrose instead of 50% dextrose. (5) Follow a strict, regular aseptic routine to care for insertion site. (6) Single port catheters to be used only for the nutritional regime. Do not draw blood samples, transfuse blood, or administer other medications. Thrombosis can occur; risk of contamination is great. Multiple port catheters (Broviac, Hickman, etc.) may be used for these additional procedures. Observe specific protocols. (7) Monitor arterial blood gases and pH, blood glucose levels, BUN, osmolality, cholesterol, serum proteins, magnesium, phosphate, prothrombin time, and electrolytes frequently during therapy. Blood ammonia levels are important especially in infants. (8) Check for glycosuria at least every 4 hours. (9) Check frequently for any signs of extravasation. (10) Observe for any signs of infection. (11) Additional insulin coverage may be required, especially when dosage is increased too rapidly or with maximum doses. (12) Decrease rate gradually over at least 24 hours to discontinue administration. Use of fluids containing 5% to 10% dextrose for several days can be helpful. (13) RDA vitamins, potassium, magnesium, phosphates, sodium, calcium, and chlorides are needed. Usually added as prescribed with aseptic technique. (14) Amino acids given without carbohydrates may cause ketone accumulation. (15) Frequently used in conjunction with IV fat emulsion as a nonprotein calorie source. Use a separate port; never mixed together in a container. (16) Tetracycline may reduce protein-sparing effects. (17) Discard any single bottle after 24 hours. Replace administration set every 24 to 48 hours.

Contraindications: Hypersensitivity to any component. Acidosis, anuria, azotemia, severe liver disease, metabolic disorders with impaired nitrogen utilization.

Incompatible with: Amobarbital (Amytal), chlorothiazide (Diuril), oxytetracycline (Terramycin), penicillins, sodium bicarbonate, sulfisoxazole (Gantrisin), thiopental (Pentothal) and many other drugs. Most incompatibilities relate to the preparation (chloride as opposed to phosphate), amount of medication added, other additives present, and thoroughness of mixing. Consult with the pharmacist before mixing any drugs in protein (amino acid) products. Only required nutritional products should be added.

Side effects: Abdominal pains, anaphylaxis, convulsions, edema at the site of injection, electrolyte imbalances, glycosuria, hyperammonemia, hyperglycemia, hyperpyrexia, metabolic acidosis and/or alkalosis, osmotic dehydration, phlebitis and thrombosis, septicemia, vasodilation, vomiting.

Antidote: Notify the physician of all side effects. An alternate brand may cause fewer problems, or amounts of additives may be adjusted to correct the problem. Many of the side effects listed will respond to a reduced rate. Some will require catheter insertion at a new site. Treat symptomatically and resuscitate as necessary.

PYRIDOSTIGMINE BROMIDE

(Mestinon, Regonol)

Usual dose: *Myasthenia gravis:* One thirtieth of the oral dose or about 2 mg. Highly individualized. Observe for cholinergic crisis.

Muscle relaxant antagonist: 10 to 20 mg as a single dose. Give atropine first (see precautions) and maintain ventilation.

Dilution: May be given undiluted. Do not add to IV solutions. May be given through Y tube or three-way stopcock of infusion set.

Rate of administration: *Myasthenia gravis:* each 0.5 mg or fraction thereof over 1 minute.

Muscle relaxant antagonist: Each 5 mg or fraction thereof over 1 minute.

Actions: An anticholinesterase muscle stimulant and antagonist of skeletal muscle relaxants. Inhibits the enzyme cholinesterase, allowing acetylcholine to accumulate at the myoneural junction. Restores normal transmission of nerve impulses and makes muscle contraction stronger and more prolonged. Has fewer side effects and longer duration of action than neostigmine (Prostigmin).

Indications and uses: (1) Treatment of myasthenia gravis during physically stressful situations when oral dosage is not practical (labor, postpartum, surgery); (2) antagonist to nondepolarizing muscle relaxants (gallamine [Flaxedil], tubocurarine [curare], etc.).

Precautions: (1) A physician should be present when this drug is used. IM route preferred. (2) Used as a curariform antagonist; administer atropine sulfate, 0.6 to 1.2 mg IV, immediately prior to pyridostigmine. *Caution:* atropine may mask symptoms of pyridostigmine overdose. Cholinergic crisis may result. Maintain a patent airway and use artificial ventilation as indicated. (3) Edrophonium (Tensilon) can differentiate between increased symptoms of myasthenia and cholinergic crisis. (4) Epinephrine and atropine should always be available. (5) Use caution in bronchial asthma, cardiac arrhythmias, and patients receiving anticholinesterase drugs. (6) Potentiates morphine, codeine, meperidine, etc., and succinylcholine (Anectine). (7) Antagonizes anesthetics (ether), ganglionic blocking agents (trimethaphan [Arfonad], etc.), and aminoglycoside antibiotics (gentamicin [Garamycin], etc.); neuromuscular block may be accentuated. (8) Potentiated by colistimethate (Coly-Mycin). (9) A peripheral nerve stimulator device can monitor effectiveness.

Contraindications: Known sensitivity to anticholinesterase agents or bromides, mechanical intestinal or urinary obstruction, urinary tract infections, patients taking mecamylamine.

Incompatible with: No specific information available. Because of potential toxicity, pyridostigmine should not be mixed with any other drug.

Side effects: *Usually caused by overdosage:* abdominal cramps, anorexia, anxiety, bradycardia, cardiac arrhythmias and arrest, cholinergic crisis, cold moist skin, convulsions, diaphoresis, diarrhea, hypotension, increased bronchial secretions, increased lacrimation, increased salivation, miosis, muscle cramps, muscle weakness, nausea, pulmonary edema, respiratory paralysis with apnea, skin rash (bromide), thrombophlebitis, vomiting.

Antidote: Atropine sulfate. If side effects occur, discontinue the drug and notify the physician. Atropine sulfate in doses of 0.6 mg IV will counteract most side effects and may be repeated every 3 to 10 minutes. Endotracheal intubation or tracheostomy is considered prophylactic in anesthesia or crisis. Artificial ventilation, oxygen therapy, cardiac monitoring, adequate suctioning, and treatment of shock or convulsions must be instituted and maintained as necessary. Pralidoxime chloride 1 to 2 Gm IV followed by 250 mg every 5 minutes may be required to reactivate cholinesterase and reverse paralysis.

PYRIDOXINE HYDROCHLORIDE   pH 2.0 to 3.8

(Beesix, Hexa-Betalin, Pyroxine, vitamin B₆)

Usual dose: 10 to 100 mg/24 hr. 1 Gm may be given in severe isoniazid poisoning. Follow with 1 Gm IM every 30 minutes to equal dose of isoniazid.

Dilution: May be given by direct IV administratoin undiluted or added to most IV solutions and given as an infusion.

Rate of administration: 50 mg or fraction thereof over 1 minute if given undiluted.

Actions: Vitamin B₆ is water soluble. It is a coenzyme, necessary for the metabolism of amino acids and fatty acids. It also aids in the conversion of tryptophan to nicotinamide and energy transformation in brain and nerve cells. Easily absorbed and utilized, metabolized by the liver, and excreted in the urine.

Indications and uses: Adjunctive therapy in treatment of hyperemesis gravidarum, irradiation sickness, vitamin B₆ deficiency, pellagra, and isoniazid poisoning. *Investigational use:* hydrazine poisoning.

Precautions: (1) Deteriorates in excessive heat, may be refrigerated. (2) Large doses in utero can cause pyridoxine dependency syndrome in the newborn. (3) May inhibit lactation. (4) Used IV only when oral dosage not acceptable. (5) An antagonist to levodopa. (6) Isoniazid is a vitam B₆ antagonist and will cause deficiency disease. (7) Deficiency can cause an abnormal EEG. (8) Excessive doses may elevate SGOT. (9) Protect from heat and light.

Contraindications: Known sensitivity.

Incompatible with: Sufficient information not available; alkaline solutions, iron salts, oxidizing solutions.

Side effects: Almost nonexistent; some slight flushing or feeling of warmth may occur. With larger doses low folic acid levels, paresthesias, somnolence, and withdrawal seizures in infants with high maternal doses may occur.

Antidote: No antidote is known or has been needed.

QUINIDINE GLUCONATE INJECTION

Usual dose: 200 mg. May be repeated as indicated to effect control of the arrhythmia. 330 mg or less is effective in most patients. Up to 1 Gm has been required. Highly individualized. Maintain with oral quinidine sulfate.

Dilution: 800 mg (10 ml) must be diluted in at least 40 ml of 5% dextrose for injection. 1 ml of properly diluted solution equals 16 mg of quinidine.

Rate of administration: 1 ml (16 mg) or fraction thereof of properly diluted solution over 1 minute. Use an infusion pump or microdrip (60 gtt/ml).

Actions: A dextroisomer of quinine. Exerts a depressing antiarrhythmic action on the heart, slowing the rate, slowing conduction, reducing myocardial contractility, and prolonging the refractory period. Increases potassium levels within the cells while it decreases sodium levels. Can have a vasodilating effect. Onset of action occurs when an effective blood concentration has been reached (15 to 30 minutes usually), and lasts 4 to 6 hours. Metabolized in the liver, most of the drug is excreted in the urine.

Indications and uses: Cardiac arrhythmias, including atrial fibrillation, atrial flutter, premature asystoles, supreventricular tachycardia, ventricular tachycardia, and paroxysmal rhythms.

Precautions: (1) Monitor patient's EKG and blood pressure continuously. Too-rapid administration may cause a marked decrease in arterial pressure. (2) Keep patient in supine position. (3) Oral or IM administration is route of choice. (4) Discontinue IV use when the normal sinus rhythm returns, over a 25% prolongation of QRS complex occurs, P waves disappear, or heart rate falls to 120 beats/min. (5) Use extreme caution in first- or second-degree blocks, extensive myocardial damage, digitalis intoxication, and impaired liver or kidney function. (6) A test dose of 200 mg IM for idiosyncrasy is desired if time permits. (7) Potentiates or is potentiated by neuromuscular blocking antibiotics (gentamicin [Garamycin], etc.), anticholinergics (atropine, etc.), thiazide diuretics, antihypertensive agents, muscle relaxants, anticoagulants, and others. Cardiac arrhythmias and other serious side effects may occur. (8) Use caution with digitalis, procainamide, and propranolol. Lower doses of both drugs may be required. (9) May cause increased urine catecholamines, an increased prothrombin time, and a positive Coombs' test. (10) Inhibited by phenobarbital, phenytoin (Dilantin), and rifampin; adjust dosage.

Contraindications: Complete heart block, known hypersensitivity to quinidine or cinchona, lactation, myasthenia gravis, aberrant impulses and abnormal rhythms due to escape mechanism.

Incompatible with: Other drugs, primary because combination is impractical due to possible side effects and need to determine effectiveness.

Side effects: *Minor:* apprehension, cramps, diaphoresis, fever, headache, nausea, rash, tinnitus, urge to defecate, urge to void, vertigo, visual disturbances, vomiting. *Major:* atrioventricular heart block, cardiac standstill, hypotension (acute), tachycardia, thrombocytopenia purpura, urticaria, ventricular fibrillation.

Antidote: Notify the physician of any side effects. If minor symptoms progress or any major side effect appears, discontinue the drug immediately and notify the physician. Use angiotension (Hypertensin) to correct hypotension and sodium lactate to block effects of quinidine on the myocardium. Treatment of toxicity is symptomatic and supportive. Hemodialysis may be indicated. Resuscitate as necessary. Depending on arrhythmia, procainamide or lidocaine is effective alternate.

RITODRINE HYDROCHLORIDE

(Yutopar)

Usual dose: 0.1 mg/min (0.33 ml/min or 20 gtt/min) initially. Gradually increase by 0.05 mg/min (0.17 ml/min or 10 gtt/min) every 10 minutes until desired result is obtained. Continue infusion until 12 hours after contractions cease, then begin oral ritodrine (approximately 30% of IV potency) immediately. Administer first oral dose 30 minutes before IV is discontinued.

Dilution: Each 150 mg (three 50 mg ampoules) must be diluted in 500 ml of one of the following solutions for infusion: 5% or 10% dextrose in water or normal saline, normal saline, 10% inverted sugar solution, Ringer's solution, or Hartmann's solution. Concentration will be 0.33 mg/ml.

Rate of administration: Specific instructions included under usual dose. Usually effective between 0.15 and 0.35 mg/min (0.50 to 1.17 ml/min or 30 to 70 gtt/min). Use of a microdrip chamber (60 gtt/ml) is required, infusion pump preferred. Estimates based on suggested dilution. Adjust if more or less diluent is used. Highly individualized based on patient's response and side effects.

Actions: A beta-adrenergic stimulator that acts to inhibit contractility of uterine smooth muscle. Increases pulse rate and widens pulse pressure moderately. Onset of action is prompt and lasts about 2 hours. Crosses the placental barrier. Primary excretion in the urine.

Indications and uses: To arrest preterm labor.

Precautions: (1) Most effective if begun as soon as diagnosis of preterm labor is established. (2) Do not use if solution is discolored or contains particulate matter or precipitate. (3) Discard solution after 48 hours. (4) Monitor uterine contractions, maternal pulse rate, blood pressure, and fetal heart rate every 5 minutes initially, every 15 to 30 minutes until stable, and hourly thereafter until infusion is discontinued. (5) Maintain adequate hydration but observe for signs of pulmonary edema (may unmask unknown cardiac disease). (6) Maintain patient in left lateral position

449

during infusion to minimize hypotension. (7) Use extreme caution if indicated in maternal mild to moderate preeclampsia, hypertension, or diabetes. (8) Evaluate fetal maturity (sonography). (9) Monitor glucose and electrolyte levels in selected patients or long-term therapy. Normal levels will be altered. (10) Corticosteroids concomitantly may precipitate pulmonary edema. (11) Inhibited by beta-adrenergic blockers (propranolol [Inderal], etc.). (12) Potentiated by other sympathomimetic amines (epinephrine [Adrenalin], dopamine [Intropin], etc.). Effects may be additive. Do not administer concurrently; allow adequate time intervals before initiating therapy with any sympathomimetic drug. (13) May precipitate hypotension with anesthetics.

Contraindications: Before the twentieth week of pregnancy, conditions during pregnancy that are hazardous to the mother or infant; that is, antepartum hemorrhage, cardiac disease (maternal), chorioamnionitis, diabetes mellitus (uncontrolled), eclampsia (or severe preeclampsia), hypersensitivity to ritodrine or its components, hyperthyroidism (maternal), intrauterine fetal death, pulmonary hypertension, preexisting maternal medical conditions adversely affected by beta-mimetic drugs (bronchial asthma treated with beta-mimetics or steroids, cardiac arrhythmias with tachycardia or digitalis intoxication), hypovolemia, hypertension (uncontrolled), and pheochromocytoma.

Incompatible with: Should be considered incompatible in solution with any other drug due to specific use, accurate rate calculation, and potential for additive toxicity.

Side effects: Anaphylaxis, anxiety, cardiac arrhythmias, chest pain, constipation, decreased diastolic pressure, diarrhea, epigastric distress, elevated systolic pressure, erythema, glycosuria, headache, hemolytic icterus, hyperventilation, ileus, jitteriness, lactic acidosis, malaise, nausea, nervousness, palpitations, pulmonary edema, pulse pressure widened, restlessness, tachycardia, tightness of the chest, tremor, vomiting.

Antidote: Keep physician informed of all side effects. Most side effects are expected and will be tolerated or treated symptomatically (note drug interactions). Marked hypotension, tachycardia, cardiac arrhythmias, and other signs of beta-adrenergic stimulation will require discontinuation of the drug. Uterine relaxation may persist for several hours, and oral therapy may be considered. A beta blocker (propranolol [Inderal]) may be required. Discontinue drug and treat anaphylaxis as indicated. At first signs of fluid overload or pulmonary edema, notify physician immediately and treat as indicated.

SECOBARBITAL SODIUM

pH 9.7 to 10.5

(Seconal sodium)

Usual dose (for adults and children): *Moderate sedation:* 1 to 1.5 mg/kg of body weight. *Hypnotic:* 2 mg/kg. *Convulsions:* 2.5 mg/kg. Any dose may be repeated in 3 to 4 hours as indicated. 250 mg is usual maximum single dose, but 500 mg is never exceeded.

Dilution: Dilute with sterile water for injection. Any desired amount of diluent may be used. 9 ml of diluent with 1 ml of secobarbital (50 mg) equals 5 mg/ml. Dilute secobarbital in powder form to a 5% solution (add 5 ml to 250 mg). Rotate ampoule gently while introducing diluent. Further dilute if desired.

Rate of administration: 50 mg or fraction thereof over 1 minute. Never exceed a rate of 50 mg or fraction thereof over 15 seconds. Titrate slowly to desired effect.

Actions: A sedative, hypnotic barbiturate of short duration with anticonvulsant effects. Secobarbital is a CNS depressant. Onset of action is prompt by IV route and lasts about 3 or 4 hours. Will effectively depress motor cortex if adequate doses are administered. Pain perception is unimpaired. Rapidly absorbed by all body tissues and excreted fairly quickly in the urine in changed form. Crosses placental barrier. Excreted in breast milk.

Indications and uses: (1) Preanesthetic sedation, (2) dental and minor surgical sedation, (3) sedation during labor, (4) control of convulsions caused by disease and drug poisoning, (5) sedation in psychotic states.

Precautions: (1) Store in refrigerator. (2) Hydrolyzes in dry or solution form when exposed to air. Use only absolutely clear solutions and discard powder or solution that has been exposed to air for 30 minutes. (3) Use only enough medication to achieve desired effect. Rapid injection rate may cause symptoms of overdose. (4) Record blood pressure, pulse, and respiration every 3 to 5 minutes. Keep patient under constant observation. (5) Maintain a patent airway. Keep equipment for artificial ventilation available. (6) Treat the cause of a convulsion. (7) May be habit forming. (8) Determine absolute patency of vein; use of large veins is preferred to prevent thrombosis. Avoid extravasation. Intraarterial injection will cause gangrene. (9) Use caution in pulmonary and cardiovascular diseases, toxemia of pregnancy, history of bleeding, impaired renal function, and depressive state after a convulsion. (10) Use extreme caution if any other CNS depressants have been given, such as alcohol, narcotic analgesics, anesthetics, antidepressants, sedatives, neuromuscular blocking antibiotics, tranquilizers, etc. Potentiation with respiratory depression may occur. (11) Inhibits effectiveness of propranolol (Inderal), corticosteroids, doxycycline (Vibramycin), oral anticoagulants, oral contraceptives, quinidine. Capable of innumerable interactions with many drugs. (12) May not drive, etc., if given on an outpatient basis. (13) May cause paradoxical excitement in children or the elderly.

Contraindications: Delivery (when maximal drug effect would be achieved at the time of delivery); history of porphyria; impaired liver function; known hypersensitivity to barbiturates; premature delivery; severe respiratory depression.

Incompatible with: Chlordiazepoxide (Librium), chlorpromazine (Thorazine), cimetidine (Tagamet), clindamycin (Cleocin), codeine, diphenhydramine (Benadryl), droperidol (Inapsine), ephedrine, erythromycin (Ilotycin), glycopyrrolate (Robinul), hydrocortisone sodium succinate (Solu-Cortef), insulin (aqueous), levarterenol (Levophed), levorphanol (Levo-Dromoran), meperidine (Demerol), methadone, penicillin G potassium, pentazocine (Talwin), phenytoin (Dilantin), phytonadione (Aquamephyton), procaine (Novocain), prochlorperazine (Compazine), promethazine (Phenergan), sodium bicarbonate, streptomycin, tetracycline, vancomycin (Vancocin).

Side effects: *Average dose:* asthma, bronchospasm, depression, dermatitis, facial edema, fever, hypotension, neonatal apnea, respiratory depression (slight), thrombocytopenic purpura. *Overdose:* apnea, coma, cough reflex depression, hypotension, laryngospasm, lowered body temperature, pulmonary edema, sluggish or absent reflexes, renal shutdown, respiratory depression.

Antidote: Notify the physician of any side effects. Symptomatic and supportive treatment is most important in overdosage. Maintain an adequate airway with artificial ventilation if indicated. Keep the patient warm. Intravenous volume expanders (dextran) will help maintain adequate circulation. Diuretics or hemodialysis will promote the elimination of the drug. Vasopressors (dopamine [Intropin], etc.) will maintain blood pressure.

SECRETIN

(Secretin-Boots)

Usual dose: *Pancreatic function testing:* 1 unit/kg of body weight as a single dose.
Diagnosis of gastrinoma (Zollinger-Ellison syndrome): 2 units/kg as a single dose.

Dilution: Each vial containing 100 (75) units must be diluted with 10 (7.5) ml of normal saline for injection. 10 units/ml.

Rate of administration: A single dose evenly distributed over 1 minute.

Actions: A polypeptide composed of many amino acids. It acts to increase the secretory function of pancreatic exocrine glands. Measuring and analyzing duodenal fluid aids in the determination of pancreatic function. Peak output occurs in 30 minutes and may continue for 2 hours. Degraded in the liver. IV secretin has a serum half-life of 18 minutes.

Indications and uses: (1) Diagnosis of chronic pancreatic dysfunction, (2) diagnosis of gastrinoma (Zollinger Ellison syndrome), (3) may aid in the diagnosis of some hepatobiliary diseases by providing cells for cytopathologic examination.

Precautions: (1) Must be refrigerated at 2° to 7° C (36° to 45° F); check expiration date. (2) Use diluted solution immediately and discard unused portion. (3) Skin testing recommended with 0.1 ml of properly diluted solution. Use a control skin test with 0.1 ml of plain normal saline (without preservatives) for injection. If the secretin causes a greater reddened area than the control area, do not give IV. (4) Pancreatic dysfunction diagnosis is accomplished by inserting a specific double-lumen gastric tube after a 12-hour fast. Correct positioning under fluoroscopic guidance is required. Aspirate gastric contents continuously to prevent passage into the duodenum. Collect duodenal contents for 10 to 20 minutes until a clear, bile-stained, uncontaminated fluid with a pH of 6.0 is obtained. Administer secretin (usually done by physician). Collect four duodenal samples in separate sterile specimen containers (one sample at 10 minutes, one at 20 minutes, one at 40 minutes, and the last at 1 hour after administration of secretin). Sometimes the samples are collected at four 20-minute intervals. (5) Gastrinoma diagnosis begins with a 12-hour fast. Draw two blood samples for fasting serum gastrin levels. Administer secretin. Collect blood samples at 1, 2, 5, 10, and 30 minutes for serum gastrin concentrations. (6) Use with extreme caution in acute pancreatitis; defer use in pregnancy if possible. (7) Safety for use in children not established. (8) Inhibited by carbonic-anhydrase inhibitors (acetazolamide [Diamox], etc.) and anticholinergics (atropine, etc.).

Contraindications: History of asthma or allergy, positive skin test to secretin, known hypersensitivity to secretin, acute pancreatitis until attack subsided.

Incompatible with: Specific information not available. Should be considered incompatible with any drug in the syringe due to specific use.

Side effects: Allergic reactions from impure preparations and/or repeat injections do occur. Skin test previous to injection of clinical dose. Thrombophlebitis can occur.

Antidote: Discontinue the drug immediately for any signs of allergic reaction. Treat anaphylaxis with epinephrine, antihistamines (diphenhydramine [Benadryl], etc.), vasopressors (dopamine [Intropin], etc.), aminophylline, and corticosteroids as indicated. Maintain a patent airway and resuscitate as necessary.

SODIUM BICARBONATE

Usual dose: Adjusted according to pH, clinical response, and fluid limitations of the patient. Available as *4.2% sodium bicarbonate solution* 500 mEq/L or 5 mEq/10 ml.
5% sodium bicarbonate solution 595 mEq/L.
7.5% sodium bicarbonate solution 892 mEq/L or 44.6 mEq/50 ml.
8.4% sodium bicarbonate solution 1,000 mEq/L or 50 mEq/50 ml.

Dilution: May be given in prepared solution. 7.5% and 8.4% solutions should be diluted with equal amount of water for injection or dilute with compatible IV solutions, depending on desired dosage and desired rate of administration.

Rate of administration: Up to 1 mEq/kg of body weight properly diluted over 1 to 3 minutes in cardiac arrest. Repeat half dose every 10 minutes if indicated by blood pH, Po_2, Pco_2, or condition. Usual rate of administration of any solution is 2 to 5 mEq/kg over 4 to 8 hours. Do not exceed 50 mEq/hr. Decrease rate markedly for neonates and children.

Actions: An alkalinizing agent and sodium salt. Helps to maintain osmotic pressure and ion balance. It is the buffering agent in blood. Bicarbonate ion elevates blood pH promptly. Excreted in the urine.

Indications and uses: (1) Metabolic acidosis as in cardiac arrest, salicylate intoxication, ketoacidoses (blood pH below 7.25); (2) hyperkalemia; (3) hyponatremia (administer with 5% sodium chloride, usually 1 part sodium bicarbonate to 3 parts sodium chloride); (4) relieve bronchospasm in status asthmaticus; (5) barbiturate or salicylate intoxication.

Precautions: (1) Use only 50 ml ampoules in cardiac arrest to prevent accidental overdose. (2) Recent practice indicates smaller doses (0.5 mEq/kg of body weight) may be appropriate in cardiac arrest and may prevent secondary alkalosis. Adequate alveolar ventilation is imperative. Evaluate patient response and blood gases. (3) Determine blood pH, Po_2, Pco_2, and electrolytes several times daily during intensive treatment and daily in most other situations. Determine base excess or deficit in infants and children. Notify physician of all results. (4) Temporary therapy in metabolic acidosis. Treatment of primary condition must be instituted. (5) Use with caution in cardiac, liver, or renal disease resulting from salt retention. (6) Rapid or excessive administration may produce alkalosis. (7) Doses in excess of 8 mEq/kg/24 hr and/or given too rapidly (10 ml/min) may cause intracranial hemorrhage in neonates and children under 2 years. (8) 4.2% solution is preferred for children.

Contraindications: Edema, hypertension, hypocalcemia, hypochloremia (from vomiting or gastrointestinal suction), impaired renal function, metabolic alkalosis, respiratory alkalosis.

Incompatible with: 5% alcohol with 5% dextrose, amino acids, ascorbic acid, atropine, calcium chloride, calcium gluconate, chlorpromazine (Thorazine), codeine, corticotropin (ACTH), dextrose solutions, dobutamine (Dobutrex), dopamine (Intropin), glycopyrrolate (Robinul), hydromorphone (Dilaudid), insulin (aqueous), isoproterenol (Isuprel), lactated Ringer's injection, levarterenol (Levophed), levorphanol (Levo-Dromoran), lincomycin (Lincocin), magnesium sulfate, meperidine (Demerol), methadone, methicillin (Staphcillin), morphine, oxytetracycline (Terramycin), penicillin G potassium, pentobarbital (Nembutal), pentazocine (Talwin), phenobarbital (Luminal), procaine (Novocain), promazine (Sparine), Ringer's injection, secobarbital (Seconal), sodium lactate injection (⅙ molar), streptomycin, tetracycline, thiopental (Pentothal), vancomycin (Vancocin), vitamin B complex with C.

Side effects: Rare when used with caution: alkalosis, hyperexcitability, hypokalemia, irritability, restlessness, tetany.

Antidote: Discontinue the drug and notify the physician of any side effect. Hypokalemia usually occurs with alkalosis. Sodium and potassium chloride must be supplemented as indicated for correction. Treatment of alkalosis often results in more alkalosis. Administration of a balanced hypotonic electrolyte solution (Isolyte H, Normosol-M, Plasma-lyte 56) with sodium and potassium chloride added may help to excrete the bicarbonate ion in the urine. Ammonium chloride may be indicated. Treat tetany as indicated.

SODIUM CHLORIDE

SODIUM CHLORIDE pH 5.5

Usual dose: Highly individualized and related to specific condition, concentration of salts in the plasma, and/or loss of body fluids.

Isotonic: (0.9%, 9 Gm of sodium chloride/L or 154 mEq of sodium and 154 mEq of chloride) 1.5 to 3 L/24 hr.

Hypotonic: (0.45%, 4.5 Gm of sodium chloride/L or 77 mEq of sodium and 77 mEq of chloride), 2 to 4 L/24 hr.

Hypertonic: (5%, 50 Gm of sodium chloride/L or 850 mEq of sodium and 850 mEq of chloride or 3% 30 Gm of sodium chloride/L or 510 mEq of sodium and 510 mEq of chloride) 200 to 400 ml/24 hr. Occasionally may have to be repeated within the 24-hour period. See precautions.

Dilution: Available as *isotonic* (10 ml, 20 ml, 30 ml, 50 ml, 100 ml, 150 ml, 250 ml, 500 ml, 1 liter); *hypotonic* (500 ml, 1 liter); or *hypertonic* (500 ml) solution in vials and/or bottles for injection or infusion and ready for use. Isotonic and hypotonic sodium chloride are frequently combined with dextrose 5% or 10%.

Rate of administration: *Isotonic and hypotonic:* A single daily dose equally distributed over 24 hours. Rate is dependent on age, weight, and clinical condition of the patient.

Hypertonic: Each 100 ml over 1 to 4 hours. Do not exceed this dose.

Actions: Sodium is the predominant cation of extracellular fluid. It controls water distribution throughout the body. Hypothalamus osmoreceptors, sensitive to osmolarity changes in the blood, control serum sodium concentration (142 mEq/L). Body fluid is lost when sodium content decreases and retained when sodium content increases. Readily absorbed in kidney tubules. Frequently exchanged for hydrogen and potassium ions. Excess excreted in urine.

Indications and uses: (1) To replace lost sodium and chloride ions in the body; to maintain electrolyte balance.

Isotonic: To replace sodium and chloride lost from vomiting because of obstructions and/or aspiration of gastrointestinal fluids.

Hypotonic: Water replacement without increase of osmotic pressure or serum sodium levels.

Hypertonic: Used only when high sodium and/or chloride content without large amounts of fluid is required. Also used in addisonian crisis and diabetic coma.

(2) As a diluent in parenteral preparations.

Precautions: (1) Use caution in circulatory insufficiency, kidney dysfunction, hypoproteinemia, elderly and debilitated individuals. (2) Maintain accurate intake and output. (3) Monitor vital signs as indicated. (4) Before and during use of hypertonic sodium chloride, determine osmolar concentrations and chloride and bicarbonate content of the serum. Observe patient continuously to prevent pulmonary edema.

Contraindications: Acidosis, congestive heart failure, hypertension, renal damage, clinical states with edema and sodium retention. 3% and 5% sodium chloride solutions are contraindicated with elevated, normal, or slightly decreased serum sodium and chloride levels.

Incompatible with: Amphotericin B (Fungizone), levarterenol (Levophed), mannitol.

Side effects: Due to sodium excess: aggravation of existing acidosis, anorexia, cellular dehydration, deep respiration, disorientation, distention, edema, hydrogen loss, hyperchloremic acidosis, hypertension, increased BUN, nausea, oliguria, potassium loss, pulmonary edema, water retention, weakness.

Antidote: Decrease the rate of infusion and notify the physician of side effects. Sodium excess can be treated by sodium restriction and/or use of diuretics or hemodialysis to remove excessive amounts. Observe the patient carefully and treat symptomatically.

SODIUM INDIGOTINDISULFONATE

(Indigo carmine)

Usual dose: 40 mg (5 ml). A single dose is all that is usually required.

Pediatric dose: Reduce dosage for children.

Dilution: May be given undiluted.

Rate of administration: 40 mg or fraction thereof over 1 minute.

Actions: A dye used to locate orifices in the body. Appears in the urine within 10 minutes after injection. Some absorption into the tissue occurs.

Indications and uses: (1) Identification of ureteral orifices during cystoscopy; (2) patency of fistulous passages in an abscess, surface, or cavity of the body.

Precautions: (1) Patients with a history of allergy should be skin tested with 0.1 ml of a 1:100 dilution. Positive reading will occur in 30 minutes if allergy is present. (2) Urine will turn a blue-green color. (3) Some skin discoloration may occur. (4) Protect from light.

Contraindications: Known sensitivity to sodium indigotindisulfonate.

Incompatible with: Any other drug in a syringe or solution.

Side effects: Rarely occur, but may include mild transient hypertension or hypersensitivity reactions including anaphylaxis.

Antidote: Mild hypertension is seldom a problem. For hypersensitivity reactions, discontinue the drug immediately, treat as necessary with antihistamines and/or epinephrine, and notify the physician. Resuscitate as necessary.

Usual dose: 500 mg to 2 Gm/24 hr or every other day.

Dilution: Should be diluted in 100 ml or more of common IV solutions including dextrose solutions in water or saline, normal saline, or Ringer's and lactated Ringer's injection.

Rate of administration: 100 ml of diluted solution over 15 to 30 minutes or a prescribed rate for larger volumes (preferred).

Actions: An antithyroid drug, sodium iodide interferes with the release of thyroid hormone into the circulation. Well distributed to all body fluids, a concentration of iodide fifty times greater than plasma level can be found in the thyroid gland. Maximum excretion occurs through the urine.

Indications and uses: (1) Thyrotoxicosis, (2) sporotrichosis.

Precautions: (1) Use only clear solutions; discard if darkened or if a precipitate is present. (2) Administer test dose for idiosyncrasy previous to therapeutic dose. (3) Observe often; side effects may be delayed several hours. (4) Adjunctive therapy. Reserpine, hydrocortisone, and other measures are necessary for successful treatment. (5) Use caution in tuberculosis.

Contraindications: Known hypersensitivity to iodides.

Incompatible with: Alkaloids, atropine, codeine, levarterenol (Levophed), levorphanol (Levo-Dromoran), meperidine (Demerol), methadone, morphine, procaine (Novocain).

Side effects: *Minor:* burning sensation of mouth and throat, cough (productive), headache, irritation of the eyes, skin rash, sneezing, swelling of the eyes. *Major:* acute iodism, angioedema, laryngeal edema, petechiae.

Antidote: Discontinue the drug and notify the physician of any side effect. Treatment is symptomatic and supportive. Treat anaphylaxis as indicated and maintain a patent airway. No specific antidote available. Mannitol as an osmotic diuretic will greatly increase the rate of iodine excretion in the urine.

SOLU-B AND SOLU-B WITH ASCORBIC ACID

(Solu-B Forte)

Usual dose: 2 ml/24 hr. May be increased to 5 ml/24 hr if indicated.

Dilution: Available in a Mix-O-Vial. Use sterile water for injection to dilute if Mix-O-Vial is not available. A minimum of 5 ml of diluent is required for direct IV use. May dilute further in 500 or 1,000 ml of IV glucose or saline for infusion. Solu-B Forte provides larger amounts of vitamins. Must be diluted in at least 1 liter and given as an infusion.

Rate of administration: Daily dose properly diluted over 5 minutes. Daily dose in prescribed infusion solution over prescribed hours, for example, 2 ml in 1,000 ml of 5% glucose in water over 8 hours.

Actions: Provides four B-complex vitamins, Solu-B with ascorbic acid adds 500 mg of ascorbic acid and doubles the amounts of B-complex vitamins. These are readily absorbable water-soluble vitamins that are essential for maintaining health. Provides daily requirements or corrects an existing deficiency.

Indications and uses: (1) Preoperative and postoperative maintenance of optimum health; (2) prolonged IV therapy; (3) increased vitamin requirements in fever, severe burns, increased metabolism, hyperthyroidism, and pregnancy; (4) deficient intestinal absorption of water-soluble vitamins; (5) prolonged or wasting diseases.

Precautions: (1) Previous injection of thiamine hydrochloride can cause sensitivity and anaphylactic shock. (2) May cause an increased prothrombin time, resulting in hemorrhage with anticoagulants. Adding ascorbic acid decreases prothrombin time. (3) Use only a clear solution.

Contraindications: Sensitivity to thiamine hydrochloride.

Incompatible with: Chlorpromazine (Thorazine), erythromycin (Erythrocin), magnesium sulfate, methicillin (Staphcillin), methylprednisolone (Solu-Medrol), procaine (Novocain), prochlorperazine (Compazine), sodium bicarbonate, tetracycline, vancomycin (Vancocin).

Side effects: Rare when administered as recommended: anaphylactic shock, feeling of warmth, flushing.

Antidote: Discontinue administration immediately and treat allergic reaction as indicated and notify the physician. Resuscitate as necessary.

STREPTOKINASE

(Kabikinase, Streptase)

Usual dose: *Coronary artery thrombi:* 20,000 IU directly into coronary artery within 6 hours of onset of symptoms of acute transmural myocardial infarction. Follow with 2,000 IU/minute for 1 hour.

Investigational use for coronary artery thrombi: 750,000 IU direct IV within 3 hours of onset of symptoms of acute transmural myocardial infarction. Follow with 250,000 IU in 30 to 60 minutes.

Deep vein thrombosis, pulmonary or arterial embolism, arterial thrombosis: Loading dose: 250,000 IU *Maintenance dose:* 100,000 IU/hour for 24 to 72 hours, depending on diagnosis. May be increased based on prothrombin time evaluations.

Arteriovenous cannula occlusion: 250,000 IU into each occluded limb of cannula.

Dilution: *All uses except cannula occlusion:* Each vial (250,000, 600,000, or 750,000 IU) must be diluted with 5 ml of normal saline for injection (preferred) or 5% dextrose for injection. Add diluent slowly, direct to sides of vial, roll and tilt gently. Do not shake. Further slowly dilute each vial to a total volume of 45 ml May be diluted to a maximum of 500 ml in 45 ml increments (preferred). Discard solution with large amounts of flocculation or any solution remaining after 24 hours. May be infused through a 0.22 or 0.45 μm filter.

Investigational use: Dilute each vial of a single dose with 5 ml of normal saline. Further dilute total single dose in 50 ml of normal saline or 5% dextrose in water. Use care in dilution, as described.

Arteriovenous cannula occlusion: Each vial (250,000 IU) must be diluted with 2 ml of sodium chloride for injection. Use care in dilution, as described.

Rate of administration: Volumetric or syringe infusion pump is required except for investigational use. Reconstituted streptokinase will alter drop size and have an impact on correct dosage with drop size mechanisms.

Coronary artery thrombi: Bolus dose over 15 to 30 seconds via coronary catheter placed by Judkins or Sones technique, directly to thrombosed site verified by selective coronary angiography. Follow with 2,000 IU/minute for 60 minutes.

Investigational IV use for coronary artery thrombi: a total dose evenly distributed over 5 to 10 minutes.

Deep vein thrombosis, pulmonary arterial embolism, arterial thrombi: Loading dose: a single dose equally distributed over 25 to 30 minutes. *Maintenance dose:*100,000 IU or more as ordered, equally distributed every hour for 24 to 72 hours. Dissolution of arterial thrombi may occur in 24 hours or less; deep vein thrombi may take up to 72 hours.

Arteriovenous cannula occlusion: A single dose slowly (do not force) into each occluded limb of cannula. Clamp for 2 hours, then aspirate contents, flush with saline, and reconnect.

Actions: An enzyme prepared from filtrates of beta-hemolytic streptococci. It converts plasminogen to plasmin, which degrades fibrin clots, fibrinogen, and other plasma proteins. This activation takes place within a thrombus as well as on the surface. Onset of action is prompt and may last up to 12 hours. End products of this activity possess an anticoagulant effect. Bleeding may be very difficult to control.

Indications and uses: (1) Lysis of coronary artery thrombi; *Investigational direct IV procedure* is indicated in patients under 65 years with no prior exposure to streptokinase, especially if heart block and/or hypotension are present; (2) lysis of acute massive pulmonary emboli if two or more lobes are involved or if hemodynamics are unstable; (3) lysis of an equivalent amount of emboli in other vessels (deep veins); (4) clearing of occluded arteriovenous cannulae as an alternative to surgical revision.

Precautions: (1) Administered only in the hospital under the direction of a physician knowledgeable in its use and with appropriate diagnostic and laboratory facilities available. Observe patient continuously. Monitor hematocrit, platelet count, activated partial thromboplastin time, thrombin time, and prothrom-

467

bin time before therapy. In 4 hours and during therapy, thrombin time or prothrombin time changes are monitored and will reflect effectiveness of treatment. Keep physician continuously informed. Request specific parameters for notifying physician after initial supervised injection. (2) For coronary catheter procedure, diagnosis of acute MI must be confirmed and the site of the coronary thrombsis confirmed with selective angiography. Concurrent heparin therapy may be required in this situation. (3) *Before direct IV investigational use,* obtain CPK in addition to above baseline blood tests. Give diphenhydramine (Benadryl) 50 mg IV prophylactically. Monitor EKG and record strips with greatest ST segment elevation initially and every 15 minutes for at least 4 hours. When thrombin time is less than twice the normal control value, initiate heparin infusion to keep partial thromboplastin time at 60 seconds. This prompt, easy treatment is a distinct advantage over catheter procedure. (4) Diagnosis of pulmonary or other emboli should be confirmed. Best results are obtained if treatment is started within 7 days of onset of emboli. Discontinue streptokinase if prothrombin time or other lysis parameters are not above $1\frac{1}{2}$ times normal in 4 hours. Excessive resistance may be present. (5) Streptokinase causes a greater alteration of hemostatic status than heparin; use care in handling patient; avoid arterial puncture, venipuncture, and IM injection. Use extreme precautionary methods (use of radial artery—not femoral; extended pressure application of up to 30 minutes) if these procedures are absolutely necessary. Minor bleeding occurs often at streptokinase insertion sites. Do not reduce or stop streptokinase, as lytic activity will be increased and cause more bleeding. (6) Use caution in presence of atrial fibrillation. Monitor for arrhythmias during therapy; atrial and ventricular arrhythmias can occur. (7) Simultaneous use of anticoagulants is not recommended except for coronary artery thrombi. Do not use either drug until the effects of the previous drug are diminished. (8) Avoid use of drugs that may alter platelet function (aspirin, indomethacin, phenylbutazone, etc.). (9) Intensive follow-up therapy with continuous infusion of heparin is indicated in all situations to prevent recurrent thrombosis. Begin in about 3 to 4 hours of completion of streptokinase, when the prothrombin time is reduced to less than twice the normal control value. (10) Do not take blood pressure in lower extremities; thrombi may be dislodged. (11) Prior sensitization to streptokinase increases the risk of allergic reaction in subsequent courses of treatment. (12) Attempt to clear arteriovenous cannulae occlusions with good syringe technique and heparinized saline before using streptokinase. Allow effect of heparin to diminish. (13) Use extreme caution in the following situations: any surgical procedure, biopsy, lumbar puncture, thoracentesis, paracentesis, multiple cutdowns, or intrarterial diagnostic procedures within 10 days; ulcerative wounds; recent trauma with possible internal injury; visceral malignancy; pregnancy and first 10 days postpartum; any lesion of gastrointestinal or genitourinary tract with a potential for bleeding (diverticulitis, ulcerative colitis); severe hypertension; acute or chronic hepatic or renal insufficiency; uncontrolled hypocoagulable state; chronic lung disease with cavitation; subacute bacterial endocarditis; rheumatic valvular disease; and any condition in which bleeding might be hazardous or difficult to manage because of location. (14) Refrigerate after initial dilution.

Contraindications: Active internal bleeding, cerebral vascular accident within 2 months, intracranial or intraspinal surgery, intracranial neoplasm, hypersensitivity to streptokinase.

Incompatible with: Specific information not available. Should be considered incompatible in syringe or solution due to hazards of use.

Side effects: Allergic reactions including anaphylaxis are not uncommon with streptokinase. Fever increase of 1° to 2° F is common. Bleeding can be life threatening.

Antidote: Notify physician of all side effects. Note even the minutest bleeding tendency. Therapy may have to be discontinued with serious bleeding and/or blood loss. Whole blood, packed red blood cells, cryoprecipitate, fresh frozen plasma, and aminocaproic acid may all be indicated. Treat minor allergic reactions symptomatically. Discontinue drug and treat anaphylaxis as indicated, resuscitate as necessary.

STREPTOZOCIN

(Zanosar)

Usual dose: 500 mg/M^2 for 5 consecutive days. Repeat every 6 weeks until maximum benefit or treatment-limiting toxicity is observed. May also give 1,000 mg/M^2 weekly for 2 doses. May then increase up to 1,500 mg/M^2 to achieve therapeutic response if significant toxicity is not observed. Overall cumulative dose to onset of response is 2000 mg/M^2. Maximal response is usually achieved with 4,000 mg/M^2 total cumulative dose.

Dilution: *Specific techniques required; see precautions.* Each 1 Gm vial must be diluted with 9.5 ml of 0.9% sodium chloride or dextrose for injection (100 mg/ml). May be further diluted in larger amounts (50 to 250 ml) of the same solutions if desired.

Rate of administration: A single dose in minimal diluent may be given over 5 to 15 minutes. Increase injection time if additional diluent is used or if indicated for patient comfort.

Actions: An alkylating agent of the nitrogen mustard group with antitumor activity, cell cycle phase non-specific. Disappears from the blood serum rapidly. Concentrates in the liver and kidneys. 20% excreted in the urine.

Indications and uses: Suppress or retard neoplastic growth in metastatic pancreatic islet cell carcinoma. Some results achieved in Hodgkin's disease, other lymphomas, melanoma, and malignant carcinoid tumors.

Precautions: (1) Follow National Study Commission on Cytotoxic Exposure guidelines for handling cytotoxic agents (see Appendix p. 528). (2) Usually administered in the hosital by or under the direction of the physician specialist. (3) Renal toxicity is dose related and cumulative and can be fatal. Monitor renal function before, weekly, and 4 weeks after each course of therapy (serial urinalysis, BUN, plasma creatinine, serum electrolytes, creatinine clearance). Reduce dose or discontinue drug if mild proteinuria occurs. Further deterioration of renal function will occur. (4)

Store in refrigerator before and after dilution. Discard within 12 hours of dilution. Contains no preservatives. (5) This drug is used to induce hypoinsulinemia diabetes mellitus in experimental animals. (6) Monitor complete blood counts and liver function tests weekly. (7) Can be used with other antineoplastic drugs in reduced doses to achieve tumor remission. (8) Will produce teratogenic effects on the fetus. Has a mutagenic potential. Discontinue breast-feeding. (9) Nausea and vomiting has occurred in all patients and can be severe. Prophylactic administration of antiemetics is recommended. (10) Do not administer vaccine or chloroquine to patients receiving antineoplastic drugs. (11) Avoid contact of streptozocin solution with the skin. (12) Potentiates or is potentiated by hepatotoxic or nephrotoxic medications and radiation therapy. (13) Observe for any signs of infection. (13) Maintain hydration.

Contraindications: Hypersensitivity to streptozocin. Severely impaired liver or renal function may be a contraindication.

Incompatible with: Consider incompatible in syringe or solution due to toxicity and specific use.

Side effects: Anemia; decreased platelet count (precipitous); diarrhea; elevated SGOT and LDH; hepatic toxicity (usually reversible); hypoalbuminemia; hypoglycemia; insulin shock; leukopenia (precipitous); nausea and vomiting (severe); proteinuria; thrombocytopenia.

Antidote: Notify physician of all side effects. Nausea and vomiting, hematological changes, and renal toxicity (proteinuria) may require dose reduction or discontinuation of the drug. There is no specific antidote. Supportive therapy as indicated will help sustain the patient in toxicity.

(Anectine, Quelicin, Sucostrin, Sux-Cert)

Usual dose: 10 to 40 mg initially for short-term muscle relaxation. Given as an infusion if muscle relaxation must be sustained over a long period of time. Highly individualized, depending on response and degree of relaxation required. Dosage ranges from 0.5 to 10 mg/min and averages 2.5 mg/min. 1 mg/kg of body weight is sufficient to cause respiratory paralysis. A test dose of 10 mg is sometimes used to test patient sensitivity and recovery time.

Dilution: May be given undiluted if short-term muscle relaxation is desired. For intermittent or continuous infusion add 1 Gm of succinylcholine to 1 liter of 5% dextrose solution or isotonic saline solution. 1 ml of diluted solution delivers 1 mg of succinylcholine.

Rate of administration: *Direct IV:* single initial dose over 30 seconds. *Intermittent or continuous infusion:* variable, depending on individual response and muscle relaxation required. Use an infusion pump or microdrip (60 gtt/ml) for accuracy. Never exceed 10 mg/min.

Actions: An ultrashort-acting skeletal muscle relaxant. Causes paralysis by interfering with neural transmission at the myoneural junction. Onset of action is within 1 or 2 minutes and lasts about 5 minutes. Complete recovery from a single dose occurs in about 10 minutes. Metabolized to succinic acid and choline. Only a small amount is excreted in the kidneys. Crosses placental barrier.

Indications and uses: (1) Skeletal muscle relaxation during operative and manipulative procedures, (2) facilitation of management of patients undergoing mechanical ventilation, (3) termination or prevention of convulsive episodes resulting from drug toxicity or electroshock therapy.

Precautions: (1) Primarily used by or under the direct observation of the anesthesiologist. (2) This drug produces apnea. Controlled artificial ventilation must be continuous and under direct observation at all times. (3) Use only freshly prepared solutions. Store in re-

frigerator. (4) Should be administered after unconsciousness is induced to reduce patient discomfort. (5)
Use caution in extensive tissue trauma, severe burns,
nerve damage, and paralysis. Hyperkalemia may
cause cardiac arrhythmias. (6) Observe for early signs
of malignant hyperthermic crisis (jaw muscle spasm,
lack of laryngeal relaxation, rigidity, and unresponsive tachycardia). (7) Use caution in anemia, cardiovascular, hepatic, pulmonary, metabolic, and renal
disorders, or malnutrition. Decreased plasma cholinesterase activity potentiates this drug. May increase
intraocular pressure. (8) Potentiated by neuromuscular blocking antibiotics (streptomycin, kanamycin,
neomycin, etc.), organic phosphate compounds (insecticides), anticholinesterase drugs (neostigmine, edrophonium, etc.), cyclophosphamide (Cytoxan), lidocaine, quinine, quinidine, and magnesium salts. Capable of innumerable other drug interactions. (9)
Inhibited by previous administration of diazepam
(Valium).

Contraindications: Hypersensitivity to succinycholine,
family history of malignant hyperthermia, genetic
disorders of plasma pseudocholinesterase, myopa-
thies associated with elevated CPK values, acute narrow angle glaucoma, penetrating eye injuries.

Incompatible with: Alkaline solutions, barbiturates (amobarbital [Amytal], methohexital [Brevital], pentobarbital [Nembutal], phenobarbital, secobarbital [Se-
conal], thiopental [Pentothal], etc.), chlorpromazine
(Thorazine), nafcillin (Unipen).

Side effects: *Minor:* bradycardia, muscular twitching,
respiratory depression. *Major:* cardiac arrhythmias,
hyperthermia, malignant hyperthermic crisis, prolonged apnea.

Antidote: Controlled artificial respiration must be continuous. Endotracheal intubation or tracheostomy is
considered prophylactic if necessary for adequate respiratory exchange. Atropine should be helpful to control bradycardia. Resuscitate as necessary. Whole
blood transfusion may restore absent cholinesterase
activity and stimulate voluntary respiration in unresponsive cases.

(Gantrisin)

Usual dose: 50 mg/kg of body weight initially, then give 100 mg/kg/24 hr, equally divided in four doses and given every 6 hours. Oral sulfonamides are preferred when possible.

Dilution: Must be diluted to a 5% solution. Add a minimum of 35 ml of sterile water for injection to the 5 ml ampoule of 40% solution. Do not add to infusion fluids. Do not use any other diluent; precipitation will result.

Rate of administration: 1 ml of properly diluted solution over 1 minute, direct IV or as an intermittent infusion through Y tube or three-way stopcock.

Actions: A wide-spectrum sulfonamide with bacteriostatic action effective against gram-negative and gram-positive organisms. Easily soluble in all body fluids; therapeutic blood levels are achieved quickly but maintained only with adequate dosage. Prevents formation of folic acid necessary for bacterial growth. Produces high urinary levels quickly and is generally easily excreted without crystal formations. Crosses placental barrier. Excreted in breast milk.

Indications and uses: Acute or chronic infections of the urinary tract and soft tissue, including meningitis.

Precautions: (1) Sensitivity studies are helpful to determine the susceptibility of the causative organisms to sulfisoxazole diolamine. (2) Use caution in impaired liver or renal function, urinary obstruction, or blood dyscrasias. (3) In prolonged therapy, blood cell counts and liver and kidney function test are recommended. (4) Not effective in viral or rickettsial infections. (5) Potentiated by acidifying agents, analgesics, vitamin C, phenothiazines, salicylates, and others. (6) Inhibited by alkalinizing agents, para-aminobenzoic acid (PABA), anesthetics (local), paraldehyde, and others. (7) Potentiates oral antidiabetics, alcohol, anticoagulants, phenytoin (Dilantin), folic acid antagonists, insulin, isoniazid, and others. Serious side effects or toxicity may result. (8) Often used in combinations with antibiotics, but the choice must be highly selec-

475

tive because of interactions. Tetracyclines and chloramphenicol are additive in some instances. (9) Encourage adequate fluid intake.

Contraindications: Infants under 2 months of age, known hypersensitivity to sulfonamides, pregnancy at term, lactation, prophyria.

Incompatible with: Amikacin (Amikin), aminophylline, ammonium chloride, ascorbic acid, cephalothin (Keflin), chloramphenicol, codeine, heparin, hydroxyzine (Vistaril), insulin (aqueous), kanamycin (Kantrex), levarterenol (Levophed), levorphanol (Levo-Dromoran), meperidine (Demerol), metaraminol (Aramine), methicillin (Staphcillin), methadone, morphine, nitrofurantoin (Ivadantin), oxytetracycline (Terramycin), phenytoin (Dilantin), procaine (Novocain), prochlorperazine (Compazine), promazine (Sparine), promethazine (Phenergan), streptomycin, tetracycline, thiopental (Pentothal), vancomycin (Vancocin), vitamin B complex with C.

Side effects: Low toxicity level, but may include anaphylaxis, blood dyscrasias, crystalluria, diarrhea, fever, headache, hematuria, hepatitis, nausea, neuropathy, pancreatitis, petechiae, purpura, rash, urticaria, vomiting.

Antidote: Notify the physician of any side effect. Drug may be discontinued depending on severity of infection and susceptibility to other drugs. Treat anaphylaxis with epinephrine, corticosteroids, antihistamines, and vasopressors as indicated.

TETRACYCLINE HYDROCHLORIDE

(Achromycin)

Usual dose: 250 to 500 mg every 12 hours. Maximum dose in 24 hours is 500 mg every 6 hours. Normal renal function is required.

Pediatric dose: 12 mg/kg of body weight/24 hr in two equal doses. May vary from 10 to 20 mg/kg/24 hr.

Dilution: Each 250 mg or fraction thereof is diluted with 5 ml of sterile water for injection. Must be further diluted with a minimum of 100 ml of 5% dextrose in water or isotonic saline for injection or preferably added to larger volumes of standard infusion solutions such as normal saline, dextrose in water or saline, or Ringer's solution.

Rate of administration: Each 100 mg or fraction thereof over a minimum of 5 minutes. Never exceed this rate. Must be completed within 12 hours of dilution.

Actions: A broad-spectrum antibiotic that is bacteriostatic against many gram-positive and gram-negative organisms. Thought to interfere with protein synthesis of microorganisms. Well distributed in most body tissues and often bound to plasma protein, tetracyclines are concentrated in the liver and excreted through the bile to urine and feces in a biologically active state. Crosses the placental barrier. Excreted in breast milk.

Indications and uses: (1) Infections caused by susceptible strains or organisms, such as rickettsiae, spirochetal agents, viruses, and many other gram-negative and gram-positive bacteria; (2) to substitute for contraindicated penicillin or sulfonamide therapy.

Precautions: (1) Initiate oral therapy as soon as possible. (2) Must be stored away from heat and light. (3) Check expiration date; outdated ampoules may cause nephrotoxicity. (4) Stable at room temperature no longer than 12 hours after dilution. (5) Buffered with ascorbic acid. (6) Sensitivity studies are necessary to determine the susceptibility of the causative organism to tetracycline. (7) Avoid prolonged use of drug. Superinfection caused by overgrowth of nonsusceptible organisms may result. (8) Use caution in impaired liver or renal function, pregnancy, postpartum, and lactation. Tetracycline serum concentrations and liver and kidney function tests are indicated. (9) May cause skeletal retardation in the fetus and infants and permanent tooth discoloration in children under 8 years, including in utero or through mother's milk. (10) Inhibits bactericidal action of penicillin, ampicillin, oxacillin, methicillin, etc. May be toxic with sulfonamides. (11) May potentiate digoxin and anticoagulants. Reduced dose of these drugs may be necessary. (12) Potentiated by alcohol, barbiturates, cimetidine (Tagamet), phenytoin (Dilantin), and other hepatotoxic drugs; severe liver damage may result. (13) Inhibited by alkalinizing agents, calcium, iron, and magnesium salts, riboflavin, sodium bicarbonate, and others. (14) Alert patient to photosensitivity skin reaction. (15) Determine patency of vein, avoid extravasation. (16) Organisms resistant to one tetracycline are usually resistant to others.

Contraindications: Known hypersensitivity to tetracyclines.

Incompatible with: Amikacin (Amikin), aminophylline, amobarbital (Amytal), amphotericin B (Fungizone), calcium salts and solutions, carabenicillin (Geopen), cefazolin (Kefzol), cephalothin (Keflin), cephapirin (Cefadyl), chloramphenicol (Chloromycetin), chlorothiazide (Diuril), dimenhydrinate (Dramamine), erythromycin (Ilotycin, Erythrocin), heparin, hyaluronidase (Wydase, etc.), hydrocortisone sodium succinate (Solu-Cortef), methicillin (Staphcillin), methohexital (Brevital), methylprednisolone (Solu-Medrol), nitrofurantoin (Ivadantin), oxacillin (Prostaphlin), penicillins, pentobarbital (Nembutal), phenobarbital (Luminal), phenytoin (Dilantin), polymyxin B (Aerosporin), prochlorperazine (Compazine), riboflavin, secobarbital (Seconal), sodium bicarbonate, sulfisoxazole (Gantrisin), thiopental (Pentothal), vitamin B complex, warfarin (Coumadin).

Side effects: Relatively nontoxic in average doses. More toxic in large doses or if given too rapidly. *Minor:* anogenital lesions, anorexia, blood dyscrasias, diar-

478

rhea, dysphagia, enterocolitis, nausea, skin rashes, vomiting. *Major:* hypersensitivity reactions, including anaphylaxis; liver damage; photosensitivity; systemic moniliasis; thrombophlebitis.

Antidote: Notify the physician of all side effects. If minor side effects are progressive or any major side effect occurs, discontinue the drug, treat allergic reaction, or resuscitate as necessary.

THEOPHYLLINE
ETHYLENEDIAMINE   pH 8.6 to 9.0

(Aminophylline)

Usual dose: Initial dose of 6 mg/kg of body weight. Follow with a continuous infusion from 0.5 to 0.7 mg/kg/hr for first 12 hours and 0.1 to 0.5 mg/kg/hr thereafter, depending on condition and response.

Pediatric dose: 6 mg/kg of body weight is maximum initial IV dose. Follow with a continuous infusion from 1.0 to 1.2 mg/kg/hr for first 12 hours and 0.8 to 1.0 mg/kg/hr thereafter, depending on condition and response.

Dilution: Only the 25 mg/ml solution may be given by direct IV administration undiluted or it can be further diluted in at least 100 or 200 ml of 5% dextrose in water and given as an infusion.

Rate of administration: A single dose over a minimum of 15 minutes. Do not exceed an average rate of 1 ml or 25 mg/min when giving direct IV or as an infusion. Discontinue primary infusion if theophylline administered by "piggyback or additive" tubing and a possible incompatibility problem exists.

Actions: An alkaloid xanthine derivative, it relaxes smooth muscle and the bronchial tubes. Cardiac output, urinary output, and sodium excretion are increased. Skeletal and cardiac muscles are stimulated, as is the CNS to a lesser degree. There is peripheral vasodilation. It decreases pulmonary artery pressure and lowers the threshold of the respiratory center to carbon dioxide. Well distributed throughout the body and excreted in a changed form in the urine. Crosses the placental barrier. Excreted in breast milk.

Indications and uses: (1) Bronchial asthma, (2) reversible bronchospasm of chronic bronchitis or emphysema, (3) *Investigational use:* apnea and bradycardia of prematurity.

Precautions: (1) Check vial carefully; must state for IV use. Minimum dilution must be 25 mg/ml, warm to room temperature. (2) Rapid administration will cause ventricular fibrillation or cardiac arrest. (3) Monitor serum levels to achieve maximum benefit with minimum risk. Each 0.6 mg/kg of body weight will increase serum theophylline by 1 μg/ml. 10 to 20 μg/ml is considered therapeutic. Beverages with caffeine may cause false high theophylline levels. (4) Long-term use in any form has a cumulative effect or may render the drug ineffective. (5) Use with caution in coronary occlusion, angina pectoris, peptic ulcer disease, renal and hepatic disease, severe hypertension, severe myocardial damage, hyperthyroidism, and glaucoma. (6) Do not use one xanthine derivative concurrently with another xanthine derivative, ephedrine, or other sympathomimetic drugs. (7) Use with extreme caution in children. Has caused fatal reactions. (8) Xanthines antagonize or potentiate or are themselves antagonized or potentiated by many drug groups. Examples are: inhibited by beta adrenergic blockers (propranolol [Inderal], etc.), hydantoins (phenytoin [Dilantin], etc.), troleandomycin (TAO); potentiated by alcohol, cimetidine (Tagamet), clindamycin (Cleocin), halothane anesthesia; potentiates erythromycin; inhibits nondepolarizing muscle relaxants (tubocurarine [Curare], etc.). (9) Crystals will form if solution pH falls below 8.0. (10) Smokers may require higher dose range. (11) Initiate oral therapy at soon as symptoms are adequately improved.

Contraindications: Known sensitivity to theophylline or ethylenediamine. Infants under 6 months of age.

Incompatible with: Acid solutions, amikacin (Amikin), ascorbic acid, cephalothin (Keflin), chloramphenicol, chlorpromazine (Thorazine), cimetidine (Tagamet), clindamycin (Cleocin), codeine, corticotropin (Acthar), dimenhydrinate (Dramamine), doxapram (Dopram), doxorubicin (Adriamycin), doxycycline (Vibramycin), epinephrine (Adrenalin), erythromycin (Ilotycin), fructose solution, hydralazine, hydroxyzine (Vistaril), insulin, invert sugar solutions, isoproterenol (Isuprel), levarterenol (Levophed), levorphanol (Levo-Dromoran), meperidine (Demerol), methadone, methicillin (Staphcillin), methylprednisolone (Solu-Medrol), morphine, nafcillin, oxytetracycline (Terramycin), penicillin G sodium and potassium, pentazocine (Talwin), phenobarbital (Luminal), phenytoin

(Dilantin), procaine, prochlorperazine (Compazine), promazine (Sparine), promethazine (Phenergan), succinylcholine (Anectine), sulfisoxazole, tetracycline (Achromycin), vancomycin (Vancocin), vitamin B complex, and vitamin B with C.

Side effects: Toxicity resulting in death may occur suddenly, especially with serum levels above 20 µg/ml. Anxiety, cardiac arrest, convulsions, delirium, dizziness, headache, nausea, peripheral vascular collapse, restlessness, temporary hypotension, ventricular fibrillation, vomiting.

Antidote: With onset of any side effect, discontinue the drug and notify the physician. For mild symptoms the physician may choose to continue the drug at a decreased rate of administration. Grand mal seizures may not respond to anticonvulsants. Do not use stimulants. Consider charcoal hemoperfusion dialysis. Resuscitate as necessary.

(Betalin S, vitamin B_1)

Usual dose: Up to 30 mg 3 times daily. Doses up to 100 mg are sometimes required.

Pediatric dose: 10 to 25 mg/24 hours.

Dilution: May be given by direct IV administration or added to most IV solutions and given as an infusion.

Rate of administration: 100 mg or fraction thereof over 5 minutes.

Actions: A water-soluble vitamin, thiamine is necessary to most metabolic processes in humans, especially carbohydrate metabolism. Many cells require its presence for growth and maturation, as well as accomplishing group formations and transfers. Found in all body tissues, stored in the liver, and excreted in urine.

Indications and uses: (1) "Wet" beriberi with myocardial failure, (2) neuritis and polyneuritis of any etiology, (3) vitamin B_1 deficiency resulting from supply or absorption.

Precautions: (1) Not commonly administered by IV route; IM route is preferred. (2) Rarely used alone, it is more often administered as a multiple B vitamin. (3) Intradermal test dose recommended in suspected sensitivity. (4) Can be refrigerated; protect from freezing, protect from light.

Contraindications: Known hypersensitivity to thiamine hydrochloride.

Incompatible with: Amobarbital (Amytal), phenobarbital (Luminal), solutions with neutral or alkaline pH, such as carbonates, citrates, barbiturates, and acetates.

Side effects: Anaphylaxis and death caused by sensitivity reaction can occur with intravenous administration.

Antidote: Discontinue the drug, treat allergic reaction or resuscitate as necessary, and notify the physician.

THIOPENTAL SODIUM

pH 10.0 to 11.0

(Pentothal Sodium)

Usual dose: Convulsions:75 to 125 mg. Up to 250 mg may be required.

Dilution: Each 500 mg ampoule of sterile thiopental powder is diluted with 20 ml of sterile water for injection (supplied) to make a 2.5% solution. Prepared solutions also available. Each 1 ml equals 25 mg. Soluble only in isotonic saline or 5% glucose in water for infusion.

Rate of administration: Each 25 mg or fraction thereof over 1 minute. Titrate slowly to desired effect.

Actions: An ultrashort-acting barbiturate and CNS depressant that produces hypnosis and anesthesia. Has potent anticonvulsant effects. Onset of action is prompt and lasts about 15 to 30 minutes. Rapidly absorbed by all body tissues. Some is retained in fatty tissue, causing sustained or delayed effect. Excreted in changed form in the urine. Crosses the placental barrier. Excreted in breast milk.

Indications and uses: Control of convulsive states. Administration for any other indication is limited to the anesthesiologist.

Precautions: (1) Usually administered by or under direct observation of a physician. (2) Use only freshly prepared clear solutions. (3) Determine absolute patency of vein. Extravasation will cause necrosis and sloughing; intraarterial injection can cause gangrene. (4) Use only enough medication to achieve desired effect. Rapid injection rate may cause symptoms of overdose. (5) Record vital signs every 3 to 5 minutes. Keep patient under constant observation. (6) Treat the cause of the convulsion. (7) Maintain a patent airway and have equipment for artificial ventilation available. (8) Reduce dosage and use caution in cardiovascular disease, hypotension, shock, medication potentiation, impaired renal or liver function, Addison's disease, myxedema, elevated blood urea, elevated intracranial pressure, asthma, and myasthenia gravis. (9) May be habit forming. (10) Use with extreme caution if any other CNS depressants have been given, such as al-

484

cohol, narcotic analgesics, anesthetics, antidepressants, sedatives, neuromuscular blocking antibiotics, tranquilizers, etc. Potentiation with respiratory depression may occur. (11) Inhibits effectiveness of propranolol (Inderal), corticosteroids, doxycycline (Vibramycin), oral anticoagulants, oral contraceptives, quinidine. Capable of innumerable interactions with many drugs. (12) May cause paradoxical excitement in children or the elderly.

Contraindications: History of porphyria, known hypersensitivity to barbiturates, status asthmaticus, suitable veins not available.

Incompatible with: Acid solutions, amikacin (Amikin), aminophylline, arginine, calcium salts, cephalothin (Keflin), cephapirin (Cefadyl), cimetidine (Tagamet), clindamycin (Cleocin), chlorpromazine (Thorazine), codeine, dimenhydrinate (Dramamine), diphenhydramine (Benadryl), doxapram (Dopram), droperidol (Inapsine), ephedrine, glycopyrrolate (Robinul), hydromorphone (Dilaudid), insulin (aqueous), levarterenol (Levophed), levorphanol (Levo-Dromoran), magnesium sulfate, meperidine (Demerol), metaraminol (Aramine), methadone, methylprednisolone (Solu-Medrol), morphine, para-aminobenzoic acid (PABA), penicillins, procaine (Novocain), prochlorperazine (Compazine), promazine (Sparine), promethazine (Phenergan), sodium bicarbonate, succinylcholine (Anectine), sulfisoxazole (Gantrisin), tetracycline, tubocurarine (curare).

Side effects: *Average dose:* asthma, bronchospasm, depression, dermatitis, facial edema, fever, hypotension, neonatal apnea, respiratory depression (slight), thrombocytopenic purpura.

Overdose: apnea, cardiac arrhythmias, coma, cough reflex depression, hypotension, hypothermia, laryngospasm, pulmonary edema, renal shutdown, respiratory depression, sluggish or absent reflexes.

Antidote: Call any side effect to the physician's attention. Symptomatic and supportive treatment is most important in overdosage. Keep the patient warm. Intravenous volume expanders (dextran) will help maintain adequate circulation. Diuretics or hemodialysis will promote the elimination of the drug. Vasopressors (dopamine [Intropin], etc.) will maintain blood pressure. For extravasation, local injection of 1% procaine will relieve pain and promote vasodilation. Local heat application may be helpful.

TICARCILLIN DISODIUM

(Ticar)

Usual dose: 150 to 300 mg/kg of body weight/24 hr in divided doses every 3, 4, or 6 hours. All dosages vary depending on the severity of the infection.

Pediatric dose: *Under 40 kg:* 50 to 300 mg/kg of body weight/24 hr in divided doses every 4, 6, or 8 hours. Do not exceed adult dose.

Neonatal dose: *Under 2,000 Gm:* age 0 to 7 days, 75 mg/kg of body weight every 12 hours. Over 7 days of age, 75 mg/kg every 8 hours.
Over 2,000 Gm: age 0 to 7 days, 75 mg/kg every 8 hours. Over 7 days of age, 100 mg/kg every 8 hours.

Dilution: Each 1 Gm or fraction thereof is diluted with 4 ml of sterile water for injection. Further dilution of each gram with an additional 10 to 20 ml or more of sterile water for injection, 5% dextrose, or normal saline is required for direct IV administration or intermittent piggyback infusion. May be added to larger volumes or standard IV fluids and given as a continuous infusion.

Rate of administration: Direct IV: 1 Gm or fraction thereof over 5 minutes or more to reduce vein irritation. *Intermittent infusion:* A single dose over 30 minutes to 2 hours. In neonate give over 10 to 20 minutes. *Continuous infusion:* At specified rate not to exceed rate and concentration of intermittent infusion.

Actions: An extended-spectrum penicillin. Bactericidal for many gram-negative and gram-positive organisms. Large doses with high blood levels are well tolerated. Excreted in the urine.

Indications and uses: Bacterial septicemia, acute and chronic infections of the respiratory tract, skin and soft tissue, intraabdominal area, female pelvis, genital tract, and urinary tract. Useful in infections complicated by impaired renal function or in patients receiving immunosuppressive or oncolytic drugs.

Precautions: (1) Stable at room temperature for at least 48 hours. (2) Sensitivity studies are indicated to determine the susceptibility of the causative organism to ticarcillin. (3) Oral probenecid will achieve higher and more prolonged blood levels. (4) Reduce daily dose commensurate with amount of renal impairment. Intervals between injections should also be increased. (5) Periodic evaluation of renal, hepatic, and hematopoietic systems is recommended in prolonged therapy. (6) Superinfection caused by overgrowth of nonsusceptible organisms can occur. (7) Electrolyte imbalance and cardiac irregularities from high sodium content are possible. (8) Slow infusion rate for pain along venipuncture site. (9) Gentamicin and tobramycin are used concurrently in severe infection. (10) Use caution in pregnancy. (11) Tetracyclines can inhibit bactericidal activity of penicillins.

Contraindications: Known penicillin or cephalosporin sensitivity.

Incompatible with: Amikacin (Amikin), colistimethate (Coly-Mycin), gentamicin (Garamycin), kanamycin (Kantrex), tobramycin (Nebcin).

Side effects: Abnormal clotting time or prothrombin time, anaphylaxis, anemia, convulsions, elevated SGOT and SGPT, eosinophilia, fever, leukopenia, nausea, neutropenia, phlebitis, pruritus, skin rash, thrombocytopenia, urticaria, vomiting.

Antidote: Notify the physician immediately of any adverse symptoms. For severe symptoms, discontinue the drug, treat allergic reaction (epinephrine, antihistamine, and corticosteroids), and resuscitate as necessary.

(Nebcin)

Usual dose: 3 mg/kg of body weight/24 hr equally divided into three or four doses. Up to 5 mg/kg may be given if indicated. Reduce to usual dose as soon as feasible. Normal renal function is necessary. Dosage is based on lean body weight plus 40% for obese patients.

Pediatric dose: 6 to 7.5 mg/kg of body weight/24 hr in 3 or 4 equally divided doses every 6 or 8 hours.

Newborn dose: 1 week of age or less: 4 mg/kg of body weight/24 hr in two equal doses every 12 hours.

Dilution: Prepared solutions equal 10 or 40 mg/ml. Further dilute each single dose in 50 to 100 ml of IV normal saline or 5% dextrose in water and administer through an additive tubing. Reduce volume of diluent proportionately for children.

Rate of administration: Each single dose, properly diluted over a minimum of 20 and a maximum of 60 minutes.

Actions: An aminoglycoside antibiotic with potential neuromuscular blocking action. Inhibits protein synthesis in bacterial cells. Bactericidal against specific gram-negative and gram-positive bacilli, including *Escherichia coli*, *Klebsiella*, *Proteus*, and *Pseudomonas*. Well distributed through all body fluids. Crosses the placental barrier. Excreted in the kidneys. Cross-allergenicity does occur between aminoglycosides.

Indications and uses: (1) Short-term treatment of serious infections caused by susceptible organisms—septicemia, meningitis, peritonitis, etc.; (2) primarily used when penicillin and other less toxic antibiotics are ineffective or contraindicated; (3) concurrent therapy with a penicillin or cephalosporin is sometimes indicated.

Precautions: (1) Use extreme caution if therapy is required over 7 to 10 days. (2) Sensitivity studies are necessary to determine the susceptibility of the causative organism to tobramycin. (3) Reduce daily dose commensurate with amount of renal impairment. Intervals between injections should also be increased. (4) Watch for decrease in urine output, rising BUN and serum creatinine, and declining creatinine clearance levels. Dosage may require decreasing. Routine serum levels and evaluation of hearing are recommended. (5) Use caution in infants, children, and elderly. (6) Potentiated by anesthetics, other neuromuscular blocking antibiotics (kanamycin, streptomycin, etc.), anticholinesterases (edrophonioum [Tensilon], etc.), antineoplastics (nitrogen mustard, cisplatin, etc), barbiturates, muscle relaxants (tubocurarine, etc.), phenothiazines (promethazine [Phenergan], etc.), procainamide, quinidine, and sodium citrate. *Apnea can occur.* (7) Ototoxicity may be potentiated by loop diuretics (ethacrynic acid [Edecrin], furosemide [Lasix], etc.). An elevated serum level of tobramycin may occur, increasing nephrotoxicity and neurotoxicity. (8) Inactivated in solution with carbenicillin and other penicillins. (9) Superinfection may occur from overgrowth of nonsusceptible organisms. (10) Maintain good hydration.

Contraindications: Known tobramycin sensitivity.

Incompatible with: Any other drug in syringe or solution. Administer separately. Note precautions.

Side effects: Occur more frequently with impaired renal function, higher doses, or prolonged administration. *Minor:* dizziness; fever; headache; increased SGOT, SGPT, and serum bilirubin; itching; lethargy; rash; roaring in the ears; urticaria; vomiting. *Major:* apnea; blood dyscrasias; cylindruria; elevated BUN, NPN, and creatinine; hearing loss; oliguria; proteinuria; tinnitus; vertigo.

Antidote: Notify the physician of all side effects. If minor side effects persist or any major symptom appears, discontinue the drug and notify the physician. Treatment is symptomatic or a reduction in dose may be required. Hemodialysis or peritoneal dialysis may be indicated. Resuscitate as necessary.

TOLAZOLINE HYDROCHLORIDE   pH 3.0 to 4.0

(Priscoline)

Usual dose: 10 to 50 mg four times every 24 hours. Initiate treatment with lower dose and increase gradually to optimal dose.

Pediatric dose: Not established at this time. Investigational use.

Dilution: May be given undiluted. May be given through Y tube or three-way stopcock of infusion set.

Rate of administration: Each 10 mg or fraction thereof over 1 minute.

Actions: An adrenergic blocking agent. Induces marked dilation of peripheral blood vessels. Increases blood flow by a threefold action: (1) direct dilation of the vessel wall, (2) sympathetic block, and (3) blocking the vasoconstrictive action of epinephrine and levarterenol (Levophed). Excreted in the urine.

Indications and uses: (1) Spastic peripheral vascular disorders; (2) Buerger's disease; (3) diabetic arteriosclerosis, gangrene; (4) endarteritis; (5) to treat sequelae of frostbite; (6) postthrombotic conditions; (7) Raynaud's disease; (8) scleroderma; (9) *investigational use:* pulmonary vasodilator in infants with acutely increased pulmonary vascular resistance.

Precautions: (1) Observe constantly during administration for flushing, which indicates optimum dose has been reached. (2) Keep patient warm, will increase effectiveness of drug. (3) Use caution in gastritis, known or suspected gastric ulcer, mitral stenosis, pregnancy and lactation. (4) May be given by intraarterial injection under specific circumstances (see literature). (5) Hazardous when given concurrently with alcohol.

Contraindications: After cerebrovascular accident, in known or suspected coronary artery disease.

Incompatible with: Ethacrynic acid (Edecrin), hydrocortisone sodium succinate (Solu-Cortef), methylprednisolone sodium succinate (Solu-Medrol).

Side effects: *Average dose:* usually mild and decrease with continued treatment; chilliness, diarrhea, epigastric discomfort, flushing, increased pilomotor activity, nausea, slight rise or fall in blood pressure, tachycardia, tingling, vomiting. *Overdose:* anginal pain, cardiac arrhythmias, exacerbations of peptic ulcer, severe hypotension or hypertension.

Antidote: Notify the physician of all side effects. If minor symptoms progress or major side effects appear, discontinue the drug immediately and notify the physician. Treat hypotension with IV fluids, a head-low position, and ephedrine if necessary. Epinephrine and levarterenol (Levophed) are contraindicated for hypotension. Further hypotension will occur. Treat all other side effects symptomatically and resuscitate as necessary.

TRIETHYLENETHIOPHOSPHORAMIDE

(Thiotepa)

Usual dose: 0.3 to 0.4 mg/kg of body weight as initial dose. Maintenance dose and frequency adjusted according to blood cell counts before and after treatment. Usually given at 1- to 4-week intervals.

Dilution: *Specific techniques required, see precautions.* Each 15 mg of drug is diluted with 1.5 ml of sterile water for injection. Shake solution gently and allow to stand until clear. May be added to IV solutions. May be given through Y tube or three-way stopcock of a free-flowing IV infusion.

Rate of administration: 60 mg or fraction thereof over 1 minute direct IV.

Actions: An alkylating agent of the nitrogen mustard group with antitumor activity. Cell cycle phase non-specific. Thought to have a radiomimetic action, which releases ethylenimine radicals to destroy actively dividing cells. Well absorbed and distributed, it is excreted unchanged in the urine.

Indications and uses: To suppress or retard neoplastic growth. Good response has been experienced in Hodgkin's disease, non-Hodgkin's lymphomas, retinoblastoma, and adenocarcinomas of the breast and ovary.

Precautions: (1) Follow guidelines for handling cytotoxic agents recommended by the National Study Commission on Cytotoxic Exposure (see Appendix, p. 528). (2) Usually administered in the hospital by or under the direction of the physician specialist. (3) Must be refrigerated before and after dilution. Potency maintained for 5 days after dilution. (4) Do not use if a precipitate is present. (5) Daily blood cell counts are necessary during initial treatment and weekly thereafter until 3 weeks after therapy is discontinued. Very toxic to hematopoietic system. (6) Dosage based on average weight in presence of edema or ascites. (7) Use caution in leukopenia, thrombocytopenia, recent radiation therapy, and infection. (8) May cause irreversible bone damage with other neoplastic drugs. (9) Will produce teratogenic effects on the fetus. Has a mutagenic potential and must be given with caution to men and women capable of conception. (10) Potentiates antiacoagulants and nondepolarizing muscle relaxants (tubocurarine [Curare], etc.). (11) Be alert for signs of bone marrow depression or infection. (12) Do not administer any vaccines or chloroquine to patients receiving antineoplastic drugs. (13) Local anesthetic at injection site may reduce pain during administration. (14) Used in combination with urokinase to treat bladder cancer. (15) Allopurinol may prevent formation of uric acid crystals. (16) Prophylactic antiemetics may increase patient comfort.

Contraindications: Hepatic, renal, or bone marrow damage unless need is greater than the risk; known hypersensitivity to triethylenethiophosphoramide.

Incompatible with: Sufficient information not available. Consider incompatible in syringe or solution with any other drug.

Side effects: *Minor:* amenorrhea, anorexia, dizziness, fever, headache, hives, hyperuricemia, nausea, pain at injection site, skin rash, throat tightness, vomiting. *Major:* anaphylaxis, bone marrow depression, hemorrhage, intestinal perforation, leukopenia, septicemia, thrombocytopenia.

Antidote: Minor side effects will be treated symptomatically if necessary. Discontinue the drug and notify the physician of major side effects. Treat allergic reaction as indicated.

TRIFLUPROMAZINE HYDROCHLORIDE

(Vesprin)

Usual dose: 1 to 3 mg. May be repeated in 4 hours. Repeat one fourth of initial dose as needed.

Dilution: Each 10 mg should be diluted with 9 ml of normal saline for injection. 1 ml of diluted solution will equal 1 mg.

Rate of administration: Each 8 mg or fraction thereof over 1 minute.

Actions: A phenothiazine derivative, said to be twice as potent as chlorpromazine (Thorazine). Primarily an antianxiety agent, it has effects on the central, autonomic, and peripheral nervous systems. Decreases anxiety and tension, relaxes muscle, produces sedation, and tranquilizes. A potent antiemetic. Onset of action is prompt and lasting. Excretion is slow through the kidneys.

Indications and uses: (1) Tranquilizer, preoperatively, postoperatively, and in obstetrics; (2) nausea and vomiting, especially after encephalograms, ventriculograms, and antineoplastic drugs.

Precautions: (1) Monitor blood pressure and pulse before administration and between doses. Keep patient in supine position. (2) Sensitive to light. Slightly yellow color does not affect potency. Discard if markedly discolored. (3) May mask diagnosis of brain tumor, drug intoxication, and intestinal obstruction. Use caution in coronary disease, severe hypertension or hypotension, and epilepsy. (4) May discolor urine pink to reddish brown. (5) Photosensitivity of skin is possible. (6) Reduce narcotic dosage by one half because of potentiation. Also potentiates other CNS depressants such as alcohol, anesthetics, barbiturates, MAO inhibitors (pargyline [Eutonyl], etc.), oral antidiabetics, insulin, anticholinergics, antihypertensives, hypnotics, muscle relaxants, and rauwolfia alkaloids. (7) Contraindicated with quinidine, epinephrine, and thiazide diuretics. (8) Capable of innumerable other interactions. (9) IV route not recommended for children. (10) Handle carefully; may cause contact dermatitis.

495

Contraindications: Known hypersensitivity to phenothiazines or other centrally acting drugs; subcortical brain damage (even if only suspected).

Incompatible with: Ascorbic acid, chlorothiazide (Diuril), levallorphan (Lorphan), pentobarbital (Nembutal), posterior pituitary extract. Incompatibilities listed under prochlorperazine should also be considered.

Side effects: Considered less toxic than prochlorperazine. Side effects are usually transient if drug is discontinued: allergic reactions (rare), agranulocytosis (rare), hypotension (usually transient), leukopenia (rare). All side effects of phenothiazines could occur, but rarely do. Extrapyramidal symptoms have not been reported. For additional possible side effects, see prochlorperazine (Compazine).

Antidote: Discontinue the drug at onset of any side effect and notify the physician. Counteract hypotension with dopamine (Intropin) and allergic reactions with antihistamines. Epinephrine is contraindicated for hypotension. Further hypotension will occur. In treating respiratory depression and unconsciousness, avoid analeptics such as doxapram (Dopram); they may cause convulsions. Resuscitate as necessary.

TRIMETHAPHAN CAMSYLATE

pH 4.9 to 5.6

(Arfonad)

Usual dose: 1 to 4 mg/min.

Pediatric dose: 100 μg (0.1 mg)/min.

Dilution: Each 500 mg (10 ml) or fraction thereof must be diluted in at least 500 ml of 5% dextrose in water and given as an IV infusion. In 500 ml, 1 mg equals 1 ml.

Rate of administration: Correct dose/minute of properly diluted solution as indicated to maintain blood pressure at the desired level. Use of an infusion pump or microdrip (60 gtt/ml) is indicated.

Actions: A ganglionic blocking agent and a potent vasodilator. Does not alter membrane potential. Liberates histamine. Will lower blood pressure in normotensive as well as hypertensive individuals. It has an extremely short duration of action. Blood pressure may return to normal within 5 to 10 minutes after trimethaphan is discontinued. Excreted by the kidneys.

Indications and uses: (1) Induce and maintain controlled hypotensive state in neurosurgery and vascular surgery, (2) hypertensive crises, (3) pulmonary edema secondary to hypertension, (4) cardiogenic shock, (5) dissecting aortic aneurysm.

Precautions: (1) Should be administered by or under the direction of the anesthesiologist. (2) Must be refrigerated. Prepare solution just prior to use, and discard any remaining portion after 24 hours. (3) Keep patient in supine position to prevent cerebral anoxia. (4) Check blood pressure every 2 minutes until stabilized at desired level. Check every 5 minutes thereafter until the drug is discontinued. (5) Adequate oxygenation and ventilation must be maintained continuously. Use artificial means if necessary. (6) Use caution in the elderly, debilitated, children, allergic individuals, and in immediate postoperative period. (7) Potentiated by antihypertensives, anesthetics (local or regional), alcohol, and thiazide diuretics. Reduced dosage of both drugs may be required to prevent additive hypotensive effect. (8) Potentiates succinylcholine (Anectine)

497

and nondepolarizing muscle relaxants (tubocurarine [Curare], etc.), prolonged apnea may result. (9) Pupillary dilation may occur with trimethaphan.

Contraindications: Anemia, blood replacement not practical, coronary or cerebrovascular insufficiency, hypovolemia, IV fluids not immediately available, MAO inhibitors in drug regime within previous 3 weeks, pregnancy, respiratory insufficiency, shock.

Incompatible with: Any other drug in syringe, solution, or infusion tubing.

Side effects: Blurring of vision, cerebral ischemia, dryness of mouth, ileus, lowering of central venous pressure, postural hypotension, respiratory depression, severe hypotension, tachycardia, urinary retention.

Antidote: Notify the physician of all side effects and discontinue the drug if indicated. Reduced central venous pressure may be a desirable effect, as in left ventricular failure. Vasopressors phenylephrine (Neo-Synephrine) or mephentermine (Wyamine) may be used to treat overdose. If ineffective, use levarterenol (Levophed). Resuscitate as necessary.

TROMETHAMINE

(Tham)

Usual dose: *Acidosis:* Required dose (ml of 0.3 M solution) equal to body weight in kilograms × base deficit in mEq/L × 1.1.

Acidosis in cardiac bypass surgery: 9 ml/kg of body weight, 500 ml is an average adult dose. Up to 1,000 ml has been used.

Acidity of ACD priming blood: Average of 60 ml to each 500 ml of stored blood is adequate. Varies from 15 to 77 ml to correct average pH of stored blood (6.80 to 6.22).

Acidosis in cardiac arrest: Initial dose of 3.5 to 6.0 ml/kg. Additional doses should be based on evaluation of base deficit.

Dilution: May be given undiluted as an infusion or added to pump oxygenator blood, other priming fluid, or ACD blood.

Rate of administration: Slow IV infusion recommended. 5 ml or less/min would deliver up to 300 ml in 1 hour. Rate dictated by patient's condition and intended use (see precautions).

Actions: Acts as a proton acceptor and actively binds hydrogen ions in metabolic acids and carbonic acid. Releases bicarbonate anions. Rapidly excreted in the urine, it has an osmotic diuretic effect, increases urine output, urine pH, and excretion of fixed acids, carbon dioxide, and electrolytes. Also capable of neutralizing acidic ions of the intracellular fluid.

Indications and uses: Prevention and correction of systemic acidosis.

Precautions: (1) Determine blood pH, Pco_2, bicarbonate, glucose, and electrolytes before, during, and after administration. (2) Avoid overdosage (total drug or too-rapid rate). Severe alkalosis and/or prolonged hypoglycemia may result. (3) Determine absolute patency of vein; necrosis may result from extravasation. (4) Reduced rate may control venospasm. (5) May severely depress respiration; oxygen and controlled respiratory equipment must always be available. (6) Use extreme caution in impaired renal function or decreased urine output. EKG monitoring and frequent serum potassium measurements are required. (7) Intended for short-term use only (1 day). (8) Severe hypoglycemia may occur in premature or full-term infants. (9) Sodium bicarbonate or sodium lactate is effective in most acidotic situations and has fewer side effects. (10) Potentiates amphetamines, ephedrine, and quinidine. (11) Inhibits lithium, methotrexate, and salicylates.

Contraindications: Hypersensitivity to tromethamine, anuria, and uremia. Pregnancy is a probable contraindication.

Incompatible with: Sufficient information not available. Should be administered alone due to specific use and potential side effects.

Side effects: Hypoglycemia, hyperkalemia, respiratory depression.

Antidote: Notify physician of all side effects. Reduced rate of infusion may prevent hypoglycemia. Use glucose if indicated. Discontinue drug immediately for hyperkalemia or extravasation. Local infiltration with 1% procaine with hyaluronidase or phentolamine may reduce tissue necrosis. Use a No. 25 needle. Symptomatic treatment is indicated. Alternate drugs are indicated (sodium bicarbonate, sodium lactate).

TRIMETHOPRIM-
SULFAMETHOXAZOLE pH 10.0

(Bactrim, Co-trimoxazole, Septra)

Usual dose: *Severe urinary tract infections and shigellosis:*
8 to 10 mg/kg of body weight in equally divided doses
every 6, 8, or 12 hours for 14 days (urinary tract infections) or 5 days (shigellosis).

Pneumocystis carinii pneumonitis: 15 to 20 mg/kg in
equally divided doses every 6 or 8 hours for up to 14
days.

Prophylaxis in neutropenic patients: 800 mg of sulfamethoxazole with 160 mg of trimethoprim (10 ml before appropriate dilution) every 12 hours.

Normal renal function is required for usual dose.

Dilution: Each 5 ml ampoule must be diluted in 125 ml
of 5% dextrose in water and given as an infusion. Reduce diluent to 75 ml for each ampoule only if fluid
restriction is required. Standard dilution must be
used within 6 hours; fluid-restriction dilution must be
used within 2 hours. Discard if cloudiness or crystallization is present.

Rate of administration: A single dose must be infused
over 60 to 90 minutes.

Actions: A broad-spectrum antibacterial and antiproto-
zoal combination agent with bacteriostatic action
that is effective against gram-positive and gram-negative organisms. Prevents formation of folic acid and
reduction of folates essential to organism growth.
Combination contains 400 mg sulfamethoxazole and
80 mg trimethoprim/5 ml. Effective ratio of sulfamethoxazole to trimethoprim is 20 to 1. Widely distributed in all body fluids and tissues including cerebral spinal fluid, sputum, and bile. Crosses placental
barrier. Onset of action is prompt, and serum levels
are maintained up to 10 hours. Metabolized in the
liver, and up to 60% is excreted in urine in 24 hours.
Excreted in breast milk.

Indications and uses: (1) Severe urinary tract infections,
(2) pneumocystis carinii pneumonitis, (3) shigellosis,
(4) prophylaxis in neutropenic patients.

Precaution: (1) Avoid rapid infusion or bolus injection. (2) Sensitivity studies are indicated to determine the susceptibility of the causative organism to trimethoprim-sulfamethoxazole. (3) Stable at room temperature; do not refrigerate. (4) Maintain adequate hydration to prevent crystalluria and stone formation. (5) CBC is required before and during therapy. Discontinue for any significant reduction in a blood-forming element. Urinalysis and renal function tests are also indicated. (6) Reduce dose by one half for creatinine clearance between 15 and 30 ml/min. (7) If extravasation occurs, discontinue and restart at a new site. May cause phlebitis. (8) Not for IM use. (9) Use caution in impaired liver or renal function, possible folate deficiency, allergic individuals, bronchial asthma, porphyria, and glucose-6-phosphate dehydrogenase (G-6PD) deficiency. (10) A sulfonamide drug; allergic reactions can occur. Use caution in patients hypersensitive to furosemide (Lasix), thiazide diuretics (chlorothiazide, etc.), sulfonylureas (tolbutamide, etc.), or carbonic anhydrase inhibitors (acetazolamide, etc.). (11) Potentiated by probenecid; sulfinpyrazone toxicity may result. (12) Will inhibit bactericidal action of penicillins and renal excretion of methotrexate. (13) Concurrent use with methenamine (Urised, etc.) may increase incidence of crystalluria and is not recommended. (14) May potentiate warfarin (Coumadin), phenytoin (Dilantin), oral hypoglycemics, and phenylbutazone (Butazolidin, etc.). (15) Inhibited by aminobenzoic acid (PABA), alkalinizing agents, thiopental (Pentothal).

Contraindications: Infants less than 2 months of age (may cause kernicterus); creatinine clearance below 15 ml/minute; hypersensitivity to trimethoprim or sulfonamides; megaloblastic anemia due to folate deficiency; pregnancy and lactation; streptococcal pharyngitis.

Incompatible with: Do not mix in syringe or solution with any other drug (manufacturer's directive).

Side effects: All side effects of sulfonamides including allergic reaction are possible. Nausea, vomiting, and rash occur most frequently. Ataxia, convulsions, tremors, and respiratory depression are symptoms of major toxicity. With high doses or administration over an extended time, bone marrow depression (leukopenia, megaloblastic anemia, and thrombocytopenia) may occur.

Antidote: Notify the physician of any side effect. Discontinue the drug if any sign of major toxicity or bone marrow depression occurs. Treat bone marrow depression with leucovorin 3 to 6 mg IM daily for 3 days or until normal hematopoiesis occurs. Peritoneal dialysis is not effective in toxicity; hemodialysis may be moderately effective in reducing serum levels. Treat anaphylaxis with epinephrine, corticosteroids, antihistamines, and vasopressors as indicated.

TUBOCURARINE CHLORIDE

(Curare)

Usual dose: *Aid to controlled respiration:* 16.5 μg (0.0165 mg)/kg of body weight. Adjust as needed.

Muscle contraction or convulsions: 0.15 mg (1 unit)/kg minus 3 mg (20 units). May repeat as necessary.

Diagnosis of myasthenia gravis: 4 to 33 μg (0.004 to 0.033 mg)/kg.

Dilution: May be given undiluted in 3 mg/ml concentration.

Myasthenia testing: dilute single dose to 4 ml with sterile normal saline for injection.

Rate of administration: A single dose over 60 to 90 seconds. Too-rapid injection will cause symptoms of overdose and histamine release resulting in severe bronchospasm and profound hypotension.

Myasthenia testing: 0.5 ml diluted medication over 2 minutes.

Actions: A short-acting skeletal muscle relaxant. Causes paralysis by interfering with neural transmission at the myoneural junction. Onset of action is within 2 or 3 minutes and lasts about 20 minutes. Complete recovery from a single dose may take another 30 minutes. Metabolized in the liver and excreted in the urine. May cause fetal malformation.

Indications and uses: (1) Muscle relaxation in severe muscle contraction or convulsion caused by disease, drugs, or electrical stimulation; (2) diagnosis of myasthenia gravis if other tests inconclusive; (3) facilitate management of patients undergoing mechanical ventilation; (4) adjunctive to general anesthesia.

Precautions: (1) Administered by or under the direction of the anesthesiologist. (2) This drug produces apnea. Controlled artificial ventilation with oxygen must be continuous and under direct observation at all times. Maintain a patent airway. (3) Repeated doses may produce cumulative effect. (4) Impaired pulmonary function or respiratory deficiencies can cause critical reactions. Use caution in impaired liver or kidney function. (5) Myasthenia gravis increases sensitivity to drug. Terminate testing process within 2 to 3 minutes with 1.5 mg of neostigmine to avoid prolonged respiratory paralysis. (6) Use only clear solutions. Faint discoloration is acceptable. (7) Potentiated by inhalant anesthetics (ether, etc.), neuromuscular blocking antibiotics (kanamycin [Kantrex], etc.), carbon dioxide, digitalis, diuretics, diazepam (Valium), and other muscle relaxants, lidocaine, MAO inhibitors, propranolol (Inderal), quinidine, and others. Markedly reduced dose of tubocurarine must be used with caution. (8) Hyperkalemia may cause cardiac arrhythmias. (9) Patient may be conscious and completely unable to communicate by any means. Tubocurarine has no analgesic properties. (10) Use of a peripheral nerve stimulator is recommended to monitor effectiveness of this drug.

Contraindications: Known sensitivity, patients in whom histamine release is definite hazard.

Incompatible with: Consider incompatible in a syringe with any other drug. Evaluation of predictable results imperative. All barbiturates.

Side effects: Airway closure caused by relaxation of epiglottis, pharynx, and tongue muscles. Allergic reactions including anaphylaxis, histamine release, profound hypotension, respiratory deficiency, respiratory failure, severe bronchospasm, and shock may occur.

Antidote: All side effects are medical emergencies. Treat symptomatically. Controlled artificial ventilation must be continuous. Edrophonium or neostigmine methylsulfate with atropine may help to reverse muscle relaxation. Not effective in all situations. Treat allergic reactions and resuscitate as necessary.

(Ureaphil, Urevert)

Usual dose: 1 to 1.5 Gm/kg of body weight. Highly individualized according to clinical condition of the patient. Do not exceed total dose of 120 Gm/24 hr. A 30% solution in 1 liter equals approximately 5,250 mOsm/L.

Pediatric dose: 0.5 Gm/kg of body weight.

Infant dose: Under 2 years: 0.1 Gm/kg of body weight may be sufficient.

Dilution: Must be diluted to a 30% solution (30 Gm/100 ml diluent) with 5% or 10% dextrose for infusion or 10% invert sugar in water. Diluent provided by some manufacturers.

30% solution: add 105 ml of recommended diluent to 40 Gm of urea. Total volume equals 135 ml (300 mg/ml).

4% solution: dilute 40 Gm of urea with 1 liter of recommended solution (40 mg/ml).

Rate of administration: 100 ml of a 30% solution is usually given over 1 or 2 hours. Do not exceed infusion rate of 1,200 mg/min (60 gtt or 4 ml of a 30% solution).

Actions: Normal degradation product of amino acids. Hypertonic urea increases blood tonicity. A greater urea concentration in the blood absorbs fluid from extravascular tissue, brain, and intraocular and cerebrospinal fluid into the blood. Effective within 15 minutes, peaks in 1 to 2 hours, and lasts 3 to 10 hours. Rebound may occur within 12 hours. Increased urea in the glomerular filtrate inhibits reabsorption of water.

Indications and uses: Reduction of intracranial pressure, cerebrospinal fluid pressure, and intraocular pressure.

Precautions: (1) Mannitol is usually the preferred drug when an osmotic diuretic is desired. (2) Use only freshly prepared solutions, discard unused portion. (3) Determine absolute patency of vein; extravasation may cause necrosis. (4) Observe infusion site; chemical phlebitis and thrombosis do occur. (5) Frequent electrolyte panels and kidney function tests necessary. Observe for early signs of hypokalemia and hyponatremia. (6) Observe urine output continuously, insert Foley catheter if necessary. (7) Use caution in pregnancy, lactation, childbearing years, and liver impairment. (8) Do not administer through same infusion set with blood. (9) Observe for reactivation of intracranial bleeding. (10) May mask symptoms of excessive blood loss. Blood replacement should be adequate. (11) Concomitant use of hypothermia increases risk of venous thrombosis and hemoglobinuria.

Contraindications: Impaired renal function (severe), active intracranial bleeding, marked dehydration, liver failure, edema of cardiac failure, lower extremity infusion in the elderly.

Incompatible with: Alkaline solutions, whole blood. Additional information not available. Should be considered incompatible in syringe or solution with any other drug because of specific indication for administration.

Side effects: Disorientation, headache, hypokalemia, hyponatremia, nausea, syncope, thrombophlebitis, vomiting.

Antidote: Notify the physician of all side effects. Treatment will probably be symptomatic. Resuscitate as necessary.

UROKINASE

(Abbokinase, Breokinase)

Usual dose: *Pulmonary embolism:* 4,400 IU/kg of body weight is given as an initial priming dose over 10 minutes. Follow by a continuous infusion of 4,400 IU/kg/hr for 12 hours. Total volume of infusion must not exceed 200 ml. Follow entire procedure with a flush of normal saline or 5% dextrose for infusion. Use a volume equal to the volume of the catheter. Keep line open with this solution at 15 ml/hr.

IV catheter clearance: 5,000 IU (1 ml of specifically diluted solution). More or less can be used. Amount should be equal to the volume of the catheter.

Dilution: Each vial (250,000 IU) must be diluted with 5.2 ml of sterile water for injection without preservatives. *For IV infusion,* each dose must be further diluted with sufficient normal saline to administer a total infusion of 195 ml. *For IV catheter clearance,* add 1 ml of the initially reconstituted drug to 9 ml of sterile water for injection without preservatives (1 ml equals 5,000 IU). Prepare immediately before using and discard any solution remaining in vial after dose removed.

Rate of administration: Initial priming dose is delivered equally distributed over 10 minutes. Follow with continuous infusion of calculated total dose over 12 hours. Use of an infusion pump capable of administering the total volume (195 ml) over 12 hours is required. Keep vein open (see usual dose).

IV catheter clearance: Confirm occlusion by gently attempting to aspirate blood with a 10 ml syringe. Slowly and gently inject specifically diluted and premeasured amount of urokinase into the catheter (usually 1 ml in a tuberculin syringe). Connect a 5 ml syringe to the catheter and wait 5 minutes. Gently aspirate to remove clot. Repeat aspiration every 5 minutes until clot clears or 30 minutes. If unsuccessful, cap catheter for 30 to 60 minutes and attempt to aspirate again. If still unsuccessful, a second dose of urokinase may be required. Maintain absolute sterility of IV system in all situations.

Actions: An enzyme obtained from human kidney cells by tissue culturing techniques. It converts plasminogen to plasmin, which degrades fibrin clots, fibrinogen, and other plasma proteins. This activation takes place within a thrombus as well as on the surface. Onset of action is prompt and may last up to 12 hours. End products of this activity possess an anticoagulant effect. Bleeding may be very difficult to control.

Indications and uses: (1) Lysis of acute massive pulmonary emboli of two or more lobes are involved or if hemodynamics are unstable, (2) restore patency of IV catheters occluded by clotted blood or fibrin (includes central venous catheters).

Precautions: (1) Administered only in the hospital under the direction of a physician knowledgeable in its use and with appropriate diagnostic and laboratory facilities available. Observe patient continuously. Monitor hematocrit, platelet count, activated partial thromboplastin time, thrombin time, and prothrombin time before therapy. In 4 hours and during therapy thrombin time or prothrombin time changes are monitored and will reflect effectiveness of treatment. Keep physician informed. Request specific parameters for notifying physician after initial supervised injection. (2) Diagnosis of pulmonary or other emboli should be confirmed. (3) Best results obtained if started within 7 days of onset of emboli. (4) A greater alteration of hemostatic status than with heparin; use care in handling patient, avoid arterial puncture, venipuncture, and IM injection. Use extreme precautionary methods (use of radial artery—not femoral; extended pressure application of up to 30 minutes) if above procedures are absolutely necessary. (5) Use caution in presence of atrial fibrillation. (6) Simultaneous use of anticoagulants is not recommended. Do not use either drug until the effects of the previous drug are diminished. Intensive follow-up therapy with heparin is indicated. Prothrombin time should be reduced to less than twice the normal control value before heparin therapy begins. (7) Avoid use of drugs that may alter platelet function (aspirin, indomethacin, phenylbutazone, etc.). (8) Do not take blood pressure in lower extremities; thrombi may be dislodged. (9) Urokinase has less potential for allergic reaction than streptokinase and is indicated if repeated therapy necessary. (10) Avoid force while attempting to clear catheters; may rupture catheter or dislodge clot into the circulation. (11) Will not dissolve drug precipitate or anything other than blood products. Use caution so as not to dislodge foreign bodies into the circulatory system. (12) Use extreme caution in the following situations: any surgical procedure, biopsy, lumbar puncture, thoracentesis, paracentesis, multiple cutdowns, or intraarterial diagnostic procedures within 10 days, ulcerative wounds, recent trauma with possible internal injury, visceral or intracranial malignancy, pregnancy and first 10 days postpartum, any lesion of gastrointestinal or genitourinary tract with a potential for bleeding (diverticulitis, ulcerative colitis), severe hypertension, acute or chronic hepatic or renal insufficiency, uncontrolled hypocoagulable state, chronic lung disease with cavitation, subacute bacterial endocarditis, rheumatic valvular disease, recent cerebral embolism, and any condition where bleeding might be hazardous or difficult to manage because of location.

Contraindications: Active internal bleeding, cerebral vascular accident within 2 months, intracranial or intraspinal surgery, intracranial neoplasm, hypersensitivity to urokinase.

Incompatible with: Specific information not available. Should be considered incompatible in solution due to specific use and hazards of use.

Side effects: Mild allergic reactions (bronchospasm, skin rash); bleeding can be life threatening.

Antidote: Notify physician of all side effects. Note even the minutest bleeding tendency. Therapy may have to be discontinued with serious bleeding and/or blood loss. Whole blood, packed red blood cells, cryoprecipitate, fresh frozen plasma, and aminocaproic acid may all be indicated. Treat minor allergic reactions symptomatically. Discontinue drug and treat anaphylaxis as indicated, resuscitate as necessary.

VANCOMYCIN HYDROCHLORIDE   pH 2.4 to 4.5
(Vancocin)

Usual dose: 500 mg every 6 hours. Maximum dosage of 3 to 4 Gm/24 hr used only in extreme situations. Normal renal function is required.

Pediatric dose: 40 mg/kg of body weight/24 hr divided into four equal doses.

Dilution: Each 500 mg is initially diluted with 10 ml of sterile water for injection. Must be further diluted with 100 to 200 ml of normal saline or 5% dextrose in water and given as an intermittent infusion. If absolutely necessary, 1 to 2 Gm may be further diluted in sufficient amounts of the same infusion fluids and given over 24 hours. Not recommended.

Rate of administration: Each 500 mg or fraction thereof, properly diluted, over 30 minutes. Preferred route of administration because of high incidence of thrombophlebitis.

Actions: A very potent antibiotic, it is bacterial against gram-positive cocci. Use limited because of ototoxic and nephrotoxic side effects. Well distributed in all body tissues and fluids including spinal fluid if the meninges are inflamed. Vancomycin is excreted in biologically active form in the urine.

Indications and uses: (1) Life-threatening gram-positive infections that do not respond or are resistant to other less toxic antibiotics, such as penicillins or cephalosporins; (2) to substitute for contraindicated penicillin therapy if absolutely necessary.

Precautions: (1) Store in refrigerator after initial dilution. Maintains potency for 2 weeks. (2) Sensitivity studies are necessary to determine the susceptibility of the causative organism to vancomycin. (3) Prolonged use of drug may result in superinfection caused by overgrowth of nonsusceptible organisms. (4) Ototoxic and nephrotoxic. Use extreme caution in impaired hearing, impaired renal function, and the elderly. (5) Blood levels of vancomycin, auditory testing, and renal function tests are necessary when this drug is used. (6) Determine absolute patency of vein. Necrosis and sloughing will result from extravasation. Rotate injection sites every 2 to 3 days. (7) Use caution with dimenhydrinate (Dramamine), which can mask ototoxicity. Other neuromuscular blocking antibiotics (kanamycin [Kantrex], etc.) and ototoxic drugs (ethacrynic acid [Edecrin], etc.) may potentiate vancomycin. (8) Observe for furry tongue, diarrhea, and foul-smelling stools.

Contraindications: Known hypersensitivity to vancomycin.

Incompatible with: Aminophylline, amobarbital (Amytal), chloramphenicol (Cloromycetin), chlorothiazide (Diuril), dexamethasone (Decadron), heparin, hydrocortisone sodium succinate (Solu-Cortef), methicillin (Staphcillin), nitrofurantoin (Ivadantin), penicillins, pentobarbital (Nembutal), phenobarbital (Luminal), phenytoin (Dilantin), prochlorperazine (Compazine), secobarbital (Seconal), sodium bicarbonate, sulfisoxazole (Gantrisin), vitamin B complex with C, warfarin (Coumadin).

Side effects: *Minor:* chills, fever, macular rashes, nausea, pain at injection site, tinnitus, urticaria. *Major:* anaphylaxis, eosinophilia, hearing loss, thrombophlebitis.

Antidote: Notify the physician of all side effects. Hearing loss may progress even if drug is discontinued. If minor side effects are progressive or any major side effect occurs, discontinue the drug, treat allergic reaction, or resuscitate as necessary.

VERAPAMIL HYDROCHLORIDE pH 4.1 to 6.0

(Calan, Isoptin)

Usual dose: 5 to 10 mg initially. 10 mg may be repeated in 30 minutes if needed to achieve appropriate response.

Pediatric dose: *Infants up to 1 year of age:* 0.1 to 0.2 mg/kg of body weight (usually 0.75 to 2 mg). Repeat in 30 minutes if indicated.

1 to 15 years of age: 0.1 to 0.3 mg/kg (usually 2 to 5 mg). Repeat in 30 minutes if indicated. Do not exceed 5 mg.

Dilution: May be given undiluted through Y tube or three-way stopcock of tubing containing dextrose 5%, sodium chloride 0.9%, or Ringer's solution for infusion.

Rate of administration: A single dose over 2 minutes for adults and children. Extend to 3 minutes in the elderly.

Actions: A calcium (and possibly sodium) ion inhibitor through slow channels. Slows conduction through SA and AV nodes, prolongs effective refractory period in the AV node, and reduces ventricular rates. Prevents reentry phenomena through the AV node. Reduces myocardial contractility, afterload, arterial pressure, vascular tone, and oxygen demand. Effective within 1 to 5 minutes. Hemodynamic effects last about 20 minutes, but antiarrhythmic effects last up to 6 hours. Does not alter total serum calcium levels. Metabolized in the liver. Excreted in urine and feces.

Indications and uses: Treatment of supraventricular tachyarrhythmias including conversion to normal sinus rhythm of paroxysmal supraventricular tachycardia (includes Wolff-Parkinson-White and Lown-Ganong-Levine syndromes) and temporary control of rapid ventricular rate in atrial flutter or atrial fibrillation.

Precautions: (1) EKG monitoring during administration is mandatory for infants and children, recommended for all others. Monitor blood pressure very closely. (2) Protect vials from light. Do not use if discolored or particulate matter present. (3) Valsalva maneuver is recommended prior to use of verapamil in all paroxysmal supraventricular tachycardias if clinically appropriate. (4) Emergency resuscitation drugs and equipment must always be available. (5) Treat heart failure with digitalis and diuretics before using verapamil. (6) Pulmonary wedge pressure above 20 mm Hg and/or ejection fraction below 20% indicates acute heart failure. (7) Monitor for side effects (AV block) and digoxin levels when used concurrently with digitalis products. Potentiates digoxin; lower dose may be appropriate. (8) Use extreme caution with oral or IV beta adrenergic blocking drugs (propranolol [Inderal], etc.) (see contraindications). Both drugs depress myocardial contractility and AV node conduction. (9) Do not administer disopyramide (Norpace) within 48 hours before or 24 hours after verapamil. (10) Caution is required in hepatic and renal disease, especially if repeated dosage is required. (11) Safety for use in pregnancy and lactation not yet established. (12) May cause excessive hypotension with other antihypertensive drugs (vasodilators and diuretics). (13) May inhibit other highly protein bound drugs (oral hypoglycemics, warfarin, etc.). Use caution.

Contraindications: Cardiogenic shock; congestive heart failure (severe) unless secondary to supraventricular tachyarrhythmia treatable with verapramil; second- or third-degree AV block; severe hypotension; sick sinus syndrome (unless functioning artificial pacemaker is in place); patients receiving IV beta adrenergic blocking drugs (propranolol [Inderal]) within 2 to 4 hours.

Incompatible with: Limited information available. No specific incompatibilities documented as yet.

Side effects: Abdominal discomfort; allergic reactions including anaphylaxis; asystole; bradycardia; dizziness; headache; heart failure; hypotension (symptomatic); increased ventricular response in atrial flutter; fibrillation (Wolff-Parkinson-White and Lown-Ganong-Levine syndromes); nausea; premature ventricular contractions; tachycardia.

Antidote: Notify physician of all side effects. Calcium chloride may reverse effects of verapamil and can be used in toxicity. Rapid ventricular response in atrial flutter/fibrillation should respond to cardioversion, procainamide and/or lidocaine. Treat bradycardia, AV block, and asystole with standard AHA protocol (atropine, isoproterenol, pacing). Levarterenol or dopamine will reverse hypotension. Treat allergic reactions or resuscitate as necessary.

VIDARABINE

(Vira-A)

Usual dose: 15 mg/kg of body weight/day for 10 days.

Dilution: Each 1 mg of vidarabine requires 2.22 ml of infusion solution to dissolve. (450 mg requires a minimum of 1 liter of fluid.) May be diluted with most intravenous solutions except biological and colloidal fluids (blood products, protein solution). Aseptic technique imperative. Shake vidarabine well before measuring dose. Warm diluent to 35° to 40° C (95° to 100° F) to facilitate solution. Thoroughly agitate diluted solution until completely clear by visual inspection. When completely clear and in solution, no further agitation is necessary.

Rate of administration: Total daily dose must be infused over 12 to 24 hours at a constant rate. Use of an infusion pump is recommended to avoid accidental overdose.

Actions: An antiviral drug obtained from fermentation cultures of *Streptomyces antibioticus*. Rapidly changed to Ara-Hx, a metabolite, and distributed in the tissues. Plasma and tissue levels are maintained by slow intravenous infusion. Excreted in the urine.

Indications and uses: Specific for treatment of herpes simplex virus encephalitis.

Precautions: (1) Confirm diagnosis by cell culture from a brain biopsy. (2) Not effective in altering morbidity in comatose patient; early diagnosis essential. (3) For IV infusion only. Avoid rapid or bolus injection. (4) Will produce teratogenic effects on the fetus. (5) Reduce dose if renal function is impaired. (6) Use caution in cerebral edema or potential fluid overload. (7) Monitor blood counts frequently during therapy. (8) Probably ineffective in the immunosuppressed patient. (9) Use of an in-line filter (0.45 μm) is required. (10) Use only freshly prepared solution; stable at room temperature 48 hours. (11) Inhibited by allopurinol.

Contraindications: Vidarabine sensitivity.

Incompatible with: Specific information not available. Do not mix with any other drug due to specific use.

Side effects: Anorexia; ataxia; confusion; decreased hematocrit, hemoglobin, white blood cells, and platelets; diarrhea; dizziness; fluid overload; hallucinations; hematemesis; malaise; nausea; pain at injection site; pruritus; rash; vomiting; weight loss.

Antidote: Notify physician of all side effects. In acute overdose monitor hematological, renal, and hepatic functions carefully. Doses over 20 mg/kg of body weight/24 hr can produce bone marrow depression. Treat allergic reaction as indicated and resuscitate as necessary.

VINBLASTINE SULFATE

pH 3.5 to 5.0

(Velban, VLB)

Usual dose: 3.7 mg/M² initially. Administered once every 7 days, increasing the dose to specific amounts (5.5, 7.4, 9.25, 11.1 mg/M²), a single step each week until the WBC is decreased to 3,000 cells/ml, remission is achieved, or a maximum dose of 18.5 mg/M² is reached. Maintenance dose is one step below any dose that causes leukopenia (3,000 cells/ml or less), once every 7 to 14 days. Usually 5.5 to 7.4 mg/M².

Pediatric dose: 2.5 mg/M² initially. Use same procedure as for adult dose using steps to 3.75, 5.0, 6.25, and 7.5 mg/M². Maintenance dose is calculated by same parameters as adult dose. Usual differs with each individual.

Dilution: *Specific techniques required, see precautions.* Each 10 mg is diluted with 10 ml of sodium chloride for injection. 1 mg equals 1 ml. Do not add to IV solutions. May be given direct IV or through Y tube or three-way stopcock of a free-flowing IV infusion.

Rate of administration: Total desired dose, properly diluted, over 1 minute.

Actions: An alkaloid of the periwinkle plant with antitumor activity. Cell cycle specific for M phase. Thought to interfere with the metabolic pathways of amino acids. Sometimes pharmacologically effective without any noticeable improvement in symptoms of malignancy. Cell energy production and synthesis of nucleic acid may also be inhibited.

Indications and uses: To suppress or retard neoplastic growth. Remission and probable cure has been achieved with bleomycin and cisplatin in testicular malignancies. Response has been noted in Hodgkin's disease, non-Hodgkin's lymphomas, breast and renal cell malignancies.

Precautions: (1) Follow guidelines for handling cytotoxic agents recommended by the National Study Commission on Cytotoxic Exposure (see Appendix, p. 528). (2) Usually administered in the hospital by or under the direction of the physician specialist. (3) Store in refrigerator before and after dilution. Potency maintained for 30 days after dilution. (4) Determine absolute patency and quality of vein and adequate circulation of extremity. Severe cellulitis may result from extravasation. Rinse syringe and needle with venous blood before withdrawal from the vein. (5) May cause corneal ulceration with accidental contact to the eye. (6) WBC must be checked before each dose. Must be above 4,000 cells/ml. (7) Sometimes used with corticosteroids and other antineoplastic drugs in reduced doses to achieve tumor remission. (8) Dosage based on average weight in presence of edema or ascites. (9) May produce teratogenic effects on the fetus. Has a mutagenic potential and must be given with caution in men and women capable of conception. (10) Inhibited by some amino acids, glutamic acid, and tryptophan. (11) Potentiates anticoagulants. (12) Potentiated by other antineoplastics. (13) Be alert for signs of bone marrow depression or infection. (14) Do not administer any vaccines or chloroquine to patients receiving antineoplastic drugs. (15) Use caution in presence of ulcerated skin areas or impaired liver function. (16) Allopurinol may prevent formation of uric acid crystals. (17) Maintain adequate hydration. (18) Prophylactic antiemetics may increase patient comfort.

Contraindications: Bacterial infection or leukopenia below 3,000 cells/ml.

Incompatible with: Specific information not available. Note precautions.

Side effects: Not always reversible: abdominal pain, alopecia, anorexia, cellulitis, constipation, convulsions, diarrhea, dizziness, extravasation, gonadal suppression, headache, hemorrhage, ileus, leukopenia (severe), malaise, mental depression, myelosuppression, nausea, numbness, oral lesions, paresthesias, peripheral neuritis, pharyngitis, reflex depression (deep tendon), skin lesions, thrombophlebitis, tumor site pain, vomiting, weakness.

Antidote: For extravasation, discontinue the drug immediately and administer into another vein. Hyaluronidase should be injected locally into extravasated area. Use a fine hypodermic needle. Moist heat may be helpful. Notify the physician of all side effects; symptomatic treatment is often indicated. Glutamic acid blocks toxicity of vinblastine, but also blocks its antineoplastic activity.

VINCRISTINE SULFATE pH 3.5 to 4.5

(Oncovin)

Usual dose: 1.4 mg/M² administered once every 7 days. Various dosage schedules have been used with caution.

Pediatric dose: 2 mg/M².

Dilution: *Specific techniques required, see precautions.* Diluent provided or each 1 mg is diluted with 10 ml of sterile water or normal saline for injection. 0.1 mg equals 1 ml (may use as little as 2 ml diluent for each 1 mg). Do not add to IV solutions. May be given direct IV or through Y tube or three-way stopcock of a free-flowing IV infusion.

Rate of administration: Total desired dose, properly diluted, over 1 minute.

Actions: An alkaloid of the periwinkle plant with antitumor activity. Cell cycle specific for the M phase. Well absorbed except in spinal fluid, it is primarily excreted through bile and feces.

Indications and uses: (1) To suppress or retard neoplastic growth; (2) good response experienced in leukemia, Hodgkin's disease, lymphosarcoma, oat cell, and others.

Precautions: (1) Follow guidelines for handling cytotoxic agents recommended by the National Study Commission on Cytotoxic Exposure (see Appendix, p. 528). (2) Usually administered in the hospital by or under the direction of the physician specialist. (3) Store in refrigerator before and after dilution. Potency maintained for 14 days after dilution. Label vial pertaining to milligrams per milliliter. (4) Determine absolute patency and quality of vein and adequate circulation of extremity. Severe cellulitis may result from extravasation. (5) Often given with corticosteroids and other antineoplastic drugs in reduced doses to achieve tumor remission. Use caution to prevent bone marrow depression. Use with asparaginase or doxorubicin not recommended. Use extreme caution in combination with radiation therapy. (6) Dosage based on average weight in presence of edema or ascites. (7) Inhibited by glutamic acid. (8) May produce teratogenic effects on the fetus. Has a mutagenic potential and must be given with caution in men and women capable of conception. (9) Do not administer any vaccine or chloroquine to patients receiving antineoplastic drugs. (10) Potentiates anticoagulants. (11) Be alert for signs of bone marrow depression or infection. (12) Use caution in preexisting neuromuscular disease or impaired liver function. (13) Allopurinol may prevent formation of uric acid crystals. (14) Maintain adequate hydration. (15) Prophylactic antiemetics may increase patient comfort. (16) Inappropriate secretion of ADH may require fluid limitation. (17) Use a stool softener to prevent impaction.

Contraindications: There are no absolute contraindications.

Incompatible with: Specific information not available. Note precautions.

Side effects: Note always reversible: abdominal pain, alopecia, ataxia, cellulitis, constipation, convulsions, cranial nerve damage, diarrhea, dysuria, extravasation, fever, footdrop, gonadal suppression, headache, hypertension, leukopenia (rare), muscle wasting, nausea, neuritic pain, oral lacerations, paralytic ileus, paresthesias, polyuria, reflex changes, sensory impairment, tingling and numbness of extremities, thrombocytopenia (rare), thrombophlebitis, upper colon impaction, uric acid nephropathy, vomiting, weakness, weight loss.

Antidote: For extravasation, discontinue the drug immediately and administer into another vein. Hyaluronidase should be injected locally into extravasated area. Use a fine hypodermic needle. Moist heat may be helpful. Notify the physician of all side effects; symptomatic treatment is often indicated. Will probably reduce dose at earliest signs of neurological toxicity (tingling and numbness of extremities). Discontinue for inappropriate ADH secretion or hyponatremia. Glutamic acid blocks toxicity of vincristine but also blocks its antineoplastic activity.

VITAMIN B WITH C

(Folbesyn)

Usual dose: 2 ml/24 hr. Larger doses may be used.

Dilution: Use only the diluent provided, which contains folic acid. Entire 2 ml of diluent must be added to the powdered vitamins. Must be added to IV solutions and given as an infusion. Soluble in most commonly used IV solutions. May be added to an infusion of over 500 ml containing tetracycline as an additive.

Rate of administration: Administer as IV solution over 4 to 8 hours.

Actions: Provides six B-complex vitamins and 300 mg of ascorbic acid. These are water-soluble vitamins, readily absorbable, and essential for maintaining health. Provides daily requirements or corrects an existing deficiency.

Indications and uses: (1) Preoperative and postoperative maintenance of optimum health; (2) prolonged IV therapy; (3) increased vitamin requirements in fever, severe burns, increased metabolism, hyperthyroidism, and pregnancy; (4) deficient intestinal absorption of water-soluble vitamins; (5) prolonged or wasting diseases.

Precautions: (1) Prepare immediately before use. Do not use if a precipitate forms. Discard any remaining solution. (2) Previous injections of thiamine hydrochloride can cause sensitivity and anaphylaxis may result, espeically with too-rapid injection. Intradermal skin test recommended in suspected sensitivity. (3) May mask blood picture and prevent diagnosis of pernicious anemia. (4) Folic acid (in diluent) not recommended for IV use in children. (5) May slightly potentiate barbiturates, salicylates, and sulfonamides.

Contraindications: Known hypersensitivity to any vitamin B compound; vitamin B_{12} deficiencies of pernicious and other megaloblastic anemias.

Incompatible with: Amikacin (Amikin), aminophylline, cephalothin (Keflin), chloramphenicol (Chloromycetin), chlorpromazine (Thorazine), clindamycin (Cleocin), erythromycin (Erythrocin), hydrocortisone sodium succinate (Solu-Cortef), hydroxyzine (Vistaril), magnesium sulfate, kanamycin (Kantrex), methicillin (Staphcillin), methylprednisolone (Solu-Medrol), nafcillin (Unipen), nitrofurantoin (Ivadantin), penicillin, procaine (Novocain), prochlorperazine (Compazine), sodium bicarbonate, sulfisoxazole, vancomycin (Vancocin), warfarin (Coumadin).

Side effects: Hypersensitivity reactions, including anaphylactic shock.

Antidote: Discontinue administration immediately and notify the physician. Treat anaphylaxis or resuscitate as necessary.

(Coumadin)

Usual dose: 40 to 60 mg initially (0.75 to 1 mg/kg of body weight). Maintenance dose is 2 to 10 mg. Dosage adjusted according to prothrombin time. Maintain with oral therapy when possible.

Dilution: Diluent provided. Each 50 mg of lyophilized powder is diluted with 2 ml. Rotate vial to dissolve completely. May not be mixed with infusion fluids. Give through Y tube or three-way stopcock of IV infusion tubing. Compatible in a syringe with sodium heparin. May be given together to accomplish immediate and long-term anticoagulation simultaneously.

Rate of administration: 25 mg (1 ml) or fraction thereof over 1 minute.

Actions: An anticoagulant that acts by depressing the formation of prothrombin and other coagulation factors in the liver. Effective anticoagulant levels are reached in 12 to 24 hours and last for about 4 days. Well-established clots are not dissolved, but growth is prevented. Does cross the placental barrier. Metabolized in the liver and excreted in changed forms in the urine.

Indications and uses: Prevention and/or treatment of all types of thromboses and emboli and situations and diseases predisposing to the formation of thromboses or emboli.

Precautions: (1) Prothrombin time must be done before initial injection. Usually repeated daily thereafter during IV therapy. Draw blood for prothrombin just prior to any heparin dose being given concomitantly. Dosage adjusted daily according to prothrombin activity. 20% of normal activity is desirable (21 to 35 seconds, with a control of 14 seconds). (2) Decrease dosage gradually. Abrupt withdrawal may precipitate increased coagulability. (3) Use with caution in hepatic or renal insufficiency, trauma involving large raw surfaces, extensive surgical procedures, hypertension, diabetes, the elderly or debilitated, or a history of allergic problems. (4) Capable of innumerable interactions. Monitor prothrombin time carefully when drugs are added or discontinued. (5) Potentiated by acidifying agents, alcohol, anabolic agents, analgesics, anesthetics, antibiotics, antineoplastics, chloral hydrate, diuretics, glucagon, hepatotoxic drugs, salicylates, skeletal muscle relaxants, thyroid preparations, vitamin B complex, and many others. Severe bleeding may result. (6) Inhibited by barbiturates, corticosteroids, benzodiazepines, digitalis, diuretics, vitamins C and K, xanthines, and many others. (7) Potentiates anticonvulsants, insulin, and others. (8) May be fatal with cinchophen, diuretics. (9) Concurrent use with streptokinase or urokinase may be hazardous.

Contraindications: Active bleeding; anesthesia (major regional block); blood dyscrasias; continuous gastrointestinal suctioning; history of bleeding, inadequate laboratory facilities; pregnancy and lactation; recent surgical procedures, especially neurosurgical, ophthalmic, and extensive traumatic procedures; subacute bacterial endocarditis; threatened abortion; vitamin C deficiency.

Incompatible with: Amikacin (Amikin), ammonium chloride, ascorbic acid, cyanocobalamin (Redisol), dextrose (any percent solution), epinephrine (Adrenalin), metaraminol (Aramine), oxytocin, promazine (Sparine), tetracycline (Achromycin), vancomycin (Vancocin), vitamin B complex with C.

Side effects: Allergic reactions (rare), alopecia (rare), bruising, epistaxis, hematuria, prothrombin time less than 20% activity, tarry stools, or any other signs of bleeding.

Antidote: Discontinue drug and notify physician of any side effects. Phytonadione (Aquamephyton) is a specific antagonist and indicated in overdose or desired warfarin sodium reversal. Will impede subsequent anticoagulant therapy.

PUBLICATIONS

Additional and more detailed information on all included drugs may be found in the following publications:

Goodman, L.S., Gilman, A., and Goodman, A.G., editors: The pharmacological basis of therapeutics, ed. 6, New York, 1980, The Macmillan Co.

Kastrup, E.K., editor: Facts and comparisons, St. Louis, 1983, Facts and Comparisons, Inc. (Updated monthly.)

King, J.C.: Guide to parenteral admixtures, St. Louis, 1980, Cutter Laboratories. (Updated quarterly.)

Mangini, R.J., editor: Mediphor drug interaction facts, St. Louis, 1983, Facts and Comparisons, Inc. (Updated quarterly.)

Manufacturer's literature.

Physicians' desk reference to pharmaceutical specialties and biologicals, ed. 37, Oradell, N.J., 1983, Medical Economics, Inc. (Updated quarterly.)

Trissel, L.A.: Handbook on injectable drugs, ed. 3, 1983, American Society of Hospital Pharmacists, Inc.

Recommendations for Handling Cytotoxic Agents*

PREAMBLE

The increasing use of cytotoxic agents and the growing awareness of potential hazards requires special attention to the procedures utilized in the handling, preparation and administration of these drugs. Equally important is the proper disposal of chemical residues and wastes. These recommendations are intended to provide information for the protection of personnel participating in the clinical process of chemotherapy. The mutagenic and carcinogenic potential of many cytotoxic agents is well established and is a possible hazard to the health of exposed individuals. It is the responsibility of institutional and private health care providers to adopt and use appropriate procedures for protection and safety.

I. Environmental Protection

1. All mixing of cytotoxic agents should be performed in a Class II, biological safety cabinet. Type A cabinets are the minimal requirement. Type A cabinets which are vented (some now classified as Type B3) are preferred.
2. Special techniques and precautions must be utilized because of the vertical (downward) laminar airflow (see Special Techniques and Precautions below).
3. The biological safety cabinet must be certified by qualified personnel annually or any time the cabinet is physically moved.
4. The biological safety cabinet should be operated with the blower on, 24 hours per day—seven days per week.
5. Drug preparations must be performed only with the view screen at the recommended access opening. Professionally accepted practices concerning the aseptic preparation of injectable products should be followed.

---

*From National Study Commission on Cytotoxic Exposure, March, 1984.

II. Operator Protection

1. Disposable surgical latex gloves are recommended for all procedures involving cytotoxic drugs. Polyvinyl chloride (PVC) gloves should not be worn while handling cytotoxic agents. Several types of PVC gloves are permeable to a variety of drugs.
2. Gloves should routinely be changed approximately every 30 minutes when working steadily with cytotoxic agents. Gloves should be removed immediately after overt contamination.
3. Double gloving is recommended for cleaning up of spills.
4. Protective barrier garments should be worn for all procedures involving the preparation and disposal of cytotoxic agents. These garments should have a closed front, long sleeves and closed cuff (either elastic or knit).
5. All potentially contaminated garments must not be worn outside the work area.

III. Compounding Procedures and Techniques

1. Hands must be washed thoroughly before gloving and after gloves are removed.
2. Care must be taken to avoid puncturing of gloves and possible self-inoculation.
3. Syringes and I.V. sets with Luer-lock fittings should be used whenever possible.
4. Vials should be vented with a hydrophobic filter to eliminate internal pressure or vacuum.
5. Before opening ampules, care should be taken to insure that no liquid remains in the tip of the ampule. A sterile, disposable alcohol dampened gauze sponge should be wrapped around the neck of the ampule to reduce aerosolization.
6. For sealed vials, final drug measurement should be performed prior to removing the needle from the stopper of the vial and after the pressure has been equalized.
7. A closed collection vessel should be available in the biological safety cabinet or the original vial may be used to hold discarded excess drug solutions.

8. Special procedures should be followed for acute exposure or spills (see Special Procedures below).
9. Cytotoxic agents which are handled within the treatment area should be properly labeled (e.g., "Chemotherapy: Dispose of Properly").

IV. Precautions for Medication Administration
1. Disposable surgical latex gloves should be worn during all cytotoxic drug administration activities.
2. Syringes and I.V. sets with Luer-lock fittings should be used whenever possible.
3. Special care must be taken in priming I.V. sets. The distal tip cover must be removed before priming. Priming should be performed into a sterile, alcohol-dampened gauze sponge, which then is disposed of appropriately.

V. Disposal Procedures
1. Place contaminated materials in a leakproof, puncture-proof container appropriately marked as hazardous waste.
2. Cytotoxic drug waste should be transported according to the institutional procedures for contaminated material.
3. There is insufficient information to recommend any single preferred method for disposal of cytotoxic drug waste.
   3.1 One method for disposal of hazardous waste is by incineration at a temperature considered sufficient by the Environmental Protection Agency (EPA) to destroy organic compounds. Incineration should be done in an EPA permitted hazardous waste incinerator.
   3.2 Another method of disposal is by burial at an EPA permitted hazardous waste site.
   3.3 A licensed hazardous waste disposal company may be consulted for information concerning available methods of disposal in the local area.

VI. Personnel Policy Recommendations
1. All personnel working with cytotoxic agents must receive special training.

2. Access to the compounding area must be limited to only necessary authorized personnel.
3. The personnel working with these agents should be observed regularly by supervisory personnel to insure compliance with procedures.
4. Acute exposure episodes must be documented. The employee must be referred for professional medical examination.

VII. Monitoring Procedures

1. Procedures to monitor the equipment and operating techniques of the personnel should be performed on a regular basis and documented. Specific methods of monitoring should be developed to meet the complexities of the function.
2. It is recommended that personnel involved in the preparation of cytotoxic agents on a full time basis be given periodic health examinations in accordance with institutional policy.

SPECIAL TECHNIQUES AND PRECAUTIONS FOR USE IN THE CLASS II BIOLOGICAL SAFETY CABINET

1. All equipment needed to complete the procedure in the Class II Biological Safety Cabinet should be placed into the cabinet before beginning and the view screen should be placed at the recommended operating position. A wait of at least two to three minutes before beginning work to allow the unit time to purge itself of airborne contaminants is recommended.
2. The proper procedures for use in the Biological Safety Cabinet are not the same as those used in the horizontal laminar hood. In many cases they seem contradictory, although in theory they are not. This is because of the nature of the airflow pattern in the Biological Safety Cabinet. Clean air descends through the work zone from the top of the cabinet toward the work surface. As it descends, the air is split, with some leaving through the rear perforation and some leaving through the front perforation. The region where the airflow splits is known as the "smoke

split" because smoke introduced into this area appears to split into two directions.

3. It is recommended that the smoke split be determined and marked on each cabinet after it is purchased even if the manufacturer states its location. This can be easily done by using an incense stick to generate smoke and moving it gently from front to rear laterally along the work surface of the cabinet near the center.

4. Routinely used large equipment should be placed in the cabinet in its normal position when the determination of the smoke split is made. The equipment should then be placed in the same position every time the cabinet is used.

5. Personnel should refrain from applying any face powder, eye make-up, rouge, fingernail polish, hairspray or other cosmetics in the work area. These cosmetics may provide a source of prolonged exposure if contaminated.

6. Eating, drinking, chewing of gum, storage of food or smoking in, around or near the Biological Safety Cabinet should be prohibited. Each of these are sources of ingestion if they are accidentally contaminated by the cytotoxic agent or other hazardous products.

7. Sterile products should be arranged in the cabinet so as to minimize the possibility of contamination. This may mean locating them in the immediate vicinity of the smoke split. If appropriate, due to quantity or configuration, the sterile items should be kept only in the center and nonsterile items on either side.

8. For additional operator protection, it is recommended that the area behind the smoke split be used whenever possible since the airflow direction in that area is away from the operator, lessening the chance of accidental exposure.

9. The least efficient area of the cabinet in terms of product and personnel protection is within three inches of the sides near the front opening. Therefore, you should not work within three inches of the sides of the cabinet.

10. Periodic evaluation of the smoke split should be performed on a routine basis. A constantly changing

smoke split location may be indicative of problems with the operation of the cabinet.

11. Entry into and exit from the cabinet should be in a direct manner perpendicular to the face of the cabinet. Rapid movements of the hands in the cabinet and laterally through the protective air barrier should be avoided.

SPECIAL PROCEDURES FOR ACUTE EXPOSURE OR SPILLS

1. Acute Exposure

1.1 Overtly contaminated gloves or outer garments should be removed and replaced immediately after an exposure.

1.2 Hands should be washed after removing gloves. Gloves are not a substitute for handwashing.

1.3 In case of skin contact with a cytotoxic drug product, the affected area should be washed thoroughly with soap and water as soon as possible. Refer to professional medical attention as soon as possible.

1.4 For eye exposure, flush affected eye with copious amounts of water. Refer to professional medical attention immediately.

2. Spills

2.1 All personnel involved in the clean-up of a spill should wear protective clothing (e.g., gloves, gowns, etc.). All clothes and other material used in the process should be treated or disposed of properly.

2.2 Double gloving should be used in the cleaning up of spills.

Index

539

545